George A. Horvath, M D

D0930253

.B. SAUNDERS COMPANY
Division of Elsevier Inc.

►00 John F. Kennedy Boulevard • Suite 1800 • Philadelphia, Pennsylvania 19103

:tp://www.theclinics.com

HE PEDIATRIC CLINICS OF NORTH AMERICA   Volume 55, Number 1
²bruary 2008   ISSN 0031-3955
ditor: Carla Holloway   ISBN-13: 978-1-4160-5790-1
     ISBN-10: 1-4160-5790-0

he ideas and opinions expressed in *The Pediatric Clinics of North America* do not necessarily reflect those of
he Publisher. The Publisher does not assume any responsibility for any injury and/or damage to persons
►r property arising out of or related to any use of the material contained in this periodical. The reader is
dvised to check the appropriate medical literature and the product information currently provided by the
nanufacturer of each drug to be administered to verify the dosage, the method and duration of adminis-
ration, or contraindications. It is the responsibility of the treating physician or other health care professional, relying on independent experience and knowledge of the patient, to determine drug dosages and
he best treatment for the patient. Mention of any product in this issue should not be construed as endorse-
ment by the contributors, editors, or the Publisher of the product or manufacturers' claims.

The Pediatric Clinics of North America (ISSN 0031-3955) is published bi-monthly by Elsevier Inc. 360 Park
Avenue South, New York, NY 10010-1710. Months of publication are February, April, June, August, October, and December. Business and Editorial Offices: 1600 John F. Kennedy Blvd., Suite 1800, Philadelphia,
PA 19103-2899. Customer Service Office: 6277 Sea Harbor Drive, Orlando, FL 32887-4800. Periodicals postage paid at New York, NY and additional mailing offices. Subscription prices are $149.00 per year (US
individuals), $315.00 per year (US institutions), $202.00 per year (Canadian individuals), $411.00 per year
(Canadian institutions), $226.00 per year (international individuals), $411.00 per year (international institutions), $72.00 per year (US students), $119.00 per year (Canadian students), and $119.00 per year (foreign
students). To receive students/resident rare, orders must be accompanied by name of affiliated institution,
date of term, and the signature of program/residency coordinator on institution letterhead. Orders will be
billed at individual rate until proof of status is received. Foreign air speed delivery is included in all Clinics
subscription prices. All prices are subject to change without notice. POSTMASTER: Send address changes
to *The Pediatric Clinics of North America*, Elsevier Journals Customer Service, 6277 Sea Harbor Drive,
Orlando, FL 32887-4800. **Customer Service: 1-800-654-2452 (US). From outside of the US, call 1-407-
563-6020. Fax: 1-407-363-9661. E-mail: JournalsCustomerService-usa@elsevier.com.**

The Pediatric Clinics of North America is also published in Spanish by McGraw-Hill Inter-americana Editores
S.A., Mexico City, Mexico; in Portuguese by Riechmann and Affonso Editores, Rua Comandante Coelho
1085, CEP 21250, Rio de Janeiro, Brazil; and in Greek by Althayia SA, Athens, Greece.

The Pediatric Clinics of North America is covered in *Index Medicus, Excerpta Medica, Current Contents, Current
Contents/Clinical Medicine, Science Citation Index, ASCA, ISI/BIOMED,* and *BIOSIS.*

Printed in the United States of America.

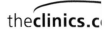

PEDIATRIC CLINIC
OF NORTH AMERIC

Pediatric Oncolo

GUEST EDIT(
Max J. Coppes, MD, PhD, M
Jeffrey S. Dome, N

February 2008 • Volume 55 • Number

SAUNDERS

An Imprint of Elsevier, Inc.
PHILADELPHIA   LONDON   TORONTO   MONTREAL   SYDNEY   TOKYC

GOAL STATEMENT

The goal of the *Pediatric Clinics of North America* is to keep practicing physicians and residents up to date with current clinical practice in pediatrics by providing timely articles reviewing the state-of-the-art in patient care.

ACCREDITATION

The *Pediatric Clinics of North America* is planned and implemented in accordance with the Essential Areas and Policies of the Accreditation Council for Continuing Medical Education (ACCME) through the joint sponsorship of the University of Virginia School of Medicine and Elsevier. The University of Virginia School of Medicine is accredited by the ACCME to provide continuing medical education for physicians.

The University of Virginia School of Medicine designates this educational activity for a maximum of 15 *AMA PRA Category 1 Credits*™. Physicians should only claim credit commensurate with the extent of their participation in the activity.

The American Medical Association has determined that physicians not licensed in the US who participate in this CME activity are eligible for 15 *AMA PRA Category 1 Credits*™.

Credit can be earned by reading the text material, taking the CME examination online at http://www.theclinics. com/home/cme, and completing the evaluation. After taking the test, you will be required to review any and all incorrect answers. Following completion of the test and evaluation, your credit will be awarded and you may print your certificate.

FACULTY DISCLOSURE/CONFLICT OF INTEREST

The University of Virginia School of Medicine, as an ACCME accredited provider, endorses and strives to comply with the Accreditation Council for Continuing Medical Education (ACCME) Standards of Commercial Support, Commonwealth of Virginia statutes, University of Virginia policies and procedures, and associated federal and private regulations and guidelines on the need for disclosure and monitoring of proprietary and financial interests that may affect the scientific integrity and balance of content delivered in continuing medical education activities under our auspices.

The University of Virginia School of Medicine requires that all CME activities accredited through this institution be developed independently and be scientifically rigorous, balanced and objective in the presentation/discussion of its content, theories and practices.

All authors/editors participating in an accredited CME activity are expected to disclose to the readers relevant financial relationships with commercial entities occurring within the past 12 months (such as grants or research support, employee, consultant, stock holder, member of speakers bureau, etc.). The University of Virginia School of Medicine will employ appropriate mechanisms to resolve potential conflicts of interest to maintain the standards of fair and balanced education to the reader. Questions about specific strategies can be directed to the Office of Continuing Medical Education, University of Virginia School of Medicine, Charlottesville, Virginia.

The authors/editors listed below have identified no financial or professional relationships for themselves or their spouse/partner:
Caitlin Allen, PhD; Lisa H. Anderson, M Div; Justin N. Baker, MD; Raymond C. Barfield, MD, PhD; Huib Caron, MD, PhD; William L. Carroll, MD; Julia C. Chishlom, MBChB, PhD, FRCPCH; Max J. Coppes, MD, PhD, MBA (Guest Editor); Ramzi N. Dagher, MD; Susan Devine, CCRP; Jeffrey S. Dome, MD (Guest Editor); R. Maarten Egeler, MD, PhD; Angelika Eggert, MD; Terry J. Fry, MD; Brenda Gibson, MD; Rupert Handgretinger, MD; Pamela S. Hinds, RN, PhD, FAAN; Johann Hitzler, FRCP(C), FAAP; Carla Holloway (Acquisitions Editor); Javier R. Kane, MD; Leontien C. Kremer, MD, PhD; Joanne Kurtzberg, MD; Arjan C. Lankester, MD, PhD; Tobey MacDonald, MD; Paul C. Nathan, MD, MSC; Kevin C. Oeffinger, MD; Robert J. Packer, MD; Julie R. Park, MD; Soonie R. Patel, MBChB, MRCP, MD; Rob Pieters, MD, MSc, PhD; Brent C. Powell, M Div; Dirk Reinhardt, PD; Jeffrey E. Rubnitz, MD, PhD; Victor M. Santana, MD; Franklin O. Smith, MD; Sheri L. Spunt, MD; Yoram Unguru, MD, MS, MA; Gilbert Vezina, MD; Paresh Vyas, FRCPath, DPHil; Karen D. Weiss, MD; and Michel C. Zwann, MD, PhD.

The authors/editors listed below identified the following professional or financial affiliations for themselves or their spouse/partner:
Paul T. Heath, MBBS, FRACP, FRCPCH is an independent contractor for Wyeth vaccines.
Naynesh Kamani, MD serves on the Advisory Board for Cryocell International, Inc., and the Speaker's Bureau for ZLB-Behring.

Disclosure of Discussion of Non-FDA Approved Uses for Pharmaceutical and/or Medical Devices:
The University of Virginia School of Medicine, as an ACCME provider, requires that all authors identify and disclose any "off label" uses for pharmaceutical and medical device products. The University of Virginia School of Medicine recommends that each physician fully review all the available data on new products or procedures prior to clinical use.

TO ENROLL

To enroll in the *Pediatric Clinics of North America* Continuing Medical Education program, call customer service at 1-800-654-2452 or visit us online at www.theclinics.com/home/cme. The CME program is available to subscribers for an additional fee of $195.00.

GUEST EDITORS

MAX J. COPPES, MD, PhD, MBA, Executive Director, Center for Cancer and Blood Disorders, Children's National Medical Center; and Professor of Oncology, Medicine, and Pediatrics, Georgetown University, Washington, DC

JEFFREY S. DOME, MD, Chief, Division of Oncology, Center for Cancer and Blood Disorders, Children's National Medical Center, Washington, DC

CONTRIBUTORS

CAITLIN ALLEN, PhD, Division of Nursing Research, St. Jude Children's Research Hospital, Memphis, Tennessee

LISA H. ANDERSON, M Div, Division of Behavioral Medicine, St. Jude Children's Research Hospital, Memphis, Tennessee

JUSTIN N. BAKER, MD, Department of Oncology; and Quality of Life Service, St. Jude Children's Research Hospital, Memphis, Tennessee

RAYMOND C. BARFIELD, MD, PhD, Department of Oncology; Division of Stem Cell Transplant; and Chair, Ethics Committee, St. Jude Children's Research Hospital, Memphis, Tennessee

HUIB CARON, MD, PhD, Professor of Pediatric Oncology, Department of Pediatric Oncology and Hematology, Emma Children's Hospital AMC, Amesterdam, the Netherlands

WILLIAM L. CARROLL, MD, Julie and Edward J. Minskoff Professor of Pediatrics and Director, Division of Pediatric Hematology/Oncology, New York University Medical Center, New York, New York

JULIA C. CHISHOLM, MBChB, PhD, FRCPCH, Consultant Paediatric Oncologist, Department of Haemotology/Oncology, Great Ormond Street Hospital, London, United Kingdom

MAX J. COPPES, MD, PhD, MBA, Executive Director, Center for Cancer and Blood Disorders, Children's National Medical Center; and Professor of Oncology, Medicine, and Pediatrics, Georgetown University, Washington, DC

RAMZI N. DAGHER, MD, Office of Oncology Drug Products, Center for Drug Evaluation and Research, Food and Drug Administration, Silver Spring, Maryland

SUSAN DEVINE, CCRP, Department of Hematology/Oncology, Hospital for Sick Children, Toronto, Ontario, Canada

R. MAARTEN EGELER, MD, PhD, Department of Pediatrics, Leiden University Medical Center, Leiden, the Netherlands

ANGELIKA EGGERT, MD, Professor of Pediatrics and Head of Pediatric Cancer Research, Department of Hematology/Oncology, University Children's Hospital Essen, Hufelandstr, Essen, Germany

TERRY J. FRY, MD, Chief, Division of Blood/Marrow Transplantation and Immunology, Center for Cancer and Blood Disorders, Children's National Medical Center; and Associate Professor of Pediatrics, George Washington University, Washington, DC

BRENDA GIBSON, MD, Department of Paediatric Haemotology, Royal Hospital for Sick Children, Glasgow, Scotland, United Kingdom

RUPERT HANDGRETINGER, MD, Chairman, Department of Hematoloyg/Oncology and General Pediatrics, Children's University Hospital, Tuebingen, Germany

PAUL T. HEATH, MBBS, FRACP, FRCPCH, Reader in Paediatric Infectious Diseases/ Honorary Consultant, Vaccine Institute and Child Health, St. George's, University of London, London, United Kingdom

PAMELA S. HINDS, RN, PhD, FAAN, Director, Division of Nursing Research; and Co-Chair, Palliative and End-of-Life Care Task Force, St. Jude Children's Research Hospital, Memphis, Tennessee

JOHANN HITZLER, FRCP(C), FAAP, Assistant Professor, Division of Hematology/ Oncology, The Hospital for Sick Children; and Developmental and Stem Cell Biology, The Hospital for Sick Children Research Institute, University of Toronto, Toronto, Ontario, Canada

NAYNESH KAMANI, MD, Chairman, Institutional Review Board, Center for Cancer and Blood Disorders, Children's National Medical Center; and Department of Pediatrics; Department of Immunology, George Washington University, Washington, DC

JAVIER R. KANE, MD, Department of Oncology; Quality of Life Service; Director, Palliative and End-of-Life Care; and Co-Chair, Palliative and End-of-Life Care Task Force, St. Jude Children's Research Hospital, Memphis, Tennessee

LEONTIEN C.M. KREMER, MD, PhD, Department of Pediatric Oncology, Emma Children's Hospital/Academic Medical Center, Amsterdam, the Netherlands

JOANNE KURTZBERG, MD, Director, Pediatric Bone Marrow and Stem Cell Transplant Program, Duke University Medical Center, Durham, North Carolina

ARJAN C. LANKESTER, MD, PhD, Pediatrician and Immunologist, Department of Pediatrics, BMT-Unit, Leiden University Medical Center, Leiden, the Netherlands

TOBEY MACDONALD, MD, Attending Oncologist and Director, Neuro-Oncology Program, Center for Cancer and Blood Disorders; and Center for Cancer Immunology Research, Children's National Medical Center, Washington, DC; Associate Professor of Pediatrics, The George Washington University School of Medicine and Health Sciences, Washington, DC

PAUL C. NATHAN, MD, MSc, Division of Hematology/Oncology, Hospital for Sick Children, Toronto, Ontario, Canada

KEVIN C. OEFFINGER, MD, Department of Pediatrics, Memorial Sloan-Kettering Cancer Center, New York, New York

ROGER J. PACKER, MD, Executive Director, Center for Neuroscience and Behavioral Medicine; Chairman, Division of Neurology; and Director, The Brain Tumor Institute, Children's National Medical Center, Washington, DC; Professor of Neurology and Pediatrics, The George Washington University School of Medicine and Health Sciences, Washington, DC

JULIE R. PARK, MD, Associate Professor of Pediatrics, Division of Hematology and Oncology, University of Washington School of Medicine, Children's Hospital and Regional Medical Center, Seattle, Washington

SOONIE R. PATEL, MBChB, MRCP, MD, Consultant Paediatrician, Paediatric Department, Mayday University Hospital, Croydon, United Kingdom

ROB PIETERS, MD, MSc, PhD, Head, Department of Pediatric Oncology and Hematology, Erasmus MC-Sophia Children's Hospital, Rotterdam, the Netherlands

BRENT C. POWELL, M Div, Division of Behavioral Medicine; and Director, Chaplain Services, St. Jude Children's Research Hospital, Memphis, Tennessee

DIRK REINHARDT, PD, Ausserplanmassiger Professor, AML-BFM Study Group, Pediatric Hematology/Oncology, Hannover Medical School, Hannover, Germany

JEFFREY E. RUBNITZ, MD, PhD, Associate Member, Department of Oncology, St. Jude Children's Research Hospital, Memphis, Tennessee

VICTOR M. SANTANA, MD, Member, Department of Oncology, St. Jude Children's Research Hospital; and Professor, Department of Pediatrics, University of Tennessee Health Sciences Center, Memphis, Tennessee

FRANKLIN O. SMITH, MD, Marjory J. Johnson Endowed Chair, Professor of Pediatrics, and Director, Division of Hematology/Oncology, University of Cincinnati College of Medicine, Cincinnati Children's Hospital Medical Center, Cincinnati, Ohio

SHERI L. SPUNT, MD, Department of Oncology; and Solid Tumor Division, St. Jude Children's Research Hospital, Memphis, Tennessee

YORAM UNGURU, MD, MS, MA, Fellow, Division of Hematology/Oncology, Center for Cancer and Blood Disorders, Children's National Medical Center, Washington, DC; Greenwall Fellow, Berman Bioethics Institute, Johns Hopkins University, Baltimore, Maryland

GILBERT VEZINA, MD, Chief, Division of Neuro-Radiology, Children's National Medical Center; and Professor of Radiology and Pediatrics, The George Washington University School of Medicine and Health Sciences, Washington, DC

PARESH VYAS, FRCPath, DPHil, Reader in Haemato-Oncology, MRC Molecular Haemotology Unit, John Radcliffe Hospital, Weatherall Institute of Molecular Medicine, University of Oxford, Headington, Oxford, United Kingdom

KAREN D. WEISS, MD, Office of Oncology Drug Products, Center for Drug Evaluation and Research, Food and Drug Administration, Silver Spring, Maryland

MICHEL C. ZWAAN, MD, PhD, Department of Pediatric Oncology/Hematology, Erasmus MC-Sophia Children's Hospital, Rotterdam, the Netherlands

CONTENTS

to pediatric oncology research and recent efforts at harmonization. The authors review the clinical trials process and the roles of the participants, highlighting the pivotal role of the clinical investigator and the research team, and briefly review the historical aspects of drug development regulations in the United States and the current regulatory paths for pediatric oncology drug development. Where relevant, historical events that underlie many of the regulations and their current applications are described, and practical examples are provided.

Physician-investigators are required to obtain informed consent from adult participants in their studies. Inclusion of children in research legally requires informed permission of a child's parent or guardian. It is increasingly recognized that a child need not assume a passive role when included in research, but that his or her active involvement should be sought, as expressed by the child's assent to partake in clinical research. This article briefly explores the history of assent and the central role of assessing a child's understanding of research and preference for participating in decisions related to their care, as necessary components of meaningful assent.

Most parents of children with cancer have dual primary goals: a primary cancer-directed goal of cure and a primary comfort-related goal of lessening suffering. Early introduction of palliative care principles and practices into their child's treatment is respectful and supportive of these goals. The Individualized Care Planning and Coordination Model is designed to integrate palliative care principles and practices into the ongoing care of children with cancer. Application of the model helps clinicians to generate a comprehensive individualized care plan that is implemented through Individualized Care Coordination processes as detailed here. Clinicians' strong desire to provide compassionate, competent, and sensitive care to the seriously ill child and the child's family can be effectively translated into clinical practice through these processes.

FORTHCOMING ISSUES

RECENT ISSUES

PEDIATRIC CLINICS
OF NORTH AMERICA

ELSEVIER
SAUNDERS

Pediatr Clin N Am 55 (2008) xv–xvi

Preface

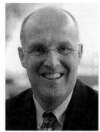 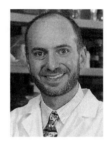

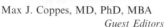

Max J. Coppes, MD, PhD, MBA   Jeffrey S. Dome, MD
Guest Editors

The field of pediatric oncology has seen tremendous advances over the past decades. Particularly impressive is the fact that, for the majority of children who are diagnosed with cancer today, the diagnosis does not carry a death sentence. Most children diagnosed with acute lymphoblastic leukemia (ALL), Wilms tumor, Hodgkin disease, non-Hodgkin lymphoma, and germ cell cancer are expected to survive and be cured following therapy. The remarkable treatment success achieved in many pediatric cancers has more recently allowed investigators to start assessing what, if any, cost is associated with long-term survival. As described in this issue of *Pediatric Clinics of North America*, the price for cancer survivors is not insignificant in many cases. Moreover, it has become evident that the fact that these children "graduate" from pediatric oncology care and become adults generates a whole new set of challenges for continued follow up and after care. Increasingly, it has become apparent that clear guidelines are needed to ensure that children cured of their cancer have access to health care services tailored to their unique needs, many of which have only recently been identified.

For some children, survival remains a major challenge. Different avenues continue being explored to improve the outcome for children with metastatic cancers (eg, osteogenic sarcoma, neuroblastoma, rhaddomyosarcoma), for many who present with a central nervous system (CNS) tumor, and for those that relapse. Investigators continue to determine how we can best use stem cell transplantation and immunotherapy, both of which are discussed in this issue, in these high risk scenarios.

0031-3955/08/$ - see front matter © 2008 Elsevier Inc. All rights reserved.
doi:10.1016/j.pcl.2007.11.005

It is obvious that not every single aspect of childhood cancer could be included in an issue such as this one. Our choice for topics was guided by several factors. First, we felt that an update on leukemia (both ALL and acute myelogenous leukemia) was warranted because leukemia is the most common form of childhood cancer. Moreover, the field of leukemia has changed considerably, mostly as a consequence of new stratification strategies, which are extensively discussed. Second, we elected to update the readers on some cancers that remain a challenge to cure (eg, CNS tumors and neuroblastoma). Finally, we elected topics that generate broad interest in the pediatric oncology community, such as how best to conduct clinical trials (by many considered standard care), the role of obtaining assent to treat children and adolescents, and the challenges to integrate palliative care early on in the management of children with cancer.

Many of the contributions in this issue are authored by colleagues from different countries. This reflects that the world of pediatric oncology is shrinking. As survival rates improve, larger clinical trials will be necessary to demonstrate further gains in outcome. This will require enhanced international dialogue and collaboration, which is exciting because there is much we can learn from each other. We can only hope that the readers will experience some of the same stimulation we felt as we communicated with the authors and read their finalized contributions.

Max J. Coppes, MD, PhD, MBA
Center for Cancer and Blood Disorders
111 Michigan Avenue
Washington, DC 20010, USA

Georgetown University
Washington, DC, USA

E-mail address: mcoppes@cnmc.org

Jeffrey S. Dome, MD
Division of Oncology
Center for Cancer and Blood Disorders
Children's National Medical Center
111 Michigan Avenue NW
Washington, DC 20010, USA

E-mail address: jdome@cnmc.org

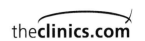

PEDIATRIC CLINICS
OF NORTH AMERICA

Pediatric Oncology

GUEST EDITORS
Max J. Coppes, MD, PhD, MBA
Jeffrey S. Dome, MD

February 2008 • Volume 55 • Number 1

SAUNDERS
An Imprint of Elsevier, Inc.
PHILADELPHIA   LONDON   TORONTO   MONTREAL   SYDNEY   TOKYO

W.B. SAUNDERS COMPANY
A Division of Elsevier Inc.

1600 John F. Kennedy Boulevard • Suite 1800 • Philadelphia, Pennsylvania 19103

http://www.theclinics.com

THE PEDIATRIC CLINICS OF NORTH AMERICA   Volume 55, Number 1
February 2008   ISSN 0031-3955
Editor: Carla Holloway   ISBN-13: 978-1-4160-5790-1
     ISBN-10: 1-4160-5790-0

The Pediatric Clinics of North America (ISSN 0031-3955) is published bi-monthly by Elsevier Inc. 360 Park Avenue South, New York, NY 10010-1710. Months of publication are February, April, June, August, October, and December. Business and Editorial Offices: 1600 John F. Kennedy Blvd., Suite 1800, Philadelphia, PA 19103-2899. Customer Service Office: 6277 Sea Harbor Drive, Orlando, FL 32887-4800. Periodicals postage paid at New York, NY and additional mailing offices. Subscription prices are $149.00 per year (US individuals), $315.00 per year (US institutions), $202.00 per year (Canadian individuals), $411.00 per year (Canadian institutions), $226.00 per year (international individuals), $411.00 per year (international institutions), $72.00 per year (US students), $119.00 per year (Canadian students), and $119.00 per year (foreign students). To receive students/resident rare, orders must be accompanied by name of affiliated institution, date of term, and the signature of program/residency coordinator on institution letterhead. Orders will be billed at individual rate until proof of status is received. Foreign air speed delivery is included in all Clinics subscription prices. All prices are subject to change without notice. POSTMASTER: Send address changes to *The Pediatric Clinics of North America*, Elsevier Journals Customer Service, 6277 Sea Harbor Drive, Orlando, FL 32887-4800. **Customer Service: 1-800-654-2452 (US). From outside of the US, call 1-407-563-6020. Fax: 1-407-363-9661. E-mail: JournalsCustomerService-usa@elsevier.com.**

The Pediatric Clinics of North America is also published in Spanish by McGraw-Hill Inter-americana Editores S.A., Mexico City, Mexico; in Portuguese by Riechmann and Affonso Editores, Rua Comandante Coelho 1085, CEP 21250, Rio de Janeiro, Brazil; and in Greek by Althayia SA, Athens, Greece.

The Pediatric Clinics of North America is covered in *Index Medicus, Excerpta Medica, Current Contents, Current Contents/Clinical Medicine, Science Citation Index, ASCA, ISI/BIOMED,* and *BIOSIS.*

Printed in the United States of America.

ELSEVIER
SAUNDERS

Pediatr Clin N Am 55 (2008) xvii

PEDIATRIC CLINICS
OF NORTH AMERICA

This issue is dedicated to Marjolein Coppes, a 14-year-old teenager with acute lymphoblastic leukemia (ALL) who is a true inspiration to her uncle, her family, and her friends.

0031-3955/08/$ - see front matter
doi:10.1016/j.pcl.2007.11.004   *pediatric.theclinics.com*

ELSEVIER
SAUNDERS

PEDIATRIC CLINICS
OF NORTH AMERICA

Pediatr Clin N Am 55 (2008) 1–20

Biology and Treatment of Acute Lymphoblastic Leukemia

Rob Pieters, MD, MSc, PhD[a,*],
William L. Carroll, MD[b]

[a]Department of Pediatric Oncology and Hematology, Erasmus MC-Sophia Children's
Hospital, Dr Molewaterplein 60, 3015GJ Rotterdam, The Netherlands
[b]Division of Pediatric Hematology/Oncology, New York University Medical Center,
160 East 32nd Street, 2nd Floor, New York, NY 10016, USA

Acute lymphoblastic leukemia (ALL), the most common type of cancer in children, is a heterogeneous disease in which many genetic lesions result in the development of multiple biologic subtypes. The etiology of ALL is characterized by the acquisition of multiple consecutive genetic alterations in the (pre)leukemic cells. In the most common genetic subtypes of ALL, the first hit occurs in utero [1], as evidenced, for example, by the presence of the *TEL/AML1* gene fusion or hyperdiploidy in neonatal blood spots on Guthrie cards. These first genetic abnormalities are, in fact, initiating preleukemic cells, not leukemic ones, because most children whose neonatal blood spots show a genetic defect typically associated with leukemia never develop leukemia. Also, such preleukemic cells harbor additional genetic abnormalities. T-cell acute lymphoblastic leukemia (T-ALL) is an exception, because the majority of genetic lesions described in T-ALL seem not to occur in the neonatal blood spots [2].

Today, with intensive multiagent chemotherapy, most children who have ALL are cured. The factors that account for the dramatic improvement in survival during the past 40 years include the identification of effective drugs and combination chemotherapy through large, randomized clinical trials, the recognition of sanctuary sites and the integration of presymptomatic central nervous system (CNS) prophylaxis, intensification of treatment using existing drugs, and risk-based stratification of treatment. The many national or institutional ALL therapy protocols in use tend to stratify patients in a multitude of different ways. Treatment results often are not published for the

---

* Corresponding author.
E-mail address: rob.pieters@erasmusmc.nl (R. Pieters).

pediatric.theclinics.com

overall patient group but rather are reported only for selected subsets of patients. This limitation hampers the comparison of outcomes in protocols. In 2000, the results of ALL trials run in the early 1990s by the major study groups were presented in a uniform way [3–12]. The 5-year event-free survival (EFS) rates seemed not to vary widely, ranging from 71% to 83% (Table 1). Overall remission rates usually were 98% or higher.

Risk-based stratification allows the tailoring of treatment according to the predicted risk of relapse. Children who have high-risk features receive aggressive treatment to prevent disease recurrence, and patients who have a good prognosis receive effective therapy but are not exposed to unnecessary treatment with associated short- and long-term side effects. Clinical factors that predict outcome and are used for stratification of patients into treatment arms are age, gender, and white blood cell count at presentation. Biologic factors with prognostic value are the immunophenotype and genotype of the leukemia cells. Another predictive factor is the rapidity of response to early therapy, such as the decrease in peripheral blood blast count in response to a week of prednisone or the decrease in bone marrow blasts after 1 to 3 weeks of multiagent chemotherapy. More recently the determination of minimal residual disease (MRD) in the bone marrow during the first months of therapy using flow cytometry or molecular techniques has been shown to have a high prognostic value and therefore is used for stratification in many contemporary trials. The detection of MRD accurately distinguishes very good responders to therapy from those who will

Table 1

Treatment results from major clinical trials in childhood acute lymphoblastic leukemia conducted in the early 1990s

Study group	Years of study	Patient number	Overall 5-year event-free survival (%)	B-lineage ALL 5-year event-free survival (%)	T-lineage ALL 5-year event-free survival (%)
DFCI-91-01	1991–1995	377	83	84	79
BFM-90	1990–1995	2178	78	80	61
NOPHO-ALL92	1992–1998	1143	78	79	61
COALL-92	1992–1997	538	77	78	71
SJCRH-13A	1991–1994	167	77	80	61
CCG-1800	1989–1995	5121	75	75	73
DCOG-ALL8	1991–1996	467	73	73	71
EORTC-58881	1989–1998	2065	71	72	64
AIEOP-91	1991–1995	1194	71	75	40
UKALL-XI	1990–1997	2090	63	63	59

Abbreviations: AIEOP, Associazione Italiana Ematologia Oncologia Pediatrica; BMF, Berlin-Frankfurt-Münster; CCG, Children's Cancer Group; COALL, Co-operative Study Group of Childhood Acute Lymphoblastic Leukemia; DCOG, Dutch Childhood Oncology Group; DFCI, Dana Farber Cancer Institute; EORTC-CLG European Organization for the Research and Treatment of Cancer; NOPHO, Nordic Society of Pediatric Haematology and Oncology; SJCHR, St. Jude Children's Research Hospital; UKALL United Kingdom Acute Lymphoblastic Leukemia.

respond poorly to therapy, irrespective of the biologic subtype of ALL and the underlying mechanism of this response [13]. In several protocols, MRD is used to stratify patients for reduction of therapy (ie, patients who are MRD negative especially at early time points) or intensification of therapy (ie, patients who are MRD positive at later time points).

Age and immunophenotype

Over the years, age has remained an independent predictor of outcome (Table 2). Children aged 1 to 9 years have the best outcome; children and adolescents aged 10 to 20 years have a slightly worse outcome, which is associated in part with a higher incidence of T-cell leukemia and a lower incidence of favorable genetic abnormalities such as *TEL/AML1* and hyperdiploidy. For adults, survival rates decrease further with increasing age. When results are corrected for differences in immunophenotype, ALL cells from older children and adults are more resistant to multiple antileukemic drugs than are cells from children in the first decade of life [14,15].

Infants diagnosed at less than 1 year of age have a relatively poor outcome that is associated with a high incidence of the unfavorable very immature proB-ALL phenotype and especially the presence of *MLL* gene rearrangements [16]. The poor outcome has led physicians in the United States, Japan, and the International Interfant collaborative group including European and non-European countries and institutes to develop specific protocols to treat infant ALL [13,17,18]. Biologic characteristics of infant ALL cells are described later in the paragraph discussing the *MLL* gene.

T-cell ALL is detected in approximately 15% of childhood ALL. It is characterized by a relative resistance to different classes of drugs when compared with B-lineage ALL [14]. T-cell ALL cells accumulate less methotrexate polyglutamates and less cytarabine triphosphate than precursor B-ALL cells [19]. With risk-adapted therapy the outcome of T-cell ALL now approaches that of B-lineage ALL in many study groups (see Table 1).

Approximately 85% of childhood ALL is of B lineage, mainly common or preB ALL. A very immature subtype characterized by the lack of CD10

Table 2
Clinical and biologic factors predicting clinical outcome

Factor	Favorable	Unfavorable
Age at diagnosis	1–9 years	< 1 or > 9 years
Sex	Female	Male
White blood cell count	Low (eg, < 50 or < 25 × 10^9/L)	High (eg, > 50 or > 25 × 10^9/L)
Genotype	Hyperdiploidy (> 50 chromosomes) t(12;21) or *TEL/AML1* fusion	Hypodiploidy (< 45 chromosomes) t(9;22) or *BCR/ABL* fusion t(4;11) or *MLL/AF4* fusion
Immunophenotype	Common, preB	ProB, T-lineage

expression (proB ALL) is associated with a high incidence of *MLL* gene rearrangements and an unfavorable outcome. Mature B-lineage ALL, defined by the presence of immunoglobulins on the cell surface, has a favorable outcome only when treated with B-non-Hodgkin lymphoma protocols.

Genetics

Hyperdiploidy

Hyperdiploidy (a DNA index > 1.16 or > 50 chromosomes per leukemia cell) is found in approximately 25% of children who have B-lineage ALL. It is associated with a favorable outcome, especially when extra copies of chromosome 4, 10 or 17 are present [20]. Hyperdiploid ALL cells have an increased tendency to undergo apoptosis, accumulate high amounts of methotrexate polyglutamates, and are highly sensitive to antimetabolites and L-asparaginase [21].

TEL/AML1

The *TEL/AML1* fusion, also found in approximately 25% of cases, is mutually exclusive with hyperdiploidy and also is associated with a favorable outcome. It is formed by a fusion of the *TEL* gene on chromosome 12 encoding for a nuclear phosphoprotein of the ETS family of transcription factors and the *AML1* gene on chromosome 21, a transcription factor gene encoding for part of the core-binding factor. The *TEL/AML1* fusion probably inhibits the transcription activity of the normal *AML1* gene involved in proliferation and differentiation of hematopoietic cells. *TEL/AML1* fusion is associated with a high chemosensitivity, especially for L-asparaginase [22]. The mechanism behind this asparaginase sensitivity remains unclear but is not caused by a low asparagines synthetase activity in the leukemic cells [23,24]. *TEL/AML1*-rearranged cells also may be more sensitive to other drugs, especially anthracyclines and etoposide [25].

Both hyperdiploidy and *TEL/AML1* occur mainly in children younger than 10 years of age with common/preB ALL and are rare above this age and in other ALL immunophenotypes.

MLL

Abnormalities of the mixed lineage leukemia (*MLL*) gene on chromosome 11q23 occur in only approximately 2% of children above the age of 1 year, although it is present in approximately 80% of infants who have ALL. All types of *MLL* gene rearrangements, such as *MLL/AF4* created by t(4;11), *MLL/ENL* created by t(11;19), and *MLL/AF9* created by t(9;11), are associated with a poor outcome in infants who have ALL [17]; in older children this poor outcome may only hold true for the presence of *MLL/AF4* [26]. The *MLL/AF9* rearrangement occurs in older infants and is characterized by a more mature pattern of immunoglobulin gene rearrangements, suggesting another pathogenesis [17,27].

The precise actions of the fusion products involving *MLL* are not known, but they are associated with abnormal expression of *HOX* genes, which may lead to abnormal growth of hematopoietic stem cells [28]. ALL cells with *MLL* gene abnormalities are highly resistant to glucocorticoids in vitro and in vivo and also to L-asparaginase [14,17,29]. These cells, however, show a marked sensitivity to the nucleoside analogues cytarabine and cladribine [30]. This sensitivity is related to a high expression of the membrane nucleoside transporter ENT1 [31]. *MLL*-rearranged ALL cells do not show a defective methotrexate polyglutamation [32] and have no overexpression of multidrug resistance proteins [33]. Methotrexate pharmacokinetics might be different in the youngest infants [34].

BCR-ABL

The translocation t(9;22) fuses the *BCR* gene on chromosome 22 to the *ABL* gene on chromosome 9 causing an abnormal *ABL* tyrosine kinase activity associated with increased proliferation and decreased apoptosis. The *BCR/ABL* fusion is found mainly in common and preB ALL. The incidence of *BCR/ABL* increases with age: it is seen in approximately 3% of children who have ALL but in approximately 25% of adults who have ALL. The presence of *BCR/ABL* predicts a poor outcome.

Children who have *BCR/ABL*-rearranged ALL or *MLL*-rearranged ALL more often show a poor response to prednisone [29,35] and have high levels of MRD after induction therapy.

Genetics in T-cell acute lymphoblastic leukemia

The prognostic value of genetic abnormalities in T-ALL is less clear [36]. Ectopic expression of *TAL-1* is caused by the translocation t(1;14) in only a few percent of T-ALL cases or, more often, by the *SIL-TAL* fusion transcript. Activation of *HOX11* by the translocations t(10;14) and t(7;10) occur in approximately 10% of T-ALL cases. Two recently described abnormalities occur frequently and exclusively in T-ALL. These are the ectopic expression of *HOX11L2*, mainly caused by the translocation t(5;14), in approximately 25% of T-ALL cases and activating mutations of the *NOTCH1* gene in 50% of T-ALL cases. *NOTCH1* mutations are not associated with a poor outcome and may be associated with a favorable outcome [37].

Others

Many other recurrent genetic and molecular genetic lesions exist in small subsets of childhood ALL such as the translocation t(1;19) leading to a *E2A-PBX1* fusion detected in less than 5% of precursor B-ALL, mainly preB ALL. Although in the past this translocation had been associated with a poor prognosis, this is not longer true with contemporary treatment protocols. Two percent of precursor B-lineage ALL cases harbor an intra-chromosomal amplification of chromosome 21 that is associated with poor survival [38]. Hypodiploidy (< 45 chromosomes) is detected in only 1% of children who have ALL and is associated with poor outcome, particularly in the low-hypodiploid (33–39 chromosomes) or near-haploid cases (23–29 chromosomes) as shown in a recent retrospective international study [39].

A discussion of all other abnormalities is beyond the scope of this article. It should be mentioned that children who have Down syndrome and ALL do not have a better outcome and perhaps even have a worse outcome than other ALL cases because they lack favorable genetic features [40,41].

Therapy

The backbone of contemporary multiagent chemotherapeutic regimens is formed by four elements: induction, CNS-directed treatment and consolidation, reinduction, and maintenance.

Induction

The goal of induction therapy is to induce morphologic remission and to restore normal hematopoiesis. Induction therapy contains at least three systemic drugs (ie, a glucocorticoid, vincristine, and L-asparaginase) and intrathecal therapy. The addition of an anthracycline as a fourth drug is matter of debate. In some protocols all patients receive an anthracycline; in other protocols it is reserved for high-risk cases. The induction phase aims to induce complete morphologic remission in 4 to 6 weeks.

Central nervous system–directed treatment and consolidation

CNS-directed therapy aims to prevent CNS relapses and to reduce the systemic minimal residual leukemia burden. CNS therapy usually is achieved by weekly or biweekly intrathecal therapy along with systemically administered drugs such as high-dose methotrexate (MTX) and 6-mercaptopurine (6-MP). Some groups rely on other drugs (eg, cyclophosphamide, cytarabine) in the consolidation phase to reduce systemic tumor burden further.

Reinduction

Reinduction therapy or delayed (re)intensification most often uses drugs comparable to those used during induction and consolidation therapy and has clearly shown its value by reducing the risk of relapse.

Maintenance

Therapy for ALL is completed by prolonged maintenance therapy for a total treatment duration of 2 years, or even longer in some protocols.

Maintenance consists of daily 6-MP and weekly MTX. In some protocols additional pulsed applications of a glucocorticoid and vincristine and intrathecal therapy are administered.

A fifth element, allogeneic stem cell transplantation (SCT), is reserved for only a small number of selected patients in first complete remission. The contribution of specific parts of treatment depends on the total therapy administered to a patient. A few important topics for which new data have been produced recently are discussed in the following sections.

Anthracyclines in induction?

It is unclear if addition of an anthracycline to a three-drug induction regimen is of benefit. Regimens that do not contain anthracycline are less myelosuppressive. Studies performed by the Children's Cancer Group, however, showed that selected patients younger than 10 years of age did not benefit from the addition of an anthracycline, whereas selected older children did [42].

Dexamethasone or prednisone?

Several recent randomized studies have shown that the substitution of prednisone (approximately 40 mg/m^2) by dexamethasone (approximately 6 mg/m^2) significantly decreases the risk of bone marrow and CNS relapses when used in what are thought to be equipotent dosages [43,44]. One Japanese study, however, did not confirm the advantage of using dexamethasone [45]. The benefit of dexamethasone may result from higher free plasma levels and a better CNS penetration or from the fact that the presumed equivalent antileukemic activity for prednisone/dexamethasone is not a 6:1 dose ratio but is higher, as some (but not all) in vitro experiments suggest [46,47]. At this dose ratio dexamethasone also results in more toxicity than prednisone [43]. In vitro, a strong cross-resistance to prednisone and dexamethasone exists in ALL cells.

Which dose intensity of which asparaginase?

Randomized studies have revealed that at the same dose schedules, the use of L-asparaginase derived from *Escherichia coli* resulted in significant better EFS and overall survival (OS) rates than when asparaginase derived from *Erwinia chrysanthemi* (Erwinase) was used [48,49]. This difference results from differences in the half-lives of the drugs, and the difference presumably would not be found if Erwinase were given in an adequate dose-intensity schedule. The dose-intensity schedule to achieve complete asparagine depletion is 5000 units/m^2 every 3 days for *E coli* asparaginase. Erwinase must be scheduled more frequently than *E coli* asparaginase to achieve the same asparagine depletion. For the pegylated type of *E coli* asparaginase (PEG-asparaginase), 2500 units/m^2 once every 2 weeks leads to the same pharmacodynamic effects. Lower doses of PEG-asparaginase (1000 units/m^2) also lead to complete asparagine depletion in serum but not in the cerebrospinal fluid [50].

Intensification of asparaginase in induction and reinduction has improved outcomes in different studies [51–53]. Also, asparaginase intolerance was an important factor predicting an inferior outcome [54,55]. Allergic reactions usually are responsible for the discontinuation of asparaginase. Allergic reactions occur mainly when the drug is readministered in reinduction several weeks after first exposure during induction. In addition, the presence of asparaginase antibodies may lead to inactivation of the drug. Consequently, many investigators favor the use of the less immunogenic PEG-asparaginase from therapy outset rather than using it only after allergic reactions have occurred. In the light of these data, pharmacodynamic monitoring of asparaginase administration may prove very important for individual children who have ALL.

Which central nervous system–directed therapy?

To clarify the role of different CNS-directed therapies, a meta-analysis was published in 2003 [56]. From this analysis it became clear that long-term intrathecal therapy leads to EFS rates comparable with those of radiotherapy. Radiotherapy seemed to be more effective than high-dose MTX in preventing CNS relapse, but intravenous MTX reduced systemic relapses, resulting in comparable EFS rates for high-dose MTX and radiotherapy. It was concluded that radiotherapy can be replaced by multiple intrathecal doses of chemotherapy and that intravenous MTX reduces systemic relapses. It is still unclear whether intrathecal triple therapy (glucocorticoid, MTX, cytarabine) has any advantage over the use of intrathecal MTX as single drug. A recent Children's Cancer Group study suggested that intrathecal triple therapy prevented CNS relapse but did not improve OS because fewer bone marrow relapses occurred when intrathecal MTX was used as a single agent [57].

The results of CNS-directed therapy depend on the treatment used. For example, the use of systemic dexamethasone reduces the incidence of CNS relapse. The comparison of different CNS preventive regimens is hampered because results are described for heterogeneous groups of patients. In several protocols, radiotherapy is still given to selected groups of high-risk patients such as those who have T-ALL with high white cell counts and children who have CNS involvement at diagnosis. Cranial radiotherapy is specifically toxic for very young children because of its detrimental effect on cognitive function.

What type of reinduction/intensification and maintenance?

Maintenance therapy consists of daily oral 6-MP and weekly intravenous or oral MTX. The intravenous administration of MTX may overcome compliance problems, but there is no evidence that it is more effective than oral

MTX. Several randomized studies have shown that the use of thioguanine offers no advantage over 6-MP in maintenance therapy [58,59]. For unknown reasons, 6-MP is more effective when administered in the evening than in the morning. Continuous adaptations of the doses of MTX and 6-MP based on peripheral blood counts are necessary to reduce the risk of relapse, on the one hand, and the risk of infections, on the other [60,61]. There are large interindividual differences in the doses that are tolerated or needed to reduce cell counts. This variability reflects pharmacogenetic differences, for instance in the status of thiopurine methyltransferase, a key enzyme that inactivates thiopurines [60,62]. Allelic differences are associated with reduced activity. Also, large intraindividual differences in doses occur (eg, because of concurrent viral infections). Recently, the major ALL study groups reached consensus on how to adjust the doses of 6-MP and MTX during maintenance so that the white blood cell count remains between 1.5 and 3.0 $\times$ 10^9/L. Routine measurements of liver function are not necessary in patients who do not have symptoms of liver dysfunction.

A meta-analysis of 42 trials showed that both longer maintenance (3 years versus 2 years) and the use of pulses of vincristine and a glucocorticoid during maintenance result in lower relapse rates but increased death rates [63]. The most important factor that has helped reduce relapses and improve survival is the use of an intensive reinduction course at the start of maintenance therapy. Several randomized studies proved the value of reinduction therapy for childhood ALL [64,65]. Attempts to omit reinduction led to a significant increase in relapse rate [66]. More than 50% of patients who were treated without reinduction did not relapse, however, illustrating that not all patients really need this intensification element. The question, of course, is how to identify these patients early on. When an intensive reinduction course is given, neither longer maintenance nor the use of vincristine/glucocorticoid pulses may contribute significantly to a better OS [63].

The results of the meta-analysis do not exclude the possibility that subgroups of patients may benefit from a longer duration of maintenance. Several study groups use longer maintenance therapy for boys than for girls. Reduction of the duration of maintenance below 2 years in a Japanese study led to an increased risk of relapse [67]. This study, however, also demonstrate that not all patients need 2 years of maintenance therapy. Again, the important question is how to identify these patients. It might be that a long maintenance therapy is less effective in high-risk leukemias with a very aggressive behavior, such as *MLL* gene–rearranged ALL, *bcr-abl*–positive ALL, and T-ALL, in which relapses occur relatively early; the more smoldering types of ALL, such as hyperdiploid and *TEL/AML1*-gene rearranged ALL, might benefit more from maintenance therapy.

A recent large, randomized study did not show a benefit for the use of pulses with vincristine and a glucocorticoid in a selected group of patients treated on a Berlin/Frankfurt/Münster regimen [68]. The benefit of these pulses therefore may be found only in studies that use no or a less intensive reinduction course, such as in the Dutch Childhood Leukemia Study Group-6 study [69] or in studies in which the upfront therapy is relatively mild.

Who should (not) be transplanted?

Autologous SCT is not effective in childhood ALL and therefore should not be performed. A collaborative study of several large study groups has shown that *BCR/ABL*-positive ALL benefits from allogeneic SCT from a matched related donor both in terms of EFS and OS [12]. For other types of donor this benefit was not proven. A comparable analysis for children who had t(4;11) could not detect a beneficial effect of SCT from any type of donor [26]. Recently, a comparison was performed between children who had very high-risk ALL in first remission who were assigned by the availability of a compatible related donor to receive SCT or to receive chemotherapy when no donor was available [70]. "Very high risk" was defined in this study by the presence of one or more of the following criteria: failure to achieve complete remission after 5 weeks' therapy, t(9;22) or t(4;11) positivity, a poor prednisone response associated with T-cell phenotype, or a white blood cell count higher than $100 \times 10^e9/L$. The 5-year disease-free survival ratewas better for the patients who received SCT from a matched related donor than for those who received chemotherapy. Only one in six of these high-risk patients had a suitable family donor, however. SCT from alternative donors resulted in an inferior outcome. Therefore the role of allogeneic SCT in first complete remission is limited in these very high-risk patients. Another recent study failed to prove a benefit for allogeneic SCT in very high-risk cases [71], whereas the Berlin/Frankfurt/Münster study group showed that high-risk T-cell ALL cases may benefit from SCT [72].

Treatment of adolescents

Four recent reports from four different countries show that outcome for adolescents who have ALL is better when these patients are treated on a pediatric rather than an adult protocol [73–76]. The 5-year EFS of patients aged 15 to 21 years was approximately 30% higher when they were treated according to a pediatric protocol (Table 3). This result could not be explained by differences in immunophenotype and genetic abnormalities, but there seemed to be large differences in the dose intensity used during treatment. The pediatric protocols contained more glucocorticoids, vincristine, L-asparaginase, MTX, and 6-MP. In addition, it is conceivable that the longer delays between different parts of treatment noted in adolescents treated according to the adult protocols might have played a role. It is possible that hematologists have a different approach in managing toxicities because they generally treat older patients who do not tolerate intensive therapy well. Also, the toxicity caused by SCT usually is accepted as part of therapy, whereas adult hematologists have less experience with glucocorticoid- and asparaginase-induced toxicities. In the Dutch study, use of the

Table 3
Outcome of adolescents treated on a pediatric or adult acute lymphoblastic leukemia protocol

Study group [reference]	Patient number	Age category (in years)	5-year event-free survival (%)
United Sates: pediatric [24]	196	16–21	64
United States: adult [24]	103	16–21	38
Dutch: pediatric [23]	47	15–18	69
Dutch: adult [23]	44	15–18	34
French: pediatric [12]	77	15–20	67
French: adult [12]	100	15–20	41
United Kingdom: pediatric [72]	61	15–17	65
United Kingdom: adult [72]	67	15–17	49

adult ALL treatment protocol resulted in both a higher relapse rate and in a higher toxic death rate for adolescents [74].

Side effects

Nearly all chemotherapy side effects seen in children treated for ALL are temporary. The single most important cause of toxic death is infections: 0.5% to 1.5% of patients die from infections during induction therapy, and between 1% and 3% die from infections while in complete remission [77]. Many toxicities result from using a combination of drugs; some, however, are drug specific. Drug-specific toxicities include neuropathy and constipation caused by vincristine, mucositis caused by MTX, diabetes, behavior disturbances, Cushingoid appearance, osteoporosis, and avascular necrosis of bone caused by glucocorticoids, and allergic reactions and thrombosis caused by asparaginase [78].

Toxicity increases with patient age. For example, children older than 10 years have a higher incidence of side effects to glucocorticoids such as avascular necrosis of bone and hyperglycemia, and pancreatitis and thromboembolic complications caused by L-asparaginase [55]. About 5% to 15% of children older than 10 years of age and adolescents experience one or more of these side effects. It has been shown that short pulses of glucocorticoids (5 days) lead to fewer side effects than more continuous schedules with the same cumulative doses of glucocorticoids.

Perspectives

New genomic techniques

The recent sequencing of the human genome and technical advances in high through-put analysis of DNA copy number and mRNA expression now allow a "molecular portrait" of leukemia. Gene-expression profiling can be helpful in classifying ALL patients, in revealing new insights into the pathways involved in different genetic subtypes of ALL, and in identifying new pathways involved in therapy resistance and new therapeutic targets [79].

The first studies using gene-expression profiling showed that known morphologic, immunophenotypic, and genetic subclasses of ALL had specific gene-expression profiles [28,80,81]. Gene-expression profiling may be even more suitable for classifying ALL cases because it takes into consideration the biologic state and genetic progression [82]. Gene-expression patterns have been revealed that are related to in vitro resistance to several classes of individual agents, to clinical outcome, and to cross-resistance to multiple antileukemic drugs [83,84]. These studies, for example, have shown that *MCL-1* overexpression is involved in glucocorticoid resistance in ALL. Modulation of *MCL-1* expression sensitizes ALL cells to glucocorticoids [85].

Bhojwani and colleagues [86] revealed that gene-expression profiles of early relapsed ALL samples were characterized by the overexpression of genes involved in cell-cycle regulation; this finding might identify attractive new targets for therapy. Armstrong [87] and Stam [88] showed high levels of wild-type *FLT3* in *MLL*-rearranged ALL. High levels of *FLT3* are related to a poor outcome [89], and inhibition of this tyrosine kinase is very effective in *MLL*-rearranged ALL cells in vitro [88] as well as in an in vivo mouse model [87]. This finding has led to the design of two different phase I/II studies of these inhibitors in *MLL*-rearranged ALL.

Genome-wide techniques to screen for mutations and amplifications and for single-nucleotide polymorphisms (SNPs) recently have revealed many recurrent genetic alterations that are important for the development of ALL [90–93] and for the sensitivity to chemotherapy. For example, polymorphisms in folate-related genes are related to the MTX sensitivity of ALL cells [94]. Mullighan and colleagues [90] used SNP arrays to reveal that childhood ALL samples show recurrent gene deletions and amplifications including somatic *PAX5* deletion, which is present in about one third of all ALL cases [90]. Overall deletions were more common than amplification, specifically deletions of genes involved in B-cell differentiation, indicating that arrested development is a key feature of leukemia transformation. In the forthcoming years, large-scale studies will analyze the profile of micro-RNAs in ALL subtypes [95] and the role of newly discovered genetic subtype-specific microRNAs in ALL.

Targeted therapies

Several new targeted therapies may contribute to a further improvement in treatment results in childhood and adolescent ALL (Table 4). The ultimate target of therapy is the leukemogenic fusion product. The best example is the *BCR/ABL* fusion product leading to an abnormal *ABL* tyrosine kinase activity. Imatinib is an effective inhibitor of this kinase [96], but resistance rapidly occurs when it is used as a single agent, mainly because of the selection or development of leukemic subclones with *BCR-ABL* point

Table 4
New targeted therapies for childhood and adolescent acute lymphoblastic leukemia

Drug	Target	Type of ALL
Imatinib	*ABL* tyrosine kinase	*BCR-ABL* fusion, *NUP214-ABL1* fusion
Dasatinib, nilotinib	*ABL* tyrosine kinase (also many mutations), *SRC* kinases	*BCR-ABL* fusion
PKC412, CEP701, other *FLT3* inhibitors	Mutated *FLT3*, wild type over-expressed *FLT3*	*MLL* gene–rearranged ALL, hyperdiploid ALL
Demethylating agents	Hypermethylation	*MLL* gene–rearranged ALL, other subtypes?
Rituximab	CD20	CD20 + (B-lineage) ALL
Epratuzumab	CD22	CD22 + (B-lineage) ALL
Gemtuzumab ozogamicin	CD33	CD33 + ALL
Alemtuzumab	CD52	CD52 + ALL
Forodesine	PNP (purine nucleoside phosphorylase)	T-ALL
Nelarabine		T-ALL

mutations. It therefore seems that imatinib must be combined with standard antileukemic agents to treat *BCR-ABL*–positive ALL effectively. A European randomized study currently is attempting to assess the efficacy and toxicity of the addition of imatinib to all chemotherapy blocks. Resistance to imatinib is caused mainly by the outgrowth of subclones with mutations in the kinase domain of *BCR-ABL* that interfere with imatinib binding. For most mutations, this resistance can be overcome with dasatinib [97] or nilotinib [98]. A pediatric phase I-II study with dasatinib is underway. The very rare subset of T-ALL with *NUP214-ABL1* fusion also may be a suitable group for targeted therapies using these compounds.

The recent finding that half of T-ALL cases have activating mutations of the *NOTCH1* gene provides a rationale for targeted therapies of the NOTCH pathway. Cleavage of the trans-membrane receptor *NOTCH1* by gamma secretase leads to release of the intracellular domain of *NOTCH1* (ICN1), followed by translocation to the nucleus and transcription activation. Inhibitors of ICN1 production and activity seemed to be toxic for T-ALL cells in vitro and have led to a clinical trial of a gamma secretase inhibitor in patients who had refractory T-ALL; however, this trial was stopped because of gastrointestinal side effects. Targeting the enzyme purine nucleoside phosphorylase in T-ALL, especially by forodesine [99], is another strategy that will be tested in childhood ALL in the forthcoming years. Nelarabine is a nucleoside analogue that is converted intracellularly to cytarabine with promising activity as single agent in T-ALL [100,101].

Overexpression of wild-type *FLT3*, especially in *MLL*-rearranged ALL and hyperdiploid ALL, also provides an opportunity for targeted therapies with *FLT3* inhibitors. Another opportunity may be found in the hypermethylation state of *MLL*-rearranged ALL, where the tumor-suppressor gene *FHIT* is silenced by hypermethylation. Re-expression leads to the killing of infant *MLL*-rearranged ALL cells, and demethylation agents have the same effect [102].

Finally, different monoclonal antibodies, directed against different antigens (CD20, CD22, and CD52), with or without conjugated toxins, are in early clinical studies in childhood ALL.

Host pharmacogenetics

There is no doubt that host polymorphisms in drug-metabolizing genes alter drug levels and target engagement. The ultimate goal of host pharmacogenetic studies is to optimize drug dosing for each patient to achieve maximum treatment efficacy with a minimum toxicity. Germline SNPs determine the toxicity of different antileukemic drugs [103]. The most extensively studied is the gene encoding for thiopurine methyltransferase (*TPMT*) involved in the metabolism of 6-MP. Genetic polymorphisms in *TPMT* correlate with enzyme activity and with both 6-MP toxicity and outcome in ALL. Many other genes are subject to genetic polymorphisms, and the development of tools such as SNP arrays facilitates the studies of many of these polymorphisms simultaneously.

Summary

More than 80% of children who have ALL are cured with contemporary intensive chemotherapy protocols. In the forthcoming decades it will be of great importance to tailor therapy for individual patients according to early response to therapy (mainly by detecting MRD) so that the intensity of therapy can be reduced or augmented. Also, more specific therapy schedules will be developed for immunophenotypic and genetic subclasses of ALL, because it now is apparent that ALL is not a single disease entity but in fact includes different diseases with differing underlying biology and clinical courses. New genomic techniques will lead to the discovery of new molecular genetic abnormalities that will provide more insights into the biology of the different ALL subtypes. New targeted therapy approaches will be developed, and it will be important to investigate how new agents can be incorporated in existing regimens.

References

[1] Greaves M. Infection, immune responses and the aetiology of childhood leukaemia. Nat Rev Cancer 2006;6(3):193–203.

[2] Fischer S, Mann G, Konrad M, et al. Screening for leukemia- and clone-specific markers at birth in children with T cell precursor ALL suggests a predominantly postnatal origin. Blood 2007;110:3036–8.

[3] Conter V, Arico M, Valsecchi MG, et al. Long-term results of the Italian Association of Pediatric Hematology and Oncology (AIEOP) acute lymphoblastic leukemia studies, 1982–1995. Leukemia 2000;14(12):2196–204.

[4] Schrappe M, Reiter A, Zimmerman M, et al. Long-term results of four consecutive trials in childhood ALL performed by the ALL-BFM study group from 1981 to 1995. Berlin-Frankfurt-Munster. Leukemia 2000;14(12):2205–22.

[5] Gaynon PS, Trigg ME, Heerema NA, et al. Children's Cancer Group trials in childhood acute lymphoblastic leukemia: 1983–1995. Leukemia 2000;14(12):2223–33.

[6] Harms DO, Janka-Schaub GE. Co-operative Study Group for Childhood Acute Lymphoblastic Leukemia (COALL): long-term follow-up of trials 82, 85, 89 and 92. Leukemia 2000; 14(12):2234–9.

[7] Kamps WA, Veerman AJ, van Wering ER, et al. Long-term follow-up of Dutch Childhood Leukemia Study Group (DCLSG) protocols for children with acute lymphoblastic leukemia, 1984–1991. Leukemia 2000;14(12):2240–6.

[8] Silverman LB, Declerck L, Gelber RD, et al. Results of Dana-Farber Cancer Institute Consortium protocols for children with newly diagnosed acute lymphoblastic leukemia (1981–1995). Leukemia 2000;14(12):2247–56.

[9] Vilmer E, Suciu S, Ferster A, et al. Long-term results of three randomized trials (58831, 58832, 58881) in childhood acute lymphoblastic leukemia: a CLCG-EORTC report. Children Leukemia Cooperative Group. Leukemia 2000;14(12):2257–66.

[10] Gustafsson G, Schmiegelow K, Forestier E, et al. Improving outcome through two decades in childhood ALL in the Nordic countries: the impact of high-dose methotrexate in the reduction of CNS irradiation. Nordic Society of Pediatric Haematology and Oncology (NOPHO). Leukemia 2000;14(12):2267–75.

[11] Pui CH, Boyett JM, Rivera GK, et al. Long-term results of total therapy studies 11, 12 and 13A for childhood acute lymphoblastic leukemia at St Jude Children's Research Hospital. Leukemia 2000;14(12):2286–94.

[12] Eden OB, Harrison G, Richards S, et al. Long-term follow-up of the United Kingdom Medical Research Council protocols for childhood acute lymphoblastic leukaemia, 1980–1997. Medical Research Council Childhood Leukaemia Working Party. Leukemia 2000;14(12):2307–20.

[13] Tomizawa D, Koh K, Sato T, et al. Outcome of risk-based therapy for infant acute lymphoblastic leukemia with or without an MLL gene rearrangement, with emphasis on late effects: a final report of two consecutive studies, MLL96 and MLL98, of the Japan Infant Leukemia Study Group. Leukemia 2007;21:2258–63.

[14] Pieters R, den Boer ML, Durian M, et al. Relation between age, immunophenotype and in vitro drug resistance in 395 children with acute lymphoblastic leukemia—implications for treatment of infants. Leukemia 1998;12(9):1344–8.

[15] Ramakers-van Woerden NL, Pieters R, Hoelzer D, et al. In vitro drug resistance profile of Philadelphia positive acute lymphoblastic leukemia is heterogeneous and related to age: a report of the Dutch and German Leukemia Study Groups. Med Pediatr Oncol 2002; 38(6):379–86.

[16] Biondi A, Cimino G, Pieters R, et al. Biological and therapeutic aspects of infant leukemia. Blood 2000;96(1):24–33.

[17] Pieters R, Schrappe M, De Lorenzo P, et al. A treatment protocol for infants younger than 1 year with acute lymphoblastic leukaemia (Interfant-99): an observational study and a multicentre randomised trial. Lancet 2007;370(9583):240–50.

[18] Hilden JM, Dinndorf PA, Meerbaum SO, et al. Analysis of prognostic factors of acute lymphoblastic leukemia in infants: report on CCG 1953 from the Children's Oncology Group. Blood 2006;108(2):441–51.

[19] Rots MG, Pieters R, Peters GJ, et al. Role of folylpolyglutamate synthetase and folylpolyglutamate hydrolase in methotrexate accumulation and polyglutamylation in childhood leukemia. Blood 1999;93(5):1677–83.

[20] Heerema NA, Sather HN, Sensel MG, et al. Prognostic impact of trisomies of chromosomes 10, 17, and 5 among children with acute lymphoblastic leukemia and high hyperdiploidy (> 50 chromosomes). J Clin Oncol 2000;18(9):1876–87.

[21] Kaspers GJ, Smets LA, Pieters R, et al. Favorable prognosis of hyperdiploid common acute lymphoblastic leukemia may be explained by sensitivity to antimetabolites and other drugs: results of an in vitro study. Blood 1995;85(3):751–6.

[22] Ramakers-van Woerden NL, Pieters R, Loonen AH, et al. TEL/AML1 gene fusion is related to in vitro drug sensitivity for L-asparaginase in childhood acute lymphoblastic leukemia. Blood 2000;96(3):1094–9.

[23] Stams WA, den Boer ML, Holleman A, et al. Asparagine synthetase expression is linked with L-asparaginase resistance in TEL-AML1-negative but not TEL-AML1-positive pediatric acute lymphoblastic leukemia. Blood 2005;105(11):4223–5.

[24] Stams WA, den Boer ML, Beverloo HB, et al. Sensitivity to L-asparaginase is not associated with expression levels of asparagine synthetase in t(12;21)+ pediatric ALL. Blood 2003;101(7):2743–7.

[25] Frost BM, Froestier E, Gustafsson G, et al. Translocation t(12;21) is related to in vitro cellular drug sensitivity to doxorubicin and etoposide in childhood acute lymphoblastic leukemia. Blood 2004;104(8):2452–7.

[26] Pui CH, Gaynon PS, Boyett JM, et al. Outcome of treatment in childhood acute lymphoblastic leukaemia with rearrangements of the 11q23 chromosomal region. Lancet 2002; 359(9321):1909–15.

[27] Jansen MW, Corral L, van der Velden VH, et al. Immunobiological diversity in infant acute lymphoblastic leukemia is related to the occurrence and type of MLL gene rearrangement. Leukemia 2007;21(4):633–41.

[28] Armstrong SA, Staunton JE, Silverman LB, et al. MLL translocations specify a distinct gene expression profile that distinguishes a unique leukemia. Nat Genet 2002;30(1):41–7.

[29] Dordelmann M, Reiter A, Borkhardt A, et al. Prednisone response is the strongest predictor of treatment outcome in infant acute lymphoblastic leukemia. Blood 1999;94(4): 1209–17.

[30] Ramakers-van Woerden NL, Beverloo HB, Veerman AJ, et al. In vitro drug-resistance profile in infant acute lymphoblastic leukemia in relation to age, MLL rearrangements and immunophenotype. Leukemia 2004;18(3):521–9.

[31] Stam RW, den Boer ML, Meijerink JP, et al. Differential mRNA expression of Ara-C-metabolizing enzymes explains Ara-C sensitivity in MLL gene-rearranged infant acute lymphoblastic leukemia. Blood 2003;101(4):1270–6.

[32] Ramakers-van Woerden NL, Pieters R, Rots MG, et al. Infants with acute lymphoblastic leukemia: no evidence for high methotrexate resistance. Leukemia 2002;16(5):949–51.

[33] Stam RW, van den Heuvel-Eibrink MM, den Boer ML, et al. Multidrug resistance genes in infant acute lymphoblastic leukemia: Ara-C is not a substrate for the breast cancer resistance protein. Leukemia 2004;18(1):78–83.

[34] Thompson PA, Murry DJ, Rosner GL, et al. Methotrexate pharmacokinetics in infants with acute lymphoblastic leukemia. Cancer Chemother Pharmacol 2007;59(6):847–53.

[35] Schrappe M, Arico M, Harbott J, et al. Philadelphia chromosome-positive (Ph+) childhood acute lymphoblastic leukemia: good initial steroid response allows early prediction of a favorable treatment outcome. Blood 1998;92(8):2730–41.

[36] Graux C, Cools J, Michaux L, et al. Cytogenetics and molecular genetics of T-cell acute lymphoblastic leukemia: from thymocyte to lymphoblast. Leukemia 2006;20(9): 1496–510.

[37] Breit S, Stanulla M, Flohr T, et al. Activating NOTCH1 mutations predict favorable early treatment response and long-term outcome in childhood precursor T-cell lymphoblastic leukemia. Blood 2006;108(4):1151–7.

[38] Moorman AV, Richards SM, Robinson HM, et al. Prognosis of children with acute lymphoblastic leukemia (ALL) and intrachromosomal amplification of chromosome 21 (iAMP21). Blood 2007;109(6):2327–30.

[39] Nachman JB, Heerema NA, Sather H, et al. Outcome of treatment in children with hypodiploid acute lymphoblastic leukemia. Blood 2007;110(4):1112–5.

[40] Bassal M, La MK, Whitlock JA, et al. Lymphoblast biology and outcome among children with Down syndrome and ALL treated on CCG-1952. Pediatr Blood Cancer 2005;44(1): 21–8.

[41] Whitlock JA, Sather HN, Gaynon P, et al. Clinical characteristics and outcome of children with Down syndrome and acute lymphoblastic leukemia: a Children's Cancer Group study. Blood 2005;106(13):4043–9.

[42] Tubergen DG, Gilchrist GS, O'Brien RT, et al. Improved outcome with delayed intensification for children with acute lymphoblastic leukemia and intermediate presenting features: a Childrens Cancer Group phase III trial. J Clin Oncol 1993;11:527–37.

[43] Bostrom BC, Sensel MR, Sather HN, et al. Dexamethasone versus prednisone and daily oral versus weekly intravenous mercaptopurine for patients with standard-risk acute lymphoblastic leukemia: a report from the Children's Cancer Group. Blood 2003;101(10): 3809–17.

[44] Mitchell CD, Richards SM, Kinsey SE, et al. Benefit of dexamethasone compared with prednisolone for childhood acute lymphoblastic leukaemia: results of the UK Medical Research Council ALL97 randomized trial. Br J Haematol 2005;129(6):734–45.

[45] Igarashi S, Manabe A, Ohara A, et al. No advantage of dexamethasone over prednisolone for the outcome of standard- and intermediate-risk childhood acute lymphoblastic leukemia in the Tokyo Children's Cancer Study Group L95-14 protocol. J Clin Oncol 2005; 23(27):6489–98.

[46] Kaspers GJ, Veerman AJ, Popp-Snijders C, et al. Comparison of the antileukemic activity in vitro of dexamethasone and prednisolone in childhood acute lymphoblastic leukemia. Med Pediatr Oncol 1996;27(2):114–21.

[47] Ito C, Evans WE, McNinch L, et al. Comparative cytotoxicity of dexamethasone and prednisolone in childhood acute lymphoblastic leukemia. J Clin Oncol 1996;14(8):2370–6.

[48] Duval M, Suciu S, Ferster A, et al. Comparison of Escherichia coli-asparaginase with Erwinia-asparaginase in the treatment of childhood lymphoid malignancies: results of a randomized European Organisation for Research and Treatment of Cancer-Children's Leukemia Group phase 3 trial. Blood 2002;99(8):2734–9.

[49] Moghrabi A, Levy DE, Asselin B, et al. Results of the Dana-Farber Cancer Institute ALL Consortium Protocol 95-01 for children with acute lymphoblastic leukemia. Blood 2007; 109(3):896–904.

[50] Appel IM, Pinheiro JP, den Boer ML, et al. Lack of asparagine depletion in the cerebrospinal fluid after one intravenous dose of PEG-asparaginase: a window study at initial diagnosis of childhood ALL. Leukemia 2003;17(11):2254–6.

[51] Pession A, Valsecchi MG, Masera G, et al. Long-term results of a randomized trial on extended use of high dose L-asparaginase for standard risk childhood acute lymphoblastic leukemia. J Clin Oncol 2005;23(28):7161–7.

[52] Rizzari C, Vasecchi MG, Arico M, et al. Effect of protracted high-dose L-asparaginase given as a second exposure in a Berlin-Frankfurt-Munster-based treatment: results of the randomized 9102 intermediate-risk childhood acute lymphoblastic leukemia study–a report from the Associazione Italiana Ematologia Oncologia Pediatrica. J Clin Oncol 2001;19(5):1297–303.

[53] Amylon MD, Shuster J, Pullen J, et al. Intensive high-dose asparaginase consolidation improves survival for pediatric patients with T cell acute lymphoblastic leukemia and advanced stage lymphoblastic lymphoma: a Pediatric Oncology Group study. Leukemia 1999;13(3):335–42.

[54] Avramis VI, Sencer C, Periclou AP, et al. A randomized comparison of native Escherichia coli asparaginase and polyethylene glycol conjugated asparaginase for treatment of children with newly diagnosed standard-risk acute lymphoblastic leukemia: a Children's Cancer Group study. Blood 2002;99(6):1986–94.

[55] Silverman LB, Gelber RD, Dalton VK, et al. Improved outcome for children with acute lymphoblastic leukemia: results of Dana-Farber Consortium Protocol 91-01. Blood 2001;97(5):1211–8.

[56] Clarke M, Gaynon P, Hann I, et al. CNS-directed therapy for childhood acute lymphoblastic leukemia: childhood ALL Collaborative Group overview of 43 randomized trials. J Clin Oncol 2003;21(9):1798–809.

[57] Matloub Y, Lindemulder S, Gaynon PS, et al. Intrathecal triple therapy decreases central nervous system relapse but fails to improve event-free survival when compared with intrathecal methotrexate: results of the Children's Cancer Group (CCG) 1952 study for standard-risk acute lymphoblastic leukemia, reported by the Children's Oncology Group. Blood 2006;108(4):1165–73.

[58] Harms DO, Gobel U, Spaar HJ, et al. Thioguanine offers no advantage over mercaptopurine in maintenance treatment of childhood ALL: results of the randomized trial COALL-92. Blood 2003;102(8):2736–40.

[59] Vora A, Mitchell CD, Lennard L, et al. Toxicity and efficacy of 6-thioguanine versus 6-mercaptopurine in childhood lymphoblastic leukaemia: a randomised trial. Lancet 2006; 368(9544):1339–48.

[60] Relling MV, Hancock ML, Boyett JM, et al. Prognostic importance of 6-mercaptopurine dose intensity in acute lymphoblastic leukemia. Blood 1999;93(9):2817–23.

[61] Lilleyman JS, Lennard L. Mercaptopurine metabolism and risk of relapse in childhood lymphoblastic leukaemia. Lancet 1994;343(8907):1188–90.

[62] McLeod HL, Relling MV, Liu Q, et al. Polymorphic thiopurine methyltransferase in erythrocytes is indicative of activity in leukemic blasts from children with acute lymphoblastic leukemia. Blood 1995;85(7):1897–902.

[63] Duration and intensity of maintenance chemotherapy in acute lymphoblastic leukaemia: overview of 42 trials involving 12,000 randomised children. Childhood ALL Collaborative Group. Lancet 1996;347(9018):1783–8.

[64] Lange BJ, Bostrom BC, Cherlow JM, et al. Double-delayed intensification improves event-free survival for children with intermediate-risk acute lymphoblastic leukemia: a report from the Children's Cancer Group. Blood 2002;99(3):825–33.

[65] Nachman JB, Sather HN, Sensel MG, et al. Augmented post-induction therapy for children with high-risk acute lymphoblastic leukemia and a slow response to initial therapy. N Engl J Med 1998;338(23):1663–71.

[66] Kamps WA, Bokkerink JP, Hahlen K, et al. Intensive treatment of children with acute lymphoblastic leukemia according to ALL-BFM-6 without cranial radiotherapy: results of Dutch Childhood Leukemia Study Group Protocol ALL-7 (1988–1991). Blood 1999; 94(4):1226–36.

[67] Toyoda Y, Manabe A, Tsuchida M, et al. Six months of maintenance chemotherapy after intensified treatment for acute lymphoblastic leukemia of childhood. J Clin Oncol 2000; 18(7):1508–16.

[68] Conter V, Valsecchi MG, Silvestri D, et al. Pulses of vincristine and dexamethasone in addition to intensive chemotherapy for children with intermediate-risk acute lymphoblastic leukaemia: a multicentre randomised trial. Lancet 2007;369(9556):123–31.

[69] Veerman AJ, Hahlen K, Kamps WA, et al. High cure rate with a moderately intensive treatment regimen in non-high-risk childhood acute lymphoblastic leukaemia. Results of protocol ALL VI from the Dutch Childhood Leukemia Study Group. J Clin Oncol 1996; 14(3):911–8.

[70] Balduzzi A, Valsecchi MG, Uderzo C, et al. Chemotherapy versus allogeneic transplantation for very-high-risk childhood acute lymphoblastic leukaemia in first complete remission: comparison by genetic randomisation in an international prospective study. Lancet 2005;366(9486):635–42.

[71] Ribera JM, Ortega JJ, Oriol A, et al. Comparison of intensive chemotherapy, allogeneic, or autologous stem-cell transplantation as postremission treatment for children with very high risk acute lymphoblastic leukemia: PETHEMA ALL-93 Trial. J Clin Oncol 2007;25(1): 16–24.

[72] Schrauder A, Reiter A, Gadner H, et al. Superiority of allogeneic hematopoietic stem-cell transplantation compared with chemotherapy alone in high-risk childhood T-cell acute lymphoblastic leukemia: results from ALL-BFM 90 and 95. J Clin Oncol 2006;24(36): 5742–9.

[73] Boissel N, Auclerc MF, Lheritier V, et al. Should adolescents with acute lymphoblastic leukemia be treated as old children or young adults? Comparison of the French FRALLE-93 and LALA-94 trials. J Clin Oncol 2003;21(5):774–80.

[74] de Bont JM, Holt B, Dekker AW, et al. Significant difference in outcome for adolescents with acute lymphoblastic leukemia treated on pediatric vs adult protocols in the Netherlands. Leukemia 2004;18(12):2032–5.

[75] Deangelo DJ. The treatment of adolescents and young adults with acute lymphoblastic leukemia. Hematology Am Soc Hematol Educ Program 2005;123–30.

[76] Ramanujachar R, Richards S, Hann I, et al. Adolescents with acute lymphoblastic leukaemia: outcome on UK national paediatric (ALL97) and adult (UKALLXII/E2993) trials. Pediatr Blood Cancer 2007;48(3):254–61.

[77] Christensen MS, Heyman M, Mottonen M, et al. Treatment-related death in childhood acute lymphoblastic leukaemia in the Nordic countries: 1992–2001. Br J Haematol 2005; 131(1):50–8.

[78] Caruso V, Iacoviello L, Di Castelnuovo A, et al. Thrombotic complications in childhood acute lymphoblastic leukemia: a meta-analysis of 17 prospective studies comprising 1752 pediatric patients. Blood 2006;108(7):2216–22.

[79] Carroll WL, Bhojwani D, Min DJ, et al. Childhood acute lymphoblastic leukemia in the age of genomics. Pediatr Blood Cancer 2006;46(5):570–8.

[80] Yeoh EJ, Ross ME, Shurtleff SA, et al. Classification, subtype discovery, and prediction of outcome in pediatric acute lymphoblastic leukemia by gene expression profiling. Cancer Cell 2002;1(2):133–43.

[81] Ross ME, Zhou X, Song G, et al. Classification of pediatric acute lymphoblastic leukemia by gene expression profiling. Blood 2003;102(8):2951–9.

[82] Schrappe M. [Medical centers–methods, purpose and benefits]. Z Arztl Fortbild Qualitatssich 2007;101(3):141–5 [in German].

[83] Holleman A, Cheok MH, den Boer ML, et al. Gene-expression patterns in drug-resistant acute lymphoblastic leukemia cells and response to treatment. N Engl J Med 2004; 351(6):533–42.

[84] Lugthart S, Cheok MH, den Boer ML, et al. Identification of genes associated with chemotherapy crossresistance and treatment response in childhood acute lymphoblastic leukemia. Cancer Cell 2005;7(4):375–86.

[85] Wei G, Twomey D, Lamb J, et al. Gene expression-based chemical genomics identifies rapamycin as a modulator of MCL1 and glucocorticoid resistance. Cancer Cell 2006;10(4): 331–42.

[86] Bhojwani D, Kang H, Moskowitz NP, et al. Biologic pathways associated with relapse in childhood acute lymphoblastic leukemia: a Children's Oncology Group study. Blood 2006;108(2):711–7.

[87] Armstrong SA, Kung AL, Mabon ME, et al. Inhibition of FLT3 in MLL. Validation of a therapeutic target identified by gene expression based classification. Cancer Cell 2003; 3(2):173–83.

[88] Stam RW, den Boer ML, Schneider P, et al. Targeting FLT3 in primary MLL-gene-rearranged infant acute lymphoblastic leukemia. Blood 2005;106(7):2484–90.

[89] Stam RW, Schneider P, de Lorenzo P, et al. Prognostic significance of high-level FLT3 expression in MLL-rearranged infant acute lymphoblastic leukemia. Blood 2007;110(7): 2774–5.

[90] Mullighan CG, Goorha S, Radtke I, et al. Genome-wide analysis of genetic alterations in acute lymphoblastic leukaemia. Nature 2007;446(7137):758–64.

[91] Lahortiga I, De Keersmaecker K, Van Vlierberghe P, et al. Duplication of the MYB oncogene in T cell acute lymphoblastic leukemia. Nat Genet 2007;39(5):593–5.

[92] van Vlierberghe P, Meijerink JP, Lee C, et al. A new recurrent 9q34 duplication in pediatric T-cell acute lymphoblastic leukemia. Leukemia 2006;20(7):1245–53.

[93] Van Vlierberghe P, van Grotel M, Beverloo HB, et al. The cryptic chromosomal deletion del(11)(p12p13) as a new activation mechanism of LMO2 in pediatric T-cell acute lympho-blastic leukemia. Blood 2006;108(10):3520–9.

[94] Cheok MH, Evans WE. Acute lymphoblastic leukaemia: a model for the pharmacogenom-ics of cancer therapy. Nat Rev Cancer 2006;6(2):117–29.

[95] Lu J, Getz G, Miska EA, et al. MicroRNA expression profiles classify human cancers. Nature 2005;435(7043):834–8.

[96] Champagne MA, Capdeville R, Krailo M, et al. Imatinib mesylate (STI571) for treatment of children with Philadelphia chromosome-positive leukemia: results from a Children's Oncology Group phase 1 study. Blood 2004;104(9):2655–60.

[97] Talpaz M, Shah NP, Kantarjian H, et al. Dasatinib in imatinib-resistant Philadelphia chromosome-positive leukemias. N Engl J Med 2006;354(24):2531–41.

[98] Kantarjian H, Giles F, Wunderle L, et al. Nilotinib in imatinib-resistan CML and Philadel-phia chromosome-positive ALL. N Engl J Med 2006;354(24):2542–51.

[99] Gandhi V, Kilpatrick JM, Plunkett W, et al. A proof-of-principle pharmacokinetic, phar-macodynamic, and clinical study with purine nucleoside phosphorylase inhibitor immucil-lin-H (BCX-1777, forodesine). Blood 2005;106(13):4253–60.

[100] Kurtzberg J, Ernst TJ, Keating MJ, et al. Phase I study of 506U78 administered on a con-secutive 5-day schedule in children and adults with refractory hematologic malignancies. J Clin Oncol 2005;23(15):3396–403.

[101] Berg SL, Blaney SM, Devidas M, et al. Phase II study of nelarabine (compound 506U78) in children and young adults with refractory T-cell malignancies: a report from the Children's Oncology Group. J Clin Oncol 2005;23(15):3376–82.

[102] Stam RW, den Boer ML, Passier MM, et al. Silencing of the tumor suppressor gene FHIT is highly characteristic for MLL gene rearranged infant acute lymphoblastic leukemia. Leukemia 2006;20(2):264–71.

[103] Kishi S, Cheng C, French D, et al. Ancestry and pharmacogenetics of antileukemic drug toxicity. Blood 2007;109(10):4151–7.

PEDIATRIC CLINICS
OF NORTH AMERICA

ELSEVIER
SAUNDERS

Pediatr Clin N Am 55 (2008) 21–51

Acute Myeloid Leukemia

Jeffrey E. Rubnitz, MD, PhD[a],*, Brenda Gibson, MD[b],
Franklin O. Smith, MD[c]

[a]Department of Oncology, St. Jude Children's Research Hospital,
MS 260, 332 N. Lauderdale, Memphis, TN 38105, USA
[b]Department of Paediatric Haematology, Royal Hospital for Sick Children,
Yorkhill, G3 8SJ, Glasgow, Scotland, UK
[c]Division of Hematology/Oncology, University of Cincinnati College of Medicine,
Cincinnati Children's Hospital Medical Center

Acute myeloid leukemia (AML) is a heterogeneous group of leukemias that arise in precursors of myeloid, erythroid, megakaryocytic, and monocytic cell lineages. These leukemias result from clonal transformation of hematopoietic precursors through the acquisition of chromosomal rearrangements and multiple gene mutations. New molecular technologies have allowed a better understanding of these molecular events, improved classification of AML according to risk, and the development of molecularly targeted therapies. As a result of highly collaborative clinical research by pediatric cooperative cancer groups worldwide, disease-free survival (DFS) has improved significantly during the past 3 decades [1–15]. Further improvements in the outcome of children who have AML probably will reflect continued progress in understanding the biology of AML and the concomitant development of new molecularly targeted agents for use in combination with conventional chemotherapy drugs.

Epidemiology and risk factors

Approximately 6500 children and adolescents in the United States develop acute leukemia each year [16]. AML comprises only 15% to 20% of these cases but accounts for a disproportionate 30% of deaths from acute leukemia. The incidence of pediatric AML is estimated to be between five and seven cases per million people per year, with a peak incidence of 11 cases

---

JER was supported, in part, by the American Lebanese Syrian Associated Charities (ALSAC).
* Corresponding author.
E-mail address: jeffrey.rubnitz@stjude.org (J.E. Rubnitz).

doi:10.1016/j.pcl.2007.11.003

per million at 2 years of age [17–19]. Incidence reaches a low point at age approximately 9 years, then increases to nine cases per million during adolescence and remains relatively stable until age 55 years. There is no difference in incidence between male and female or black and white populations [16]. There is, however, evidence suggesting that incidence is highest in Hispanic children, intermediate in black children (5.8 cases per million), and slightly lower in white children (4.8 cases per million) [20–23]. The French-American-British (FAB) classification subtypes of AML are equally represented across ethnic and racial groups with the exception of acute promyelocytic leukemia (APL), which has a higher incidence among children of Latin and Hispanic ancestry.

During the years between 1977 and 1995, the overall incidence of AML remained stable, but there was a disturbing increase in the incidence of secondary AML as the result of prior exposure to chemotherapy and radiation [24–30]. This risk remains particularly high among individuals exposed to alkylating agents (cyclophosphamide, nitrogen mustard, ifosfamide, melphalan, and chlorambucil) and intercalating topoisomerase II inhibitors, including the epipodophyllotoxins (etoposide).

Most children who have de novo AML have no identifiable predisposing environmental exposure or inherited condition, although a number of environmental exposures, inherited conditions, and acquired disorders are associated with the development of AML. Myelodysplastic syndrome and AML reportedly are associated with exposure to chemotherapy and ionizing radiation and also to chemicals that include petroleum products and organic solvents (benzene), herbicides, and pesticides (organophosphates) [31–36].

A large number of inherited conditions predispose children to the development of AML. Among these are Down syndrome, Fanconi anemia, severe congenital neutropenia (Kostmann syndrome), Shwachman-Diamond syndrome, Diamond-Blackfan syndrome, neurofibromatosis type 1, Noonan syndrome, dyskeratosis congenita, familial platelet disorder with a predisposition to AML (FDP/AML), congenital amegakaryocytic thrombocytopenia, ataxia-telangiectasia, Klinefelter's syndrome, Li-Fraumeni syndrome, and Bloom syndrome [37–40].

Finally, AML has been associated with several acquired conditions including aplastic anemia [41,42], myelodysplastic syndrome, acquired amegakaryocytic thrombocytopenia [43,44], and paroxysmal nocturnal hemoglobinuria.

Pathogenesis

AML is the result of distinct but cooperating genetic mutations that confer a proliferative and survival advantage and that impair differentiation and apoptosis [45–47]. This multistep mechanism for the pathogenesis of AML is supported by murine models [48,49], the analysis of leukemia in twins [50–53], and the analysis of patients who have FDP/AML syndrome

[54]. Mutations in a number of genes that confer a proliferative and/or survival advantage to cells but do not affect differentiation (Class I mutations) have been identified in AML, including mutations of *FLT3*, *ALM*, oncogenic *Ras* and *PTPN11*, and the *BCR/ABL* and *TEL/PDGFβR* gene fusions. Similarly, gene mutations and translocation-associated fusions that impair differentiation and apoptosis (Class II mutations) in AML include the *AML/ETO* and *PML/RARα* fusions, *MLL* rearrangements, and mutations in *CEBPA*, *CBF*, *HOX* family members, *CBP/P300*, and co-activators of *TIF1*. AML results when hematopoietic precursor cells acquire both Class I and Class II genetic abnormalities. Although only one cytogenetic or molecular abnormality has been reported in many cases of AML, new molecular tools now are identifying multiple genetic mutations in such cases.

Accumulating data suggest that the leukemic stem cell arises at different stages of differentiation and involves heterogeneous, complex patterns of abnormality in myeloid precursor cells [55–60]. The leukemic stem cell, also called the "self-renewing leukemia-initiating cell," is located within both the CD34$^+$ and CD34$^-$ cell compartments and is rare (0.2–200 per 10^6 mononuclear cells) [61–64]. A recent study of pediatric AML suggested that patients who have *FLT3* abnormalities in less mature CD34$^+$ CD38$^-$ precursor cells are less likely to survive than patients who have *FLT3* mutations in more mature CD34$^+$ CD38$^+$ cells (11% versus 100% at 4 years; $P = .002$) [65]. Although sample sizes in this study were small, this result demonstrates the heterogeneity of genetic abnormalities in various stem cell compartments and suggests a worse outcome when less mature precursor cells harbor these abnormalities.

Clinical presentation and diagnosis

The presentation of childhood AML reflects signs and symptoms that result from leukemic infiltration of the bone marrow and extramedullary sites. Replacement of normal bone marrow hematopoietic cells results in neutropenia, anemia, and thrombocytopenia. Children commonly present with signs and symptoms of pancytopenia, including fever, fatigue, pallor, bleeding, bone pain, and infections. Disseminated intravascular coagulation may be observed at presentation of all AML subtypes but is much more frequent in childhood APL. Infiltration of extramedullary sites can result in lymphadenopathy, hepatosplenomegaly, chloromatous tumors (myeloblastomas and granulocytic sarcomas), disease in the skin (leukemia cutis), orbit, and epidural space, and, rarely, testicular involvement. The central nervous system is involved at diagnosis in approximately 15% of cases [66]. Patients who have high white blood cells counts may present with signs or symptoms of leukostasis, most often affecting the lung and brain.

A diagnosis is suggested by a complete blood cell count showing pancytopenia and blast cells and is confirmed by examination of the bone marrow. The diagnosis and subtype classification of AML is based on morphologic, cytochemical, cytogenetic, and fluorescent in situ hybridization analyses, flow cytometric immunophenotyping, and molecular testing (eg, *FLT3* mutation analysis).

Treatment of childhood acute myeloid leukemia

The prognosis of children who have AML has improved greatly during the past 3 decades (Fig. 1). Rates of complete remission (CR) as high as 80% to 90% and overall survival (OS) rates of 60% now are reported (Table 1) [1]. This success reflects the use of increasingly intensive induction chemotherapy followed by postremission treatment with additional anthracyclines and high-dose cytarabine or myeloablative regimens followed by stem cell transplantation (SCT). The drugs used in the treatment of AML have changed little, but refinement of their delivery and striking advances in supportive care have allowed administration of optimally intensive therapy with less morbidity and mortality. Better postrelapse salvage therapy also has contributed to the improvement in OS.

Treatment of AML in children generally is based on an anthracycline, cytarabine, and etoposide regimen given as a minimum of four cycles of chemotherapy. A recent report compared the results of anthracycline, cytarabine, and etoposide regimens used by 13 national study groups [1]. The regimens differed in many ways, including the cumulative doses of drugs, the choice of anthracycline, the number and intensity of blocks of treatment, and the intrathecal chemotherapy used for central nervous system (CNS) prophylaxis. Treatment generally was risk stratified, although the definition of risk groups varied, as did the indications for SCT. Despite the varying strategies, results are relatively similar (see Table 1) [2]. Many groups now

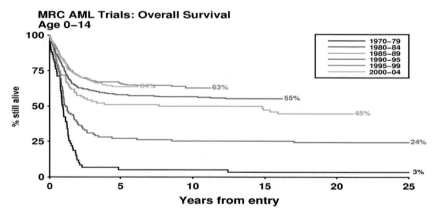

Fig. 1. Overall survival of children younger than 15 years of age who had acute myeloid leukemia treated in MRC trials during the past 3 decades.

achieve CR rates of 80% to 90%, relapse rates of 30% to 40%, event-free survival (EFS) rates of 50%, and OS rates of 60% [3–15].

Because of the small number of pediatric patients who have AML, many important questions have not been addressed in the context of randomized trials. The unresolved issues include the optimal intensity of chemotherapy, the optimal anthracycline, the optimal dose of cytarabine, the cumulative dose of anthracycline that minimizes cardiotoxicity without compromising outcome, the role of allogeneic SCT in first CR, and the use of risk-directed therapy.

Induction and consolidation therapy

The most favorable outcomes are achieved by the use of a relatively high cumulative dose of either anthracycline or cytarabine (see Table 1) [1,2]. The schedule and timing of intensification also are important. The Children's Cancer Group (CCG) reported that intensively timed induction therapy (the second cycle delivered 10 days after the first cycle) was more advantageous than standard therapy (the second cycle delivered 14 or more days after the first cycle, dependent on bone marrow status and cell-count recovery) [4,67]. Both the CR and EFS rates were significantly higher with intensively timed dosing, regardless of postremission therapy, suggesting that the depth of remission may profoundly affect survival. The benefit derived from early intensification, whether achieved by time sequencing or by adjusting cytarabine and etoposide doses to achieve a targeted plasma level, may be lost, however, if prolonged neutropenia and thrombocytopenia cause unacceptable delays in subsequent treatment [9,13]. The intensification of early therapy beyond a certain threshold therefore is unlikely to improve outcome and may even be detrimental to OS [13].

In a Medical Research Council (MRC) study, an additional course of postremission chemotherapy (four versus five courses in total) provided no advantage to patients already receiving intensive treatment [5], suggesting a plateau in the benefit of conventional postremission chemotherapy. If such a plateau is confirmed, it is likely that any additional antileukemic effect will have to come from alternative approaches, such as targeted or cellular therapies.

Certain anthracyclines are favored for their perceived greater antileukemic effect and/or their lower cardiotoxicity, but no anthracycline agent has been demonstrated to be superior. The MRC found daunorubicin and mitoxantrone to be equally efficacious but mitoxantrone to be more myelosuppressive [5]. Idarubicin is used commonly because in vitro and preclinical studies suggest that it offers a greater clinical benefit because of its faster cellular uptake, increased retention, and lower susceptibility to multidrug resistant glycoprotein [68,69]. In addition, its main metabolite, idarubicinol, has a prolonged plasma half-life (54 hours) and has antileukemic activity in the cerebrospinal fluid [70]. In the Berlin-Frankfurt-Münster (BFM) AML 93

Table 1
Outcome data from 13 national groups for patients younger than 15 years of age who had acute myeloid leukemia

Study (years of enrollment)	Number of patients enrolled	Non-responders (%)	Early death rate (%)	Complete response (%)	% 5-Year event-free survival (SE)	% 5-Year overall survival (SE)	Death rate in complete response (%)	Cumulative doses of ara-C, etoposide, and anthracyclines[a]	% of total number of patients who underwent allogeneic stem cell transplantation
AIEOP92 (1992–2001)	160	5	6	89	54 (4)	60 (4)	7	No strict protocol guidelines	29
AML-BFM93 (1993–1998)	427	10	7	83	51 (3)	58 (2)	4	41.1 g/m^2 950 mg/m^2 300–400 mg/m^2	7
CCG2891 (1989–1995)	750	18	4	78	34 (3)	47 (4)	15	14.6 g/m^2 1100 mg/m^2 180 mg/m^2	25
DCOG-ANLL 92/94 (1992–1998)	78	8	10	82	42 (6)	42 (6)	16	33.2 g/m^2 950 mg/m^2 400 mg/m^2	27
EORTC-CLG 58,921 (1993–2000)	166	13	2	84	48 (4)	62 (4)	6	23.32–29.32 g/m^2 1350 mg/m^2 380 mg/m^2	20
GATLA-AML90 (1990–1997)	179	11	20	70	31 (4)	41 (4)	7	41.1 g/m^2 1450 mg/m^2 300 mg/m^2	3
LAME91 (1991–1998)	247	5	4	91	48 (4)	62 (4)	6	9.8–13.4 g/m^2 400 mg/m^2 460 mg/m^2	30

Study								Cumulative dose	
NOPHO-AML93 (1993–2001)	223	5	2	92	50 (3)	66 (3)	2	49.6–61.3 g/m² 1600 mg/m² 300–375 mg/m²	25
PINDA-92 (1992–1998)	151	5	26	68	36	36	4	7.64 g/m² 450 mg/m² 350 mg/m²	—
POG8821 (1988–1993)	511	19	4	77	31 (2)	42 (2)	8	55.7 g/m² 2250 mg/m² 360 mg/m²	13
PPLLSG98 (1998–2002)	104	13	8	80	47 (5)	50 (5)	10	7.0–15.1 g/m² 450–950 mg/m² 420–600 mg/m²	Not reported
St. Jude-AML91 (1991–1997)	62	16	3	79	44 (15)	57 (11)	?	3.8 g/m² 1200 g/m² 270 mg/m²	Not given
UK MRC AML10 (1988–1995)	303	3	4	93	49	58	10	10.6 g/m² 500–1500 mg/m² 550 mg/m²	20
UK MRC AML12 (1995–2002)	455	4	4	92	56	66	6	4.6–34.6 g/m² 1500 mg/m² 300–610 mg/m²	8

Abbreviations: AIEOP, Associazione Italiana Ematologia Oncologia Pediatrica; BFM, Berlin-Frankfurt-Münster; CCG, Children's Cancer Group; DCOG, Dutch Childhood Oncology Group; EORTC-CLG, European Organization for the Research and Treatment of Cancer–Children Leukemia Group; GATLA, The Argentine Group for the Treatment of Acute Leukemia; LAME, Leucemie Aigue Myeloblastique Enfant); NOPHO, Nordic Society of Pediatric Haematology and Oncology; PINDA, the National Program for Antineoplastic Drugs for Children; POG, Pediatric Oncology Group; PPLLSG, Polish Pediatric Leukemia/Lymphoma Study Group; UK MRC, United Kingdom Medical Research Council.

[a] Cumulative dose of anthracyclines was calculated by applying the following arbitrary conversion factors to obtain daunorubicin equivalents: idarubicin, 5×; mitoxantrone, 5×; doxorubicin, 1×. Some groups (Leucemie Aique Myeloide Enfant and the Medical Research Council in the United Kingdom) also administered amsacrine, which is not included in calculated total anthracycline exposure.

trial, induction therapy with idarubicin, cytarabine, and etoposide (AIE) resulted in significantly greater blast-cell clearance at day 15 than induction with daunorubicin, cytarabine, and etoposide (ADE) ($P = .01$) but did not improve 5-year OS (51% with AIE versus 50% with ADE; $P = .72$) or EFS (60% for AIE versus 57% for ADE; $P = .55$) [71]. Similarly, the Australian and New Zealand Children's Cancer Study Group reported that idarubicin and daunorubicin were equally efficacious, but idarubicin was more toxic [72]. The addition of cyclosporin A to induction chemotherapy to inhibit P-glycoprotein–mediated anthracycline efflux did not prolong the duration of remission or improve OS in children [73].

Another important question is whether the cumulative dose of anthracyclines can be reduced safely without compromising survival. Although cumulative doses above 375 mg/m^2 increase the risk of cardiotoxicity, EFS is lower in protocols that use lower doses of anthracycline [1,2]. Optimal results may be achievable with a cumulative dose of approximately 375 to 550 mg/m^2 if high-dose cytarabine is used in postremission therapy [1,2]. The full impact of cardiotoxicity, particularly late cardiotoxicity, also is poorly defined. In the MRC AML10 protocol, which delivered a high cumulative anthracycline dose (550 mg/m^2), 9 of 341 registered patients died of acute cardiotoxicity (all after a cumulative dose of 300 mg/m^2); 7 of the 9 deaths occurred during an episode of sepsis. Subclinical deficits in cardiac function would have gone undetected in the absence of cardiac monitoring [74]. Minimizing cardiotoxicity is important, however, and cardioprotectant agents and liposomal anthracyclines with reduced cardiotoxicity are being tested.

The use of high-dose cytarabine in postremission therapy seems to be important in improving survival, but the optimal dose has not been determined. Core binding factor (CBF) leukemias may respond particularly well to multiple courses of high-dose cytarabine [75].

Central nervous system–directed therapy

The impact of CNS involvement on EFS is not well defined [8,9,11,13,76,77]. Most pediatric clinical trial groups use intrathecal chemotherapy for CNS prophylaxis, employing either one or three agents and various doses. Not all pediatric groups routinely use intrathecal CNS prophylaxis [9], however, and few adult groups do. The correlation between the type of CNS treatment given and the incidence of CNS relapse is not clear. The CNS relapse rate seems to be around 2% for isolated CNS relapse and between 2% and 9% for combined CNS and bone marrow relapse [2,4–10]. The low rate of CNS relapse may reflect both the use of intrathecal chemotherapy and the CNS protection afforded by high-dose cytarabine and by idarubicin, both of which can penetrate the CNS [70]. Cranial irradiation, because of its sequelae, is not widely used as prophylaxis. It is used currently only by the BFM Study Group, which observed an increase in CNS and systemic relapse in patients who did not receive cranial irradiation in the AML BFM 87 trial [78]. The current AML BFM 98 trial is exploring reduction of the dose of cranial irradiation to limit late sequelae. The necessity of cranial irradiation for patients who have CNS involvement at presentation or CNS relapse is unproven. Many groups reserve cranial irradiation for patients whose CNS is not cleared of leukemic cells by intrathecal and intensive systemic chemotherapy [4,11,13].

Maintenance therapy

Maintenance therapy is no longer used in the treatment of AML, having failed to demonstrate benefit except in BFM studies. Patients who have APL, however, do seem to benefit from antimetabolite maintenance treatment given with all-trans retinoic acid (ATRA). In patients who have non-APL AML, maintenance treatment showed no benefit in two randomized studies (Leucemie Aigue Myeloblastique Enfant 91 and CCG 213); these studies even suggested that maintenance therapy may be deleterious when intensive chemotherapy is used and may contribute to clinical drug resistance and treatment failure after relapse [9,79].

Stem cell transplantation

SCT is the most successful curative treatment for AML; it produces a strong graft-versus-leukemia effect and can cure even relapsed AML. Its potential benefit, however, must be weighed against the risk of transplantation-related mortality and the late sequelae of transplantation. SCT has become a less attractive option as the outcomes of increasingly intensive chemotherapy and postrelapse salvage therapy have improved. Furthermore, although SCT is reported to provide a survival advantage for patients in first CR, studies so far have used matched sibling donors, who are available to only about one in four patients. Although experienced groups have reported comparable outcomes with alternative donors, it is too early to determine whether their wider use will result in greater transplantation-related mortality.

The role of allogeneic SCT, particularly whether it should be done during first CR or reserved for second remission, remains the most controversial issue in pediatric AML. Competing factors, particularly risk group, may tip the balance in favor of SCT or intensive chemotherapy. Most groups agree that children who have APL, AML and Down syndrome or AML and the t(8;21) or inv(16) are not candidates for SCT in first CR, but opinions differ about patients in the standard-risk and high-risk categories. The trend in Europe [79] is to reduce the use of SCT in first CR, but in the United States [80] SCT in first CR is supported. Both views have been reported recently [80–82].

In the absence of randomized, controlled trials comparing allogeneic SCT with postremission intensive chemotherapy, "biologic randomization" or "donor versus no donor" studies are accepted as the least biased comparison methods, but even these are open to criticism. Much of the trial data used to support the benefits of SCT and intensive chemotherapy are old and do not reflect current improvements in SCT and intensive chemotherapy. A meta-analysis [83] of studies enrolling patients younger than 21 years of age between 1985 and 2000 that recommended SCT if a histocompatible family donor were available found that SCT from a matched sibling donor reduced the risk of relapse significantly and improved DFS and OS.

The MRC AML10 (included in the meta-analysis) and AML12 studies combined (relapse risk did not differ between the trials; $P = .3$) showed a significant reduction in relapse risk ($2P = 0.02$) but no significant improvement in DFS ($2P = 0.06$) or OS ($2P = 0.1$) [5]. MRC AML10 is typical of a number of trials in which SCT significantly reduced the risk of relapse, but the resulting improvement in survival was not statistically significant (68% versus 59%; $P = .3$). The small number of pediatric patients in AML10 hinders meaningful interpretation, but at 7 years' follow-up SCT recipients (children and adults) who had a suitable donor showed a significant reduction in relapse risk (36%, versus 52% in patients who did not have a suitable donor; $P = .0001$) and a significant improvement in DFS (50%, versus 42% in patients who did not have a suitable donor; $P = .001$) but no significant improvement in OS (55% versus 50%; $P = .1$) [84]. The reduction in relapse risk was seen in all risk and age groups, but the significant benefit in DFS was seen only in the cytogenetic intermediate-risk group (50% versus 39%; $P = .004$). The 86 children who had a donor, 61 of whom (71%) underwent SCT, had no survival advantage, and children who did not undergo SCT were salvaged more easily [5].

The lack of benefit found for pediatric SCT in the MRC trials mirrors the experience of the BFM [3,85]. CCG trial 2891, however, showed a significant survival advantage for patients who underwent allogeneic SCT versus autologous SCT (60% versus 53%; $P = .002$) or chemotherapy (60% versus 48%; $P = .05$) as postremission treatment, although autologous SCT provided no advantage over intensive chemotherapy [86]. The benefit was most marked in patients who had received intensively timed induction chemotherapy. The CCG analysis was not a true intent-to-treat comparison, however. Although it included patients whether or not they received SCT, it did not include all patients who lacked a donor; instead, it included only patients who lacked a donor and who were randomly assigned to autologous SCT instead of chemotherapy [86], and favorable cytogenetics were overrepresented among patients who had a donor (38% versus 23%). The MRC AML10 (5-year OS, 58%) and CCG 2891 (5-year OS, 47%; 49% for the intensive arm) studies enrolled patients during approximately the same time period, although the patient populations may not have been comparable. It is possible that the improved outcomes achieved by intensive chemotherapy may diminish the role of SCT in first CR of AML and that SCT provides a benefit only when compared with relatively less intensive treatment.

Randomized studies analyzed according to intent to treat have failed to show that autologous SCT provides a survival advantage over intensive chemotherapy [87–89], and a meta-analysis concluded that data were insufficient to determine whether autologous SCT is superior to nonmyeloablative chemotherapy [83].

The controversy continues. In some groups, all patients who have a matched sibling donor proceed to SCT, whereas in others SCT is reserved for patients at high risk, although high risk is not defined consistently. In the MRC, SCT has not been demonstrated to reduce the risk of relapse even in children at high risk [90]. Unless it is demonstrated to reduce the risk of relapse, transplantation can offer no benefit. SCT may have a role in the treatment of pediatric AML in first CR if the graft-versus-leukemia effect can be expanded by pre- and posttransplantation graft manipulation, which may include the use of killer-cell immunoglobulin receptor–incompatible donors and donor lymphocyte infusions.

There is also a need to improve risk-group stratification and to identify better the children who may benefit from SCT. This goal may be achieved by identifying better prognostic indicators and by using minimal residual disease (MRD) monitoring, both of which are discussed in later sections.

Special subgroups

Acute myeloid leukemia in children who have Down syndrome

Children who have Down syndrome who develop AML generally do so between 1 and 4 years of age. This subset of cases of AML is very responsive to therapy but carries a significant risk of early mortality. Children treated during the past decade have had a reported EFS estimate of 83% [91], with relapse rates as low as 3% [92]. The recommendation is to limit the cumulative anthracycline dose to 240 to 250 mg/m^2 [93] or to reduce overall dose intensity rather than the absolute dose [94].

Acute promyelocytic leukemia

Children who have APL are treated with special APL protocols that combine ATRA with intensive chemotherapy. Although ATRA can cause considerable (but manageable) toxicity in some children, this approach induces a stable and continuous remission without the early hemorrhagic deaths that previously characterized this type of leukemia. APL is the only subtype of AML in which maintenance chemotherapy is believed to be of benefit [95]. SCT in first CR is not indicated for a disease that responds so well to chemotherapy. Regimens increasingly based on alternatives to traditional chemotherapy, including ATRA and arsenic trioxide, are being tested [96].

Relapsed acute myeloid leukemia

After relapse, chemotherapy alone is unlikely to be curative, and the survival rate is only 21% to 33% in recent reports [77,97–101]. In these reports, the length of first remission was the best predictor of survival

[97–100]. Various remission induction regimens, including fludarabine plus cytarabine and mitoxantrone plus cytarabine, seem to give similar results. The addition of liposomal daunorubicin to fludarabine plus cytarabine is being tested currently to try to improve CR rates while minimizing cardiotoxicity. It is important to reduce the toxicity of reinduction to a level that allows SCT to proceed, because children who receive SCT can have a 5-year survival probability of 60% (56% after early relapse; 65% after late relapse) [102].

The targeted immunotherapy agents gemtuzumab ozogamicin and clofarabine have shown activity against relapsed AML. Gemtuzumab ozogamicin has been shown to be safe and well tolerated in children and, as a single agent, has induced responses in 30% of patients who have recurrent $CD33^+$ AML [103]. Clofarabine has demonstrated activity against refractory and relapsed AML [104]. Both of these drugs may be more useful when given in combination with other chemotherapeutic agents.

A second allograft seems to offer a benefit to patients who experience relapse after SCT during first CR. Despite a high rate of transplantation-related mortality and second relapse, more than one third of patients are reported to be long-term survivors. Patients who undergo SCT during remission may have an even better outcome [105]. Therefore every effort should be made to induce remission before the second SCT.

Prognostic factors

Although clinical measures of tumor burden, such as leukocyte count and hepatosplenomegaly, largely have been replaced by genetic factors in the risk-classification schemes of contemporary treatment protocols, several clinical features are still prognostically important. In both adult and pediatric patients who have AML, age at diagnosis is associated inversely with the probability of survival [106,107]. In an analysis of 424 patients less than 21 years of age, an age greater than 10 years at diagnosis was significantly associated with a worse outcome, even after controlling for cytogenetics, leukocyte count, and FAB subtype [107]. The effect of age was important only among patients treated in contemporary trials, reinforcing the view that the effect of any prognostic factor ultimately depends on the therapy given. Two recent studies suggest that another clinically apparent feature—ethnicity—may be an important predictor of outcome [108,109]. Among more than 1600 children who had AML treated on the CCG 2891 and 2961 trials, black children treated with chemotherapy had a significantly worse outcome than white children treated with chemotherapy, a disparity that the authors suggest may reflect pharmacogenetic differences [109]. Body mass index, another easily measured clinical feature, also may affect the outcome of children who have AML [110]. In the CCG 2961 trial, underweight and overweight patients were less likely to survive than normoweight patients because of a greater risk of treatment-related death [110].

In addition to clinical features, certain pathologic features, such as M0 and M7 subtypes, seem to carry prognostic importance in AML [111,112]. The present authors and others have demonstrated that non–Down syndrome patients who have megakaryoblastic leukemia have significantly worse outcomes than patients who have other subtypes of AML [111,113,114]. The EFS estimates for patients who have megakaryoblastic leukemia treated in the CCG 2891 trial or in the St. Jude trial were only 22% and 14%, respectively [111,113]. In the St. Jude study [111] and in a report from the European Group for Blood and Marrow Transplantation [115], patients who underwent SCT during first remission had a better outcome than those who received chemotherapy, suggesting that SCT should be recommended for these patients. A study by French investigators, however, suggested that children who had megakaryoblastic leukemia with the t(1;22), but without Down syndrome, had a better outcome than similar children who did not have the t(1;22), indicating that this subgroup may not need transplantation [114]. In addition, the BFM study group reported an improved outcome for patients who had megakaryoblastic leukemia treated in recent, more intensive trials [116]. SCT did not provide a benefit to patients treated in these trials. Thus, the role of SCT for patients who have megakaryoblastic leukemia remains controversial.

Conventional cytogenetic studies have demonstrated that the karyotype of leukemic blast cells is one of the best predictors of outcome [117,118]. An analysis of more than 1600 patients enrolled in the MRC AML 10 trial revealed that t(8;21) and inv(16) were associated with a favorable outcome (5-year OS estimates, 69% and 61%, respectively), whereas a complex karyotype, -5, del(5q), -7, and abnormalities of 3q predicted a poor outcome [117]. On the basis of these observations, the MRC investigators proposed a cytogenetics-based risk classification system that is used by many cooperative groups today [117]. Among the 340 patients in the MRC study who were less than 15 years old, those with a favorable karyotype had a 3-year survival estimate of 78%, compared with 55% for the intermediate-risk group and 42% for the high-risk group. Other cooperative groups have confirmed the MRC findings, with slightly different results for some subgroups that probably reflect differences in therapy. For example, in the Pediatric Oncology Group 8821 trial, patients who had t(8;21) had a 4-year OS estimate of 52% and those who had inv(16) had an estimate of 75% [118]. Similarly, among adults who had AML treated in Cancer and Leukemia Group B trials, patients who had these karyotypes had a better outcome than others and had a particularly good outcome when treated with multiple courses of high-dose cytarabine [75,119,120].

Because both t(8;21) and inv(16) disrupt the CBF, they are often referred to as "CBF leukemias" and are grouped together in risk-classification systems. Several studies, however, have demonstrated that CBF leukemia is a heterogeneous group of diseases in adults and therefore probably is heterogeneous in children as well [121,122]. An analysis of 312 adults who had CBF AML demonstrated that, although CR and relapse rates were similar for patients who had t(8;21) and inv(16), OS was significantly worse for those who had t(8;21), primarily because of a lower salvage rate after relapse [121]. In addition, race was prognostically important among patients who had t(8;21), whereas sex and secondary cytogenetic changes were predictive of outcome among patients who had inv(16). A similar analysis of 370 adults who had CBF AML confirmed the heterogeneity of this type of AML and confirmed the poor outcome after relapse among patients who had t(8;21) [122]. Not surprisingly, in both studies, outcome depended on treatment intensity.

Other prognostically important cytogenetic abnormalities include rearrangements of the *MLL* gene, located at chromosome band 11q23. The abnormality is usually a reciprocal translocation between *MLL* and one of more than 30 other genes in distinct chromosomal loci [123]. *MLL* rearrangements are seen in as many as 20% of cases of AML, although the reported frequency varies among studies [124,125]. In general, children and adults whose leukemic cells contain 11q23 abnormalities are considered at intermediate risk, and their outcome does not differ significantly from that of patients without these translocations (3-year OS estimate, 50% in the MRC AML 10 trial) [117]. Some studies, however, suggest that t(9;11) confers a favorable outcome [124]. Among patients treated for AML at St. Jude, those who had t(9;11) had a better outcome (5-year EFS estimate, 65%) than did patients in all other cytogenetic or molecular subgroups. This finding may be attributable to the use of epipodophyllotoxins and cladribine, both of which are effective against monoblastic leukemia.

In the MRC AML 10 study mentioned previously, monosomy 7 was associated with a particularly poor outcome (5-year OS, 10%) but was detected in only 4% of cases [117].

Because of the rarity of this abnormality, an international collaborative study was undertaken to characterize further the impact of -7 and del(7q) in children and adolescents who have AML [126]. In this study, which included 172 patients who had -7 (with or without other abnormalities) and 86 patients who had del(7q) (also with or without other changes), patients who had -7 had lower CR rates (61% versus 89%) and worse outcome (5-year survival, 30% versus 51%) than those who had del(7q). Patients who had del(7q) and a favorable genetic abnormality had a good outcome (5-year survival, 75%), suggesting that the del(7q) does not alter the impact of the favorable feature. By contrast, patients who had -7 and inv(3), -5/del(5q), or +21 had a dismal outcome (5-year survival, 5%) that was not improved by SCT [126].

During the past 10 years, molecular studies have demonstrated heterogeneity within cytogenetically defined subgroups of AML and have identified new, prognostically important subgroups. Mutations of *c-kit*, *ras*, and *FLT3* have been detected in cases of childhood and adult AML; *c-kit* mutations may be particularly important in cases of CBF leukemia [127–131]. Several studies demonstrated that among adult patients who had t(8;21), those who had mutations at *c-kit* codon 816 had a significantly higher relapse rate and worse outcome than those who had wild-type *c-kit* [127–129]. In some studies, mutations of *c-kit* also seem to confer a worse outcome among patients who have inv(16) [132]. Although *c-kit* mutations have been detected in 3% to 11% of pediatric AML cases, their prognostic impact is uncertain [130,133]. One study found *c-kit* mutations in 37% of cases of CBF leukemia, but these cases did not differ from others in outcome [130]. In contrast, the Japanese Childhood AML Cooperative Study Group found that *c-kit* mutations, in 8 of 46 patients who had t(8;21), were associated with significantly worse OS, DFS, and relapse rates [131].

The impact of *FLT3* mutations in childhood and adult AML has been established by dozens of studies, only a few of which are summarized here. In one of the first studies reported, the estimated 5-year OS rate was only 14% for adult patients who had internal tandem duplications (ITD) of *FLT3*, and the presence of these mutations was the strongest prognostic factor in multivariate analysis [134]. Similarly, in an analysis of 106 adults who had AML treated in MRC trials, 13 of the 14 patients who had *FLT3* ITD died within 18 months of diagnosis [135]. A subsequent study of 854 patients treated in the MRC AML trials demonstrated a *FLT3* ITD, present in 27% of cases, was associated with an increased risk of relapse and a lower probability of DFS, EFS, and OS [136]. Other reports have confirmed the presence of *FLT* ITD in 20% to 30% of adult AML cases, but some studies suggest that its negative prognostic impact may depend on the absence of the wild-type allele or the ratio of the mutant to the wild-type allele [137–139].

Studies of childhood AML identify *FLT3* ITD in only 10% to 15% of cases, but still it is associated with a poor outcome [140–143]. Among 91 pediatric patients who had AML treated in CCG trials, the 8-year EFS estimate was only 7% for patients who had *FLT3* ITD, whereas among 234 patients treated on Dutch AML protocols, the 5-year EFS for these patients estimate was only 29% [140,141]. In both studies, multivariate analysis demonstrated that *FLT3*-ITD was the strongest predictor of relapse. A more recent study of 630 patients treated in contemporary CCG trials confirmed the poor outcome associated with *FLT3* ITD and demonstrated that survival decreased with an increasing allelic ratio of *FLT* ITD to *FLT3* wild-type [143]. The estimated progression-free survival was considerably lower with a ratio greater than 0.4 than with a lower ratio (16% versus 72%). CCG investigators also compared the outcome of patients who had *FLT3* ITD in CD34$^+$/CD33$^-$ precursors with that of patients who had the mutated gene in only the more mature CD34$^+$/CD33$^+$ progenitors [65]. Patients who had the mutation in the less mature precursors had dramatically worse outcomes, confirming the heterogeneity within *FLT3* ITD–positive cases of AML and suggesting that only a subset of these patients have a poor prognosis. Data from studies by the Pediatric Oncology Group suggest that gene expression profiles also may be used to identify patients who have a good prognosis despite *FLT3* mutations [144].

Other molecular alterations reported to be prognostic factors in AML include expression of ATP-binding cassette transporters [145–147], *CEBPA* mutations [148,149], *DCC* expression [150], secretion of vascular endothelial growth factor [151], expression of apoptosis-related genes [152–154], expression of *BAALC* [155], expression of *ERG* [156,157], *NPM1* mutations [158–160], partial tandem duplications (PTD) of the *MLL* gene [161,162], and global gene expression patterns [163–167]. The clinical relevance of these alterations has been reviewed comprehensively [168] and is discussed only briefly here. Mutations of the nucleophosmin member 1 (*NPM1*) gene have been detected in about 50% of cases of adult AML with a normal karyotype [159] but occur much less commonly in childhood AML [160]. In both populations, *NPM1* mutations are associated with *FLT3* ITD; however, in patients who have wild-type *FLT3*, *NPM1* mutations are associated with a favorable outcome [168]. *MLL* PTD occur in about 5% to 10% of adult AML cases and, like *NPM1* mutations, commonly are associated with *FLT3* ITD [168]. *MLL* PTD seem to be an adverse prognostic factor, but it is not clear whether the negative impact is related to the association with *FLT3* ITD. High expression of the *BAALC* gene and the *ERG* gene are additional factors that have independent negative prognostic significance among adult patients who have a normal karyotype, whereas mutations of the *CEBPA* gene are associated with a favorable outcome [168]. A risk-classification scheme for adults who have a normal AML karyotype that incorporates the status of *FLT3*, *NPM1*, *BAALC*, *MLL*, and *CEBPA* has been proposed and may be used in future clinical trials [168]. *MLL* PTD, *BAALC*, and *CEBPA* have not been studied extensively in childhood AML. Nevertheless, it is likely that forthcoming pediatric clinical trials will use gene-expression profiling to identify important prognostic subgroups that may benefit from more intensive or novel therapies [144,169].

Minimal residual disease

The heterogeneity within cytogenetically and even molecularly defined subgroups indicates that other methods are needed to optimize risk classification. Many studies of ALL and AML have demonstrated the prognostic importance of early response to therapy (ie, reduction or elimination of leukemic cells in the bone marrow), which may be a more powerful predictor of outcome than genetic features [170]. Response to therapy can be measured by morphologic [171,172] or cytogenetic [173] examination of bone marrow, but these methods cannot detect levels of residual leukemia below 1% (1 leukemic cell in 100 mononuclear bone marrow cells). In contrast, MRD assays provide objective and sensitive measurement of low levels of leukemic cells [170,174] in childhood [175–178] and adult [179–183] AML. Methods of assessing MRD include DNA-based polymerase chain reaction

(PCR) analysis of clonal antigen-receptor gene rearrangements (applicable to less than 10% of AML cases), RNA-based PCR analysis of leukemia-specific gene fusions (applicable to less than 50% of AML cases), and flow cytometric detection of aberrant immunophenotype (applicable to more than 90% of AML cases). Among 252 children evaluated for MRD in the CCG-2961 trial, occult leukemia (defined as more than 0.5% bone marrow blast cells with an aberrant phenotype) was detected in 16% of the children considered to be in remission [176]. Multivariate analysis demonstrated that patients who had detectable MRD were 4.8 times more likely to experience relapse ($P < .0001$) and 3.1 times more likely to die ($P < .0001$) than patients who were MRD negative. A study at St. Jude Children's Research Hospital yielded similar findings: the 2-year survival estimate for patients who had detectable MRD at the end of induction therapy was 33%, compared with 72% for MRD-negative patients ($P = .022$) [177]. Recent studies in adults have confirmed that the level of residual leukemia cells detected immunophenotypically after induction or consolidation therapy is associated strongly with the risk of relapse [181–183].

Quantitative reverse transcription PCR assays of leukemia-specific fusion transcripts is an alternative method of MRD detection that can be used in AML cases that harbor these gene fusions [113,184–190]. Several studies have indicated that quantification of *AML1-ETO* and *CBFβ-MYH11* fusion transcripts at the time of diagnosis and during therapy is a useful predictor of outcome. Similarly, there is emerging evidence that quantitative PCR assessment of *WT1* transcripts also may prove useful for monitoring MRD and predicting outcome in patients who have AML [191–193].

Pharmacogenomics of therapy for acute myeloid leukemia

Patient factors, such as pharmacodynamics and pharmacogenomics, significantly affect the outcome of treatment in many types of cancer, including AML [194,195]. The effect of such factors is demonstrated clearly by the chemosensitivity and excellent outcome of AML in children who have Down syndrome, who have cure rates of 80% to 100% [196]. Increased levels of cystathionine-β-synthetase (CBS), a high frequency of *CBS* genetic polymorphisms, low levels of cytidine deaminase, and altered expression of other *GATA1* target genes in these patients' leukemic blast cells contribute to the high cure rates [197–200]. Polymorphisms or altered expression of other proteins involved in cytarabine metabolism, such as deoxycytidine kinase, DNA polymerase, and *es* nucleoside transporter, also may play a role in leukemic blast cell sensitivity to this agent [201–203]. In addition, polymorphisms may influence toxicity. For example, homozygous deletions of the glutathione *S*-transferase theta (*GSTT1*) gene have been reported to be associated with a higher frequency of early toxic death and a lower likelihood of survival [204,205]. Recently, polymorphisms of the *XPD* gene (*XPD751*), which is involved in DNA repair, were shown to be associated with a lower likelihood of survival and a higher risk of therapy-related leukemia in elderly patients who had AML [206]. *XPD751* does not seem to influence outcome in children who have AML, however [207].

Complications and supportive care

At the time of diagnosis, patients who have AML may have life-threatening complications, including bleeding, leukostasis, tumor lysis syndrome, and infection. The first three are managed through the use of platelet transfusions, leukapheresis or exchange transfusion, aggressive hydration, oral phosphate binders and recombinant urate oxidase, and the prompt initiation of chemotherapy. Infectious complications at the time of diagnosis and during therapy remain a major cause of morbidity and mortality [74,208–211]. Viridans streptococci, which commonly colonize the oral, gastrointestinal, and vaginal mucosa, are particularly troublesome in patients undergoing therapy for AML [208,210,212,213]. Because of the high risk of sepsis, most clinicians agree that all patients who have AML and who have febrile neutropenia should be hospitalized and treated with broad-spectrum intravenous antibiotics, such as a third- or fourth-generation cephalosporin, as well as vancomycin. Patients who have evidence of sepsis or infection with *Pseudomonas aeruginosa* should receive an aminoglycoside, and patients who have severe abdominal pain, evidence of typhlitis, or known infection with *Bacillus cereus* should be treated with a carbapenem (imipenem or meropenem) rather than a cephalosporin. In addition, patients who have AML are at high risk of fungal infection [213] and therefore should receive empiric antifungal therapy with traditional amphotericin B, lipid formulations of amphotericin B, an azole (voriconazole or posaconazole), or an echinocandin (caspofungin or micafungin). Cytokines such as granulocyte-macrophage colony stimulating factor and granulocyte colony-stimulating factor also should be considered in cases of proven sepsis or fungal infection, but there is little evidence that their prophylactic use significantly reduces morbidity [214–216].

Because of the high incidence of bacterial and fungal infections, the present authors recently tested several prophylactic antimicrobial regimens in 78 children receiving chemotherapy for AML at St. Jude Children's Research Hospital. Oral cephalosporins were ineffective, but intravenous cefepime completely prevented viridans streptococcal sepsis and reduced the odds of bacterial sepsis by 91%. Similarly, intravenous vancomycin given with oral ciprofloxacin reduced the odds of viridans streptococcal sepsis by 98% and the odds of any bacterial sepsis by 94%. All patients received antifungal prophylaxis with oral voriconazole, which contributed to a low rate of disseminated fungal infection (1.0/000 patient-days). Most important, there were no deaths from bacterial or fungal infection among patients who received prophylactic antibiotics and voriconazole. Because of the relatively small number of patients studied, these prophylactic antibiotic regimens must be evaluated in a multi-institutional setting before recommendations can be made.

Future directions

As a result of highly collaborative clinical trials, the outcome for children who have AML has improved continuously over the past several decades, but approximately half of all children diagnosed as having AML still die of the disease or of complications of treatment. Further advances will require a greater understanding of the biology of AML, improved risk stratification and risk-directed therapies, improved treatment of high-risk disease, and the development of molecularly targeted agents or better cellular therapies. Targeted therapies may cause less toxicity, but they may be clinically applicable only to well-defined molecular subgroups, as with the use of ATRA and arsenic trioxide for APL [95,217]. Agents under investigation include gemtuzumab ozogamicin [218], proteasome inhibitors [219,220], histone deacetylase inhibitors [221,222], and tyrosine kinases inhibitors [223–225]. Clofarabine, a purine nucleoside analogue that was designed to integrate the qualities of fludarabine and cladribine, also has activity against AML [226–228]. Recently, cellular therapy with haploidentical natural killer cells has been shown to exert antitumor activity with minimal toxicity in patients who have relapsed AML [229]. Timely evaluation of these and other therapies will require novel clinical trial designs with new statistical models that allow the testing of new treatment approaches in increasingly small subgroups of patients. In addition, future clinical trials will require international collaboration among the pediatric cooperative oncology groups.

Acknowledgments

The authors thank Sharon Naron for expert editorial review.

References

[1] Kaspers G, Creutzig U. Pediatric AML: long term results of clinical trials from 13 study groups worldwide. Leukemia 2005;19:2025–146.

[2] Kaspers GJ, Creutzig U. Pediatric acute myeloid leukemia: international progress and future directions. Leukemia 2005;19(12):2025–9.

[3] Creutzig U, Zimmermann M, Ritter J, et al. Treatment strategies and long-term results in paediatric patients treated in four consecutive AML-BFM trials. Leukemia 2005;19(12):2030–42.

[4] Smith FO, Alonzo TA, Gerbing RB, et al. Long-term results of children with acute myeloid leukemia: a report of three consecutive phase III trials by the Children's Cancer Group: CCG 251, CCG 213 and CCG 2891. Leukemia 2005;19(12):2054–62.

[5] Gibson BE, Wheatley K, Hann IM, et al. Treatment strategy and long-term results in paediatric patients treated in consecutive UK AML trials. Leukemia 2005;19(12):2130–8.

[6] Pession A, Rondelli R, Basso G, et al. Treatment and long-term results in children with acute myeloid leukaemia treated according to the AIEOP AML protocols. Leukemia 2005;19(12):2043–53.

[7] Kardos G, Zwaan CM, Kaspers GJ, et al. Treatment strategy and results in children treated on three Dutch Childhood Oncology Group acute myeloid leukemia trials. Leukemia 2005; 19(12):2063–71.

[8] Entz-Werle N, Suciu S, van der Werff ten Bosch J, et al. Results of 58872 and 58921 trials in acute myeloblastic leukemia and relative value of chemotherapy vs allogeneic bone marrow transplantation in first complete remission: the EORTC Children Leukemia Group report. Leukemia 2005;19(12):2072–81.

[9] Perel Y, Auvrignon A, Leblanc T, et al. Treatment of childhood acute myeloblastic leukemia: dose intensification improves outcome and maintenance therapy is of no benefit— multicenter studies of the French LAME (Leucemie Aigue Myeloblastique Enfant) Cooperative Group. Leukemia 2005;19(12):2082–9.

[10] Lie SO, Abrahamsson J, Clausen N, et al. Long-term results in children with AML: NOPHO-AML Study Group–report of three consecutive trials. Leukemia 2005;19(12):2090–100.

[11] Ravindranath Y, Chang M, Steuber CP, et al. Pediatric Oncology Group (POG) studies of acute myeloid leukemia (AML): a review of four consecutive childhood AML trials conducted between 1981 and 2000. Leukemia 2005;19(12):2101–16.

[12] Dluzniewska A, Balwierz W, Armata J, et al. Twenty years of Polish experience with three consecutive protocols for treatment of childhood acute myelogenous leukemia. Leukemia 2005;19(12):2117–24.

[13] Ribeiro RC, Razzouk BI, Pounds S, et al. Successive clinical trials for childhood acute myeloid leukemia at St Jude Children's Research Hospital, from 1980 to 2000. Leukemia 2005;19(12):2125–9.

[14] Armendariz H, Barbieri MA, Freigeiro D, et al. Treatment strategy and long-term results in pediatric patients treated in two consecutive AML-GATLA trials. Leukemia 2005;19(12): 2139–42.

[15] Quintana J, Advis P, Becker A, et al. Acute myelogenous leukemia in Chile PINDA protocols 87 and 92 results. Leukemia 2005;19(12):2143–6.

[16] Smith MA, Ries LAG, Gurney JG, et al. Leukemia. In: Ries LAG, Smith MA, Gurney JG, et al, editors. Cancer incidence and survival among children and adolescents: United States SEER Progam 1975–1995. NIH Pub. No. 99–4649. Bethesda (MD): National Cancer Institute, SEER Program; 1999. p. 17–34.

[17] Glavel J, Goubin A, Auclerc MF, et al. Incidence of childhood leukaemia and non-Hodgkin's lymphoma in France: National Registry of Childhood Leukaemia and Lymphoma, 1990–1999. Eur J Cancer Prev 2004;13:97–103.

[18] Hjalgrim LL, Rostgaard K, Schmiegelow K, et al. Age- and sex-specific incidence of childhood leukemia by immunophenotype in the Nordic countries. J Natl Cancer Inst 2003; 95(20):1539–44.

[19] Xie Y, Davies SM, Xiang Y, et al. Trends in leukemia incidence and survival in the United States (1973–1998). Cancer 2003;97(9):2229–35.

[20] Gurney JG, Severson RK, Davis S, et al. Incidence of cancer in children in the United States. Sex-, race-, and 1-year age-specific rates by histologic type. Cancer 1995;75(8):2186–95.

[21] Bhatia S, Neglia JP. Epidemiology of childhood acute myelogenous leukemia [see comments]. J Pediatr Hematol Oncol 1995;17(2):94–100.

[22] Ross JA, Davies SM, Potter JD, et al. Epidemiology of childhood leukemia, with a focus on infants. Epidemiol Rev 1994;16(2):243–72.

[23] Sandler DP, Ross JA. Epidemiology of acute leukemia in children and adults. Semin Oncol 1997;24(1):3–16.

[24] Linassier C, Barin C, Calais G, et al. Early secondary acute myelogenous leukemia in breast cancer patients after treatment with mitoxantrone, cyclophosphamide, fluorouracil and radiation therapy. Ann Oncol 2000;11(10):1289–94.

[25] Micallef IN, Lillington DM, Apostolidis J, et al. Therapy-related myelodysplasia and secondary acute myelogenous leukemia after high-dose therapy with autologous hematopoietic progenitor-cell support for lymphoid malignancies. J Clin Oncol 2000;18(5):947–55.

[26] Smith MA, McCaffrey RP, Karp JE. The secondary leukemias: challenges and research directions. J Natl Cancer Inst 1996;88(7):407–18.

[27] Sandoval C, Pui CH, Bowman LC, et al. Secondary acute myeloid leukemia in children previously treated with alkylating agents, intercalating topoisomerase II inhibitors, and irradiation. J Clin Oncol 1993;11(6):1039–45.

[28] Relling MV, Yanishevski Y, Nemec J, et al. Etoposide and antimetabolite pharmacology in patients who develop secondary acute myeloid leukemia. Leukemia 1998;12(3):346–52.

[29] Pui CH, Ribeiro RC, Hancock ML, et al. Acute myeloid leukemia in children treated with epipodophyllotoxins for acute lymphoblastic leukemia. N Engl J Med 1991;325(24):1682–7.

[30] Le Deley MC, Leblanc T, Shamsaldin A, et al. Risk of secondary leukemia after a solid tumor in childhood according to the dose of epipodophyllotoxins and anthracyclines: a case-control study by the Societe Francaise d'Oncologie Pediatrique. J Clin Oncol 2003;21(6):1074–81.

[31] Korte JE, Hertz-Picciotto I, Schulz MR, et al. The contribution of benzene to smoking-induced leukemia. Environ Health Perspect 2000;108(4):333–9.

[32] McBride ML. Childhood cancer and environmental contaminants. Can J Public Health 1998;89(Suppl 1):S53–68.

[33] Yin SN, Hayes RB, Linet MS, et al. An expanded cohort study of cancer among benzene-exposed workers in China. Benzene Study Group. Environ Health Perspect 1996;104(Suppl 6):1339–41.

[34] Yin SN, Hayes RB, Linet MS, et al. A cohort study of cancer among benzene-exposed workers in China: overall results. Am J Ind Med 1996;29(3):227–35.

[35] Linet MS, Bailey PE. Benzene, leukemia, and the Supreme Court. J Public Health Policy 1981;2(2):116–35.

[36] Mills PK, Zahm SH. Organophosphate pesticide residues in urine of farmworkers and their children in Fresno County, California. Am J Ind Med 2001;40(5):571–7.

[37] Rosenberg PS, Greene MH, Alter BP. Cancer incidence in persons with Fanconi anemia. Blood 2003;101(3):822–6.

[38] German J. Bloom's syndrome. XX. The first 100 cancers. Cancer Genet Cytogenet 1997; 93(1):100–6.

[39] Bader JL, Miller RW. Neurofibromatosis and childhood leukemia. J Pediatr 1978;92(6): 925–9.

[40] Bader-Meunier B, Tchernia G, Mielot F, et al. Occurrence of myeloproliferative disorder in patients with Noonan syndrome. J Pediatr 1997;130(6):885–9.

[41] Socie G, Henry-Amar M, Bacigalupo A, et al. Malignant tumors occurring after treatment of aplastic anemia. European Bone Marrow Transplantation-Severe Aplastic Anaemia Working Party. N Engl J Med 1993;329(16):1152–7.

[42] Imashuku S, Hibi S, Nakajima F, et al. A review of 125 cases to determine the risk of myelodysplasia and leukemia in pediatric neutropenic patients after treatment with recombinant human granulocyte colony-stimulating factor. Blood 1994;84(7):2380–1.

[43] Xue Y, Zhang R, Guo Y, et al. Acquired amegakaryocytic thrombocytopenic purpura with a Philadelphia chromosome. Cancer Genet Cytogenet 1993;69(1):51–6.

[44] Geissler D, Thaler J, Konwalinka G, et al. Progressive preleukemia presenting amegakaryocytic thrombocytopenic purpura: association of the 5q- syndrome with a decreased megakaryocytic colony formation and a defective production of Meg-CSF. Leuk Res 1987;11(8):731–7.

[45] Gilliland DG. Molecular genetics of human leukemia. Leukemia 1998;12(Suppl 1):S7–12.

[46] Dash A, Gilliland DG. Molecular genetics of acute myeloid leukaemia. Best Pract Res Clin Haematol 2001;14(1):49–64.

[47] Gilliland DG, Tallman MS. Focus on acute leukemias. Cancer Cell 2002;1(5):417–20.

[48] Castilla LH, Garrett L, Adya N, et al. The fusion gene Cbfb-MYH11 blocks myeloid differentiation and predisposes mice to acute myelomonocytic leukaemia. Nat Genet 1999;23:144–6.

[49] Higuchi M, O'Brien D, Kumaravelu P, et al. Expression of a conditional AML1-ETO oncogene bypasses embryonic lethality and establishes a murine model of human t(8;21) acute myeloid leukemia. Cancer Cell 2002;1(1):63–74.

[50] Ford AM, Ridge SA, Cabrera ME, et al. In utero rearrangements in the trithorax-related oncogene in infant leukaemias. Nature 1993;363:358–60.

[51] Gill Super HJ, Rothberg PG, Kobayashi H, et al. Clonal, nonconstitutional rearrangements of the MLL gene in infant twins with acute lymphoblastic leukemia: in utero chromosome rearrangement of 11q23. Blood 1994;83(3):641–4.

[52] Megonigal MD, Rappaport EF, Jones DH, et al. t(11;22)(q23;q11.2) In acute myeloid leukemia of infant twins fuses MLL with hCDCrel, a cell division cycle gene in the genomic region of deletion in DiGeorge and velocardiofacial syndromes. Proc Natl Acad Sci U S A 1998;95(11):6413–8.

[53] Wiemels JL, Ford AM, Van Wering ER, et al. Protracted and variable latency of acute lymphoblastic leukemia after TEL-AML1 gene fusion in utero. Blood 1999;94(3): 1057–62.

[54] Song WJ, Sullivan MG, Legare RD, et al. Haploinsufficiency of CBFA2 causes familial thrombocytopenia with propensity to develop acute myelogenous leukaemia. Nat Genet 1999;23(2):166–75.

[55] Bonnet D, Dick JE. Human acute myeloid leukemia is organized as a hierarchy that originates from a primitive hematopoietic cell. Nat Med 1997;3(7):730–7.

[56] Caligiuri MA, Strout MP, Gilliland DG. Molecular biology of acute myleloid leukemia. Semin Oncol 1997;24:32–44.

[57] Sabbath KD, Ball ED, Larcom P, et al. Heterogeneity of clonogenic cells in acute myeloblastic leukemia. J Clin Invest 1985;75:746–53.

[58] Lapidot T, Sirard C, Vormoor J, et al. A cell initiating human acute myeloid leukaemia after transplantation into SCID mice. Nature 1994;367(6464):645–8.

[59] Mehrotra B, George TI, Kavanau K, et al. Cytogenetically aberrant cells in the stem cell compartment (CD34+lin-) in acute myeloid leukemia. Blood 1995;86(3):1139–47.

[60] Sirard C, Lapidot T, Vormoor J, et al. Normal and leukemic SCID-repopulating cells (SRC) coexist in the bone marrow and peripheral blood from CML patients in chronic phase, whereas leukemic SRC are detected in blast crisis. Blood 1996;87(4):1539–48.

[61] Hope KJ, Jin L, Dick JE. Human acute myeloid leukemia stem cells. Arch Med Res 2003; 34(6):507–14.

[62] Hope KJ, Jin L, Dick JE. Acute myeloid leukemia originates from a hierarchy of leukemic stem cell classes that differ in self-renewal capacity. Nat Immunol 2004;5(7):738–43.

[63] Warner JK, Wang JC, Hope KJ, et al. Concepts of human leukemic development. Oncogene 2004;23(43):7164–77.

[64] Terpstra W, Prins A, Ploemacher RE, et al. Long-term leukemia-initiating capacity of a CD34-subpopulation of acute myeloid leukemia. Blood 1996;87(6):2187–94.

[65] Pollard JA, Alonzo TA, Gerbing RB, et al. FLT3 internal tandem duplication in CD34+/. Blood 2006;108(8):2764–9.

[66] Pui CH, Dahl GV, Kalwinsky DK, et al. Central nervous system leukemia in children with acute nonlymphoblastic leukemia. Blood 1985;66(5):1062–7.

[67] Woods WG, Kobrinsky N, Buckley JD, et al. Time-sequential induction therapy improves postremission outcome in acute myeloid leukemia: a report from the Children's Cancer Group. Blood 1996;87(12):4979–89.

[68] Carella AM, Berman E, Maraone MP, et al. Idarubicin in the treatment of acute leukemias. An overview of preclinical and clinical studies. Haematologica 1990;75(2):159–69.

[69] Berman E, McBride M. Comparative cellular pharmacology of daunorubicin and idarubicin in human multidrug-resistant leukemia cells. Blood 1992;79(12):3267–73.

[70] Reid JM, Pendergrass TW, Krailo MD, et al. Plasma pharmacokinetics and cerebrospinal fluid concentrations of idarubicin and idarubicinol in pediatric leukemia patients: a Children's Cancer Study Group report. Cancer Res 1990;50(20):6525–8.

[71] Creutzig U, Ritter J, Zimmermann M, et al. Idarubicin improves blast cell clearance during induction therapy in children with AML: results of study AML-BFM 93. AML-BFM Study Group. Leukemia 2001;15(3):348–54.

[72] O'Brien TA, Russell SJ, Vowels MR, et al. Results of consecutive trials for children newly diagnosed with acute myeloid leukemia from the Australian and New Zealand Children's Cancer Study Group. Blood 2002;100(8):2708–16.

[73] Becton D, Dahl GV, Ravindranath Y, et al. Randomized use of cyclosporin A (CsA) to modulate P-glycoprotein in children with AML in remission: Pediatric Oncology Group Study 9421. Blood 2006;107(4):1315–24.

[74] Riley LC, Hann IM, Wheatley K, et al. Treatment-related deaths during induction and first remission of acute myeloid leukaemia in children treated on the Tenth Medical Research Council acute myeloid leukaemia trial (MRC AML10). The MCR Childhood Leukaemia Working Party. Br J Haematol 1999;106(2):436–44.

[75] Byrd JC, Dodge RK, Carroll A, et al. Patients with t(8;21)(q22;q22) and acute myeloid leukemia have superior failure-free and overall survival when repetitive cycles of high-dose cytarabine are administered. J Clin Oncol 1999;17(12):3767–75.

[76] Abbott BL, Rubnitz JE, Tong X, et al. Clinical significance of central nervous system involvement at diagnosis of pediatric acute myeloid leukaemia: a single institution's experience. Leukemia 2003;17(11):2090–6.

[77] Johnston DL, Alonzo TA, Gerbing RB, et al. Risk factors and therapy for isolated central nervous system relapse of pediatric acute myeloid leukemia. J Clin Oncol 2005;23(36): 9172–8.

[78] Creutzig U, Ritter J, Zimmermann M, et al. Does cranial irradiation reduce the risk for bone marrow relapse in acute myelogenous leukemia? Unexpected results of the Childhood Acute Myelogenous Leukemia Study BFM-87. J Clin Oncol 1993;11(2):279–86.

[79] Wells RJ, Woods WG, Buckley JD, et al. Treatment of newly diagnosed children and adolescents with acute myeloid leukemia: a Children's Cancer Group study. J Clin Oncol 1994;12(11):2367–77.

[80] Creutzig U, Reinhardt D. Current controversies: which patients with acute myeloid leukaemia should receive a bone marrow transplantation? A European view. Br J Haematol 2002; 118(2):365–77.

[81] Chen AR, Alonzo TA, Woods WG, et al. Current controversies: which patients with acute myeloid leukaemia should receive a bone marrow transplantation? An American view. Br J Haematol 2002;118(2):378–84.

[82] Wheatley K. Current controversies: which patients with acute myeloid leukaemia should receive a bone marrow transplantation? A statistician's view. Br J Haematol 2002;118(2): 351–6.

[83] Bleakley M, Lau L, Shaw PJ, et al. Bone marrow transplantation for paediatric AML in first remission: a systematic review and meta-analysis. Bone Marrow Transplant 2002; 29(10):843–52.

[84] Burnett AK, Wheatley K, Goldstone AH, et al. The value of allogeneic bone marrow transplant in patients with acute myeloid leukaemia at differing risk of relapse: results of the UK MRC AML 10 trial. Br J Haematol 2002;118(2):385–400.

[85] Creutzig U, Reinhardt D, Zimmermann M, et al. Intensive chemotherapy versus bone marrow transplantation in pediatric acute myeloid leukemia: a matter of controversies. Blood 2001;97(11):3671–2.

[86] Woods WG, Neudorf S, Gold S, et al. A comparison of allogeneic bone marrow transplantation, autologous bone marrow transplantation, and aggressive chemotherapy in children with acute myeloid leukemia in remission. Blood 2001;97(1):56–62.

[87] Stevens RF, Hann IM, Wheatley K, et al. Marked improvements in outcome with chemotherapy alone in paediatric acute myeloid leukemia: results of the United Kingdom Medical Research Council's 10th AML trial. MRC Childhood Leukaemia Working Party. Br J Haematol 1998;101(1):130–40.

[88] Ravindranath Y, Yeager AM, Chang MN, et al. Autologous bone marrow transplantation versus intensive consolidation chemotherapy for acute myeloid leukemia in childhood. Pediatric Oncology Group. N Engl J Med 1996;334(22):1428–34.

[89] Amadori S, Testi AM, Arico M, et al. Prospective comparative study of bone marrow transplantation and postremission chemotherapy for childhood acute myelogenous leukemia. The Associazione Italiana Ematologia ed Oncologia Pediatrica Cooperative Group. J Clin Oncol 1993;11(6):1046–54.

[90] Gibson B, Hann I, Webb I, et al. Should stem cell transplantation (SCT) be recommended for a child with AML in 1st CR. Blood 2007;106:171.

[91] Zeller B, Gustafsson G, Forestier E, et al. Acute leukaemia in children with Down syndrome: a population-based Nordic study. Br J Haematol 2005;128(6):797–804.

[92] Ao A, Hills R, Stiller C, et al. Treatment for myeloid leukaemia of Down syndrome: population-based experience in the UK and results from the Medical Research Council AML10 and AML 12 trials. Br J Haematol 2005;132:576–83.

[93] Creutzig U, Ritter J, Vormoor J, et al. Myelodysplasia and acute myelogenous leukemia in Down's syndrome. A report of 40 children of the AML-BFM Study Group. Leukemia 1996;10(11):1677–86.

[94] Gamis AS, Woods WG, Alonzo TA, et al. Increased age at diagnosis has a significantly negative effect on outcome in children with Down syndrome and acute myeloid leukemia: a report from the Children's Cancer Group Study 2891. J Clin Oncol 2003;21(18): 3415–22.

[95] Testi AM, Biondi A, Lo CF, et al. GIMEMA-AIEOP AIDA protocol for the treatment of newly diagnosed acute promyelocytic leukemia (APL) in children. Blood 2005;106:447–53.

[96] Ravindranath Y, Gregory J, Feusner J. Treatment of acute promyelocytic leukemia in children: arsenic or ATRA. Leukemia 2004;18(10):1576–7.

[97] Webb DK, Wheatley K, Harrison G, et al. Outcome for children with relapsed acute myeloid leukaemia following initial therapy in the Medical Research Council (MRC) AML 10 trial. MRC Childhood Leukaemia Working Party. Leukemia 1999;13(1):25–31.

[98] Stahnke K, Boos J, Bender-Gotze C, et al. Duration of first remission predicts remission rates and long-term survival in children with relapsed acute myelogenous leukemia. Leukemia 1998;12(10):1534–8.

[99] Aladjidi N, Auvrignon A, Leblanc T, et al. Outcome in children with relapsed acute myeloid leukemia after initial treatment with the French Leucemie Aique Myeloide Enfant (LAME) 89/91 protocol of the French Society of Pediatric Hematology and Immunology. J Clin Oncol 2003;21(23):4377–85.

[100] Wells RJ, Adams MT, Alonzo TA, et al. Mitoxantrone and cytarabine induction, high-dose cytarabine, and etoposide intensification for pediatric patients with relapsed or refractory acute myeloid leukemia: Children's Cancer Group Study 2951. J Clin Oncol 2003;21(15): 2940–7.

[101] Rubnitz JE, Razzouk BI, Lensing S, et al. Prognostic factors and outcome of recurrence in childhood acute myeloid leukemia. Cancer 2007;109(1):157–63.

[102] Abrahamsson J, Clausen N, Gustafsson G, et al. Improved outcome after relapse in children with acute myeloid leukaemia. Br J Haematol 2007;136(2):222–36.

[103] Zwaan CM, Reinhardt D, Corbacioglu S, et al. Gemtuzumab ozogamicin: first clinical experiences in children with relapsed/refractory acute myeloid leukemia treated on compassionate-use basis. Blood 2003;101(10):3868–71.

[104] Jeha S, Gandhi V, Chan KW, et al. Clofarabine, a novel nucleoside analog, is active in pediatric patients with advanced leukemia. Blood 2004;103(3):784–9.

[105] Meshinchi S, Leisenring WM, Carpenter PA, et al. Survival after second hematopoietic stem cell transplantation for recurrent pediatric acute myeloid leukemia. Biol Blood Marrow Transplant 2003;9(11):706–13.

[106] Appelbaum FR, Gundacker H, Head DR, et al. Age and acute myeloid leukemia. Blood 2006;107(9):3481–5.

[107] Razzouk BI, Estey E, Pounds S, et al. Impact of age on outcome of pediatric acute myeloid leukemia: a report from 2 institutions. Cancer 2006;106(11):2495–502.

[108] Rubnitz JE, Lensing S, Razzouk BI, et al. Effect of race on outcome of white and black children with acute myeloid leukemia: the St. Jude experience. Pediatr Blood Cancer 2007;48(1):10–5.

[109] Aplenc R, Alonzo TA, Gerbing RB, et al. Ethnicity and survival in childhood acute myeloid leukemia: a report from the Children's Oncology Group. Blood 2006;108(1):74–80.

[110] Lange BJ, Gerbing RB, Feusner J, et al. Mortality in overweight and underweight children with acute myeloid leukemia. J Am Med Assoc 2005;293(2):203–11.

[111] Athale UH, Razzouk BI, Raimondi SC, et al. Biology and outcome of childhood acute megakaryoblastic leukemia: a single institution's experience. Blood 2001;97(12):3727–32.

[112] Barbaric D, Alonzo TA, Gerbing R, et al. Minimally differentiated acute myeloid leukemia (FAB AML-10) is associated with an adverse outcome in children: a report from the Children's Oncology Group, studies CCG-2891 and CCG-2961. Blood 2007;109(6):2314–21.

[113] Barnard D, Alonzo TA, Gerbing R, et al. Comparison of childhood myelodysplastic syndrome, AML FAB M6 or M7, CCG 2891: report from the Children's Oncology Group. Pediatr Blood Cancer 2007;49:17–22.

[114] Dastugue N, Lafage-Pochitaloff M, Pages MP, et al. Cytogenetic profile of childhood and adult megakaryoblastic leukemia (M7): a study of the Groupe Francais de Cytogenetique Hematologique (GFCH). Blood 2002;100(2):618–26.

[115] Garderet L, Labopin M, Gorin NC, et al. Hematopoietic stem cell transplantation for de novo acute megakaryocytic leukemia in first complete remission: a retrospective study of the European Group for Blood and Marrow Transplantation (EBMT). Blood 2005; 105(1):405–9.

[116] Reinhardt D, Diekamp S, Langebrake C, et al. Acute megakaryoblastic leukemia in children and adolescents, excluding Down's syndrome: improved outcome with intensified induction treatment. Leukemia 2005;19(8):1495–6.

[117] Grimwade D, Walker H, Oliver F, et al. The importance of diagnostic cytogenetics on outcome in AML: analysis of 1,612 patients entered into the MRC AML 10 trial. The Medical Research Council Adult and Children's Leukaemia Working Parties. Blood 1998;92(7):2322–33.

[118] Raimondi SC, Chang MN, Ravindranath Y, et al. Chromosomal abnormalities in 478 children with acute myeloid leukemia: clinical characteristics and treatment outcome in a cooperative Pediatric Oncology Group study-POG 8821. Blood 1999;94(11):3707–16.

[119] Bloomfield CD, Lawrence D, Byrd JC, et al. Frequency of prolonged remission duration after high-dose cytarabine intensification in acute myeloid leukemia varies by cytogenetic subtype. Cancer Res 1998;58(18):4173–9.

[120] Byrd JC, Mrozek K, Dodge RK, et al. Pretreatment cytogenetic abnormalities are predictive of induction success, cumulative incidence of relapse, and overall survival in adult patients with de novo acute myeloid leukemia: results from Cancer and Leukemia Group B (CALGB 8461). Blood 2002;100(13):4325–36.

[121] Marcucci G, Mrozek K, Ruppert AS, et al. Prognostic factors and outcome of core binding factor acute myeloid leukemia patients with t(8;21) differ from those of patients with inv(16): a Cancer and Leukemia Group B Study. J Clin Oncol 2006;24:5705–17.

[122] Appelbaum F, Kopecky KJ, Tallman M, et al. The clinical spectrum of adult acute myeloid leukaemia associated with core binding factor translocations. Br J Haematol 2006;135: 165–73.

[123] Dimartino JF, Cleary ML. Mll rearrangements in haematological malignancies: lessons from clinical and biological studies. Br J Haematol 1999;106(3):614–26.

[124] Rubnitz JE, Raimondi SC, Tong X, et al. Favorable impact of the t(9;11) in childhood acute myeloid leukemia. J Clin Oncol 2002;20(9):2302–9.

[125] Schoch C, Schnittger S, Klaus M, et al. AML with 11q23/MLL abnormalities as defined by the WHO classification: incidence, partner chromosomes, FAB subtype, age distribution,

and prognostic impact in an unselected series of 1897 cytogenetically analyzed AML cases. Blood 2003;102(7):2395–402.

[126] Hasle H, Alonzo TA, Auvrignon A, et al. Monosomy 7 and deletion 7q in children and adolescents with acute myeloid leukemia: an international retrospective study. Blood 2007;109(11):4641–7.

[127] Cairoli R, Beghini A, Grillo G, et al. Prognostic impact of c-KIT mutations in core binding factor leukemias: an Italian retrospective study. Blood 2007;107:3463–8.

[128] Schnittger S, Kohl T, Haferlach T, et al. KIT-D816 mutations in AML1-ETO-positive AML are associated with impaired event-free and overall survival. Blood 2006;107:1791–9.

[129] Paschka P, Marcucci G, Ruppert AS, et al. Adverse prognostic significance of KIT muta-tions in adult acute myeloid leukemia with inv(16) and t(8;21): a Cancer and Leukemia Group B Study. J Clin Oncol 2006;24(24):3904–11.

[130] Goemans BF, Zwaan CM, Miller M, et al. Mutations in KIT and RAS are frequent events in pediatric core-binding factor acute myeloid leukemia. Leukemia 2005;19(9):1536–42.

[131] Shimada A, Taki T, Tabuchi K, et al. KIT mutations, and not FLT3 internal tandem duplication, are strongly associated with a poor prognosis in pediatric acute myeloid leuke-mia with t(8;21); a study of the Japanese Childhood AML Cooperative Study Group. Blood 2006;107:1806–9.

[132] Boissel N, Leroy H, Brethon B, et al. Incidence and prognostic impact of c-Kit, FLT3, and Ras gene mutations in core binding factor acute myeloid leukemia (CBF-AML). Leukemia 2006;20(6):965–70.

[133] Meshinchi S, Stirewalt DL, Alonzo TA, et al. Activating mutations of RTK/ras signal transduction pathway in pediatric acute myeloid leukemia. Blood 2003;102(4):1474–9.

[134] Kiyoi H, Naoe T, Nakano Y, et al. Prognostic implication of FLT3 and N-RAS gene mutations in acute myeloid leukemia. Blood 1999;93(9):3074–80.

[135] Abu-Duhier FM, Goodeve AC, Wilson GA, et al. FLT3 internal tandem duplication mutations in adult acute myeloid leukaemia define a high-risk group. Br J Haematol 2000;111(1):190–5.

[136] Kottaridis PD, Gale RE, Frew ME, et al. The presence of a FLT3 internal tandem duplication in patients with acute myeloid leukemia (AML) adds important prognostic information to cytogenetic risk group and response to the first cycle of chemotherapy: analysis of 854 patients from the United Kingdom Medical Research Council AML 10 and 12 trials. Blood 2001;98(6):1752–9.

[137] Whitman SP, Archer KJ, Feng L, et al. Absence of the wild-type allele predicts poor prog-nosis in adult de novo acute myeloid leukemia with normal cytogenetics and the internal tandem duplication of FLT3: a cancer and leukemia group B study. Cancer Res 2001; 61(19):7233–9.

[138] Schnittger S, Schoch C, Dugas M, et al. Analysis of FLT3 length mutations in 1003 patients with acute myeloid leukemia: correlation to cytogenetics, FAB subtype, and prognosis in the AMLCG study and usefulness as a marker for the detection of minimal residual disease. Blood 2002;100(1):59–66.

[139] Thiede C, Steudel C, Mohr B, et al. Analysis of FLT3-activating mutations in 979 patients with acute myelogenous leukemia: association with FAB subtypes and identification of subgroups with poor prognosis. Blood 2002;99(12):4326–35.

[140] Zwaan CM, Meshinchi S, Radich JP, et al. FLT3 internal tandem duplication in 234 children with acute myeloid leukemia: prognostic significance and relation to cellular drug resistance. Blood 2003;102(7):2387–94.

[141] Meshinchi S, Woods WG, Stirewalt DL, et al. Prevalence and prognostic significance of Flt3 internal tandem duplication in pediatric acute myeloid leukemia. Blood 2001;97(1): 89–94.

[142] Iwai T, Yokota S, Nakao M, et al. Internal tandem duplication of the FLT3 gene and clinical evaluation in childhood acute myeloid leukemia. The Children's Cancer and Leukemia Study Group, Japan. Leukemia 1999;13(1):38–43.

[143] Meshinchi S, Alonzo TA, Stirewalt DL, et al. Clinical implications of FLT3 mutations in pediatric AML. Blood 2006;108(12):3654–61.

[144] Lacayo NJ, Meshinchi S, Kinnunen P, et al. Gene expression profiles at diagnosis in de novo childhood AML patients identify FLT3 mutations with good clinical outcomes. Blood 2004;104(9):2646–54.

[145] Leith CP, Kopecky KJ, Chen IM, et al. Frequency and clinical significance of the expression of the multidrug resistance proteins MDR1/P-glycoprotein, MRP1, and LRP in acute myeloid leukemia: a Southwest Oncology Group Study. Blood 1999;94(3):1086–99.

[146] Legrand O, Simonin G, Beauchamp-Nicoud A, et al. Simultaneous activity of MRP1 and Pgp is correlated with in vitro resistance to daunorubicin and with in vivo resistance in adult acute myeloid leukemia. Blood 1999;94(3):1046–56.

[147] den Boer ML, Pieters R, Kazemier KM, et al. Relationship between major vault protein/lung resistance protein, multidrug resistance-associated protein, P-glycoprotein expression, and drug resistance in childhood leukemia. Blood 1998;91(6):2092–8.

[148] Preudhomme C, Sagot C, Boissel N, et al. Favorable prognostic significance of CEBPA mutations in patients with de novo acute myeloid leukemia: a study from the Acute Leukemia French Association (ALFA). Blood 2002;100(8):2717–23.

[149] Frohling S, Schlenk RF, Stolze I, et al. CEBPA mutations in younger adults with acute myeloid leukemia and normal cytogenetics: prognostic relevance and analysis of cooperating mutations. J Clin Oncol 2004;22(4):624–33.

[150] Inokuchi K, Yamaguchi H, Hanawa H, et al. Loss of DCC gene expression is of prognostic importance in acute myelogenous leukemia. Clin Cancer Res 2002;8(6):1882–8.

[151] De Bont ES, Fidler V, Meeuwsen T, et al. Vascular endothelial growth factor secretion is an independent prognostic factor for relapse-free survival in pediatric acute myeloid leukemia patients. Clin Cancer Res 2002;8(9):2856–61.

[152] Kohler T, Schill C, Deininger MW, et al. High Bad and Bax mRNA expression correlate with negative outcome in acute myeloid leukemia (AML). Leukemia 2002;16(1):22–9.

[153] Karakas T, Miething CC, Maurer U, et al. The coexpression of the apoptosis-related genes Bcl-2 and Wt1 in predicting survival in adult acute myeloid leukemia. Leukemia 2002;16(5): 846–54.

[154] Del Poeta G, Venditti A, Del Principe MI, et al. Amount of spontaneous apoptosis detected by Bax/Bcl-2 ratio predicts outcome in acute myeloid leukemia (AML). Blood 2003;101(6): 2125–31.

[155] Baldus CD, Thiede C, Soucek S, et al. BAALC expression and FLT3 internal tandem duplication mutations in acute myeloid leukemia patients with normal cytogenetics: prognostic implications. J Clin Oncol 2006;24(5):790–7.

[156] Marcucci G, Maharry K, Whitman SP, et al. High expression levels of the ETS-related gene, ERG, predict adverse outcome and improve molecular risk-based classification of cytogenetically normal acute myeloid leukemia: a Cancer and Leukemia Group B Study. J Clin Oncol 2007;25(22):3337–43.

[157] Marcucci G, Baldus CD, Ruppert AS, et al. Overexpression of the ETS-related gene, ERG, predicts a worse outcome in acute myeloid leukemia with normal karyotype: a Cancer and Leukemia Group B study. J Clin Oncol 2005;23(36):9234–42.

[158] Boissel N, Renneville A, Biggio V, et al. Prevalence, clinical profile, and prognosis of NPM mutations in AML with normal karyotype. Blood 2005;106(10):3618–20.

[159] Thiede C, Koch S, Creutzig E, et al. Prevalence and prognostic impact of NPM1 mutations in 1485 adult patients with acute myeloid leukemia (AML). Blood 2006;107(10): 4011–20.

[160] Brown P, McIntyre E, Rau R, et al. The incidence and clinical significance of nucleophosmin mutations in childhood AML. Blood 2007;110(3):979–85.

[161] Schnittger S, Kinkelin U, Schoch C, et al. Screening for MLL tandem duplication in 387 unselected patients with AML identify a prognostically unfavorable subset of AML. Leukemia 2000;14(5):796–804.

[162] Dohner K, Tobis K, Ulrich R, et al. Prognostic significance of partial tandem duplications of the MLL gene in adult patients 16 to 60 years old with acute myeloid leukemia and normal cytogenetics: a study of the Acute Myeloid Leukemia Study Group Ulm. J Clin Oncol 2002;20(15):3254–61.

[163] Yagi T, Morimoto A, Eguchi M, et al. Identification of a gene expression signature associated with pediatric AML prognosis. Blood 2003;102(5):1849–56.

[164] Valk PJ, Verhaak RG, Beijen MA, et al. Prognostically useful gene-expression profiles in acute myeloid leukemia. N Engl J Med 2004;350(16):1617–28.

[165] Bullinger L, Dohner K, Bair E, et al. Use of gene-expression profiling to identify prognostic subclasses in adult acute myeloid leukemia. N Engl J Med 2004;350(16):1605–16.

[166] Radmacher MD, Marcucci G, Ruppert AS, et al. Independent confirmation of a prognostic gene-expression signature in adult acute myeloid leukemia with a normal karyotype: a Cancer and Leukemia Group B study. Blood 2006;108(5):1677–83.

[167] Wilson CS, Davidson GS, Martin SB, et al. Gene expression profiling of adult acute myeloid leukemia identifies novel biologic clusters for risk classification and outcome prediction. Blood 2006;108(2):685–96.

[168] Mrozek K, Marcucci G, Paschka P, et al. Clinical relevance of mutations and gene-expression changes in adult acute myeloid leukemia with normal cytogenetics: are we ready for a prognostically prioritized molecular classification? Blood 2007;109(2):431–48.

[169] Ross ME, Mahfouz R, Onciu M, et al. Gene expression profiling of pediatric acute myelogenous leukemia. Blood 2004;104(12):3679–87.

[170] Campana D. Determination of minimal residual disease in leukaemia patients. Br J Haematol 2003;121(6):823–38.

[171] Creutzig U, Zimmermann M, Ritter J, et al. Definition of a standard-risk group in children with AML. Br J Haematol 1999;104(3):630–9.

[172] Kern W, Haferlach T, Schoch C, et al. Early blast clearance by remission induction therapy is a major independent prognostic factor for both achievement of complete remission and long-term outcome in acute myeloid leukemia: data from the German AML Cooperative Group (AMLCG) 1992 Trial. Blood 2003;101(1):64–70.

[173] Marcucci G, Mrozek K, Ruppert AS, et al. Abnormal cytogenetics at date of morphologic complete remission predicts short overall and disease-free survival, and higher relapse rate in adult acute myeloid leukemia: results from Cancer and Leukemia Group B study 8461. J Clin Oncol 2004;22(12):2410–8.

[174] Szczepanski T, Orfao A, van DV, et al. Minimal residual disease in leukaemia patients. Lancet Oncol 2001;2(7):409–17.

[175] Sievers EL, Lange BJ, Buckley JD, et al. Prediction of relapse of pediatric acute myeloid leukemia by use of multidimensional flow cytometry. J Natl Cancer Inst 1996;88(20):1483–8.

[176] Sievers EL, Lange BJ, Alonzo TA, et al. Immunophenotypic evidence of leukemia after induction therapy predicts relapse: results from a prospective Children's Cancer Group study of 252 patients with acute myeloid leukemia. Blood 2003;101(9):3398–406.

[177] Coustan-Smith E, Ribeiro RC, Rubnitz JE, et al. Clinical significance of residual disease during treatment in childhood acute myeloid leukaemia. Br J Haematol 2003;123(2):243–52.

[178] Langebrake C, Creutzig U, Dworzak M, et al. Residual disease monitoring in childhood acute myeloid leukemia by multiparameter flow cytometry: the MRD-AML-BFM Study Group. J Clin Oncol 2006;24(22):3686–92.

[179] San Miguel JF, Martinez A, Macedo A, et al. Immunophenotyping investigation of minimal residual disease is a useful approach for predicting relapse in acute myeloid leukemia patients. Blood 1997;90(6):2465–70.

[180] San Miguel JF, Vidriales MB, Lopez-Berges C, et al. Early immunophenotypical evaluation of minimal residual disease in acute myeloid leukemia identifies different patient risk groups and may contribute to postinduction treatment stratification. Blood 2001;98(6):1746–51.

[181] Buccisano F, Maurillo L, Gattei V, et al. The kinetics of reduction of minimal residual disease impacts on duration of response and survival of patients with acute myeloid leukemia. Leukemia 2006;20(10):1783–9.

[182] Feller N, van der Pol MA, van Stijn A, et al. MRD parameters using immunophenotypic detection methods are highly reliable in predicting survival in acute myeloid leukaemia. Leukemia 2004;18(8):1380–90.

[183] Kern W, Voskova D, Schoch C, et al. Determination of relapse risk based on assessment of minimal residual disease during complete remission by multiparameter flow cytometry in unselected patients with acute myeloid leukemia. Blood 2004;104(10):3078–85.

[184] Tobal K, Newton J, Macheta M, et al. Molecular quantitation of minimal residual disease in acute myeloid leukemia with t(8;21) can identify patients in durable remission and predict clinical relapse. Blood 2000;95(3):815–9.

[185] Schnittger S, Weisser M, Schoch C, et al. New score predicting for prognosis in PML-RARA+, AML1-ETO+, or CBFBMYH11+ acute myeloid leukemia based on quantification of fusion transcripts. Blood 2003;102(8):2746–55.

[186] Buonamici S, Ottaviani E, Testoni N, et al. Real-time quantitation of minimal residual disease in inv(16)-positive acute myeloid leukemia may indicate risk for clinical relapse and may identify patients in a curable state. Blood 2002;99(2):443–9.

[187] Guerrasio A, Pilatrino C, De Micheli D, et al. Assessment of minimal residual disease (MRD) in CBFbeta/MYH11-positive acute myeloid leukemias by qualitative and quantitative RT-PCR amplification of fusion transcripts. Leukemia 2002;16(6):1176–81.

[188] Viehmann S, Teigler-Schlegel A, Bruch J, et al. Monitoring of minimal residual disease (MRD) by real-time quantitative reverse transcription PCR (RQ-RT-PCR) in childhood acute myeloid leukemia with AML1/ETO rearrangement. Leukemia 2003;17(6):1130–6.

[189] Krauter J, Gorlich K, Ottmann O, et al. Prognostic value of minimal residual disease quantification by real-time reverse transcriptase polymerase chain reaction in patients with core binding factor leukemias. J Clin Oncol 2003;21(23):4413–22.

[190] Perea G, Lasa A, Aventin A, et al. Prognostic value of minimal residual disease (MRD) in acute myeloid leukemia (AML) with favorable cytogenetics [t(8;21) and inv(16)]. Leukemia 2006;20:87–94.

[191] Trka J, Kalinova M, Hrusak O, et al. Real-time quantitative PCR detection of WT1 gene expression in children with AML: prognostic significance, correlation with disease status and residual disease detection by flow cytometry. Leukemia 2002;16(7):1381–9.

[192] Cilloni D, Gottardi E, De Micheli D, et al. Quantitative assessment of WT1 expression by real time quantitative PCR may be a useful tool for monitoring minimal residual disease in acute leukemia patients. Leukemia 2002;16(10):2115–21.

[193] Lapillonne H, Renneville A, Auvrignon A, et al. High WT1 expression after induction therapy predicts high risk of relapse and death in pediatric acute myeloid leukemia. J Clin Oncol 2006;24(10):1507–15.

[194] Evans WE, Relling MV. Moving towards individualized medicine with pharmacogenomics. Nature 2004;429(6990):464–8.

[195] Monzo M, Brunet S, Urbano-Ispizua A, et al. Genomic polymorphisms provide prognostic information in intermediate-risk acute myeloblastic leukemia. Blood 2006;107(12):4871–9.

[196] Gamis AS. Acute myeloid leukemia and Down syndrome evolution of modern therapy—state of the art review. Pediatr Blood Cancer 2005;44(1):13–20.

[197] Ge Y, Jensen T, James SJ, et al. High frequency of the 844ins68 cystathionine-beta-synthase gene variant in Down syndrome children with acute myeloid leukemia. Leukemia 2002;16(11):2339–41.

[198] Ge Y, Stout ML, Tatman DA, et al. GATA1, cytidine deaminase, and the high cure rate of Down syndrome children with acute megakaryocytic leukemia. J Natl Cancer Inst 2005;97(3):226–31.

[199] Ge Y, Dombkowski AA, Lafiura KM, et al. Differential gene expression, GATA1 target genes, and the chemotherapy sensitivity of Down syndrome megakaryocytic leukemia. Blood 2006;107(4):1570–81.

[200] Taub JW, Ge Y. Down syndrome, drug metabolism and chromosome 21. Pediatr Blood Cancer 2005;44(1):33–9.

[201] Galmarini CM, Thomas X, Calvo F, et al. In vivo mechanisms of resistance to cytarabine in acute myeloid leukaemia. Br J Haematol 2002;117(4):860–8.

[202] Gati WP, Paterson AR, Belch AR, et al. Es nucleoside transporter content of acute leukemia cells: role in cell sensitivity to cytarabine (AraC). Leuk Lymphoma 1998; 32(1–2):45–54.

[203] Galmarini CM, Thomas X, Graham K, et al. Deoxycytidine kinase and cN-II nucleotidase expression in blast cells predict survival in acute myeloid leukaemia patients treated with cytarabine. Br J Haematol 2003;122(1):53–60.

[204] Davies SM, Robison LL, Buckley JD, et al. Glutathione S-transferase polymorphisms and outcome of chemotherapy in childhood acute myeloid leukemia. J Clin Oncol 2001;19(5): 1279–87.

[205] Naoe T, Tagawa Y, Kiyoi H, et al. Prognostic significance of the null genotype of glutathione S- transferase-T1 in patients with acute myeloid leukemia: increased early death after chemotherapy. Leukemia 2002;16(2):203–8.

[206] Allan JM, Smith AG, Wheatley K, et al. Genetic variation in XPD predicts treatment outcome and risk of acute myeloid leukemia following chemotherapy. Blood 2004;104(13): 3872–7.

[207] Mehta PA, Alonzo TA, Gerbing RB, et al. XPD Lys751Gln polymorphism in the etiology and outcome of childhood acute myeloid leukemia: a Children's Oncology Group report. Blood 2006;107(1):39–45.

[208] Okamoto Y, Ribeiro RC, Srivastava DK, et al. Viridans streptococcal sepsis: clinical features and complications in childhood acute myeloid leukemia. J Pediatr Hematol Oncol 2003;25(9):696–703.

[209] Creutzig U, Zimmermann M, Reinhardt D, et al. Early deaths and treatment-related mortality in children undergoing therapy for acute myeloid leukemia: analysis of the multicenter clinical trials AML-BFM 93 and AML-BFM 98. J Clin Oncol 2004;22(21): 4384–93.

[210] Lehrnbecher T, Varwig D, Kaiser J, et al. Infectious complications in pediatric acute myeloid leukemia: analysis of the prospective multi-institutional clinical trial AML-BFM 93. Leukemia 2004;18(1):72–7.

[211] Rubnitz JE, Lensing S, Zhou Y, et al. Death during induction therapy and first remission of acute leukemia in childhood: the St. Jude experience. Cancer 2004;101(7):1677–84.

[212] Gamis AS, Howells WB, DeSwarte-Wallace J, et al. Alpha hemolytic Streptococcal infection during intensive treatment for acute myeloid leukemia: a report from the Children's Cancer Group Study CCG-2891. J Clin Oncol 2000;18(9):1845–55.

[213] Sung L, Lange BJ, Gerbing RB, et al. Microbiologically documented infections and infection-related mortality in children with acute myeloid leukemia. Blood 2007;110: 3532–9.

[214] Godwin JE, Kopecky KJ, Head DR, et al. A double-blind placebo-controlled trial of granulocyte colony-stimulating factor in elderly patients with previously untreated acute myeloid leukemia: a Southwest Oncology Group study (9031). Blood 1998;91(10):3607–15.

[215] Heil G, Hoelzer D, Sanz MA, et al. A randomized, double-blind, placebo-controlled, phase III study of filgrastim in remission induction and consolidation therapy for adults with de novo acute myeloid leukemia. The International Acute Myeloid Leukemia Study Group. Blood 1997;90(12):4710–8.

[216] Amadori S, Suciu S, Jehn U, et al. Use of glycosylated recombinant human G-CSF (lenograstim) during and/or after induction chemotherapy in patients 61 years of age and older with acute myeloid leukemia: final results of AML-13, a randomized phase 3 study

of the European Organisation for Research and Treatment of Cancer and Gruppo Italiano Malattie Ematologiche dell'Adulto (EORTC/GIMEMA) Leukemia Groups. Blood 2005; 106:27–34.

[217] George B, Mathews V, Poonkuzhali B, et al. Treatment of children with newly diagnosed acute promyelocytic leukemia with arsenic trioxide: a single center experience. Leukemia 2004;18(10):1587–90.

[218] Burnett A, Kell WJ, Goldstone A, et al. The addition of gemtuzumab ozogamicin to induction chemotherapy for AML improves disease free survival without extra toxicity: preliminary analysis of 1115 patients in the MRC AML15 trial. Blood 2006;108:13.

[219] Guzman ML, Swiderski CF, Howard DS, et al. Preferential induction of apoptosis for primary human leukemic stem cells. Proc Natl Acad Sci U S A 2002;99(25):16220–5.

[220] Adams J. The proteasome: a suitable antineoplastic target. Nat Rev Cancer 2004;4(5): 349–60.

[221] Insinga A, Monestiroli S, Ronzoni S, et al. Inhibitors of histone deacetylases induce tumor-selective apoptosis through activation of the death receptor pathway. Nat Med 2005;11(1): 71–6.

[222] Nebbioso A, Clarke N, Voltz E, et al. Tumor-selective action of HDAC inhibitors involves TRAIL induction in acute myeloid leukemia cells. Nat Med 2005;11(1):77–84.

[223] Levis M, Allebach J, Tse KF, et al. A FLT3-targeted tyrosine kinase inhibitor is cytotoxic to leukemia cells in vitro and in vivo. Blood 2002;99(11):3885–91.

[224] Brown P, Meshinchi S, Levis M, et al. Pediatric AML primary samples with FLT3/ITD mutations are preferentially killed by FLT3 inhibition. Blood 2004;104(6):1841–9.

[225] Smith BD, Levis M, Beran M, et al. Single-agent CEP-701, a novel FLT3 inhibitor, shows biologic and clinical activity in patients with relapsed or refractory acute myeloid leukemia. Blood 2004;103(10):3669–76.

[226] Parker WB, Shaddix SC, Chang CH, et al. Effects of 2-chloro-9-(2-deoxy-2-fluoro-beta-D-arabinofuranosyl)adenine on K562 cellular metabolism and the inhibition of human ribonucleotide reductase and DNA polymerases by its 5'-triphosphate. Cancer Res 1991; 51(9):2386–94.

[227] Xie KC, Plunkett W. Deoxynucleotide pool depletion and sustained inhibition of ribonucleotide reductase and DNA synthesis after treatment of human lymphoblastoid cells with 2-chloro-9-(2-deoxy-2-fluoro-beta-D-arabinofuranosyl) adenine. Cancer Res 1996;56(13): 3030–7.

[228] Gandhi V, Kantarjian H, Faderl S, et al. Pharmacokinetics and pharmacodynamics of plasma clofarabine and cellular clofarabine triphosphate in patients with acute leukemias. Clin Cancer Res 2003;9(17):6335–42.

[229] Miller JS, Soignier Y, Panoskaltsis-Mortari A, et al. Successful adoptive transfer and in vivo expansion of human haploidentical NK cells in patients with cancer. Blood 2005; 105(8):3051–7.

ELSEVIER
SAUNDERS

PEDIATRIC CLINICS
OF NORTH AMERICA

Pediatr Clin N Am 55 (2008) 53–70

Acute Leukemias in Children with Down Syndrome

Michel C. Zwaan, MD, PhD[a],*, Dirk Reinhardt, PD[b],
Johann Hitzler, FRCP(C), FAAP[c,d],
Paresh Vyas, FRCPath, DPHil[e]

[a]*Department of Pediatric Oncology/Hematology, Erasmus MC/Sophia Children's Hospital,
Dr Molewaterplein 60, 3015GJ Rotterdam, The Netherlands*
[b]*Acute Myeloid Leukemia–Berlin-Frankfurt-Münster Study Group, Pediatric Hematology/
Oncology, Hannover Medical School, Carl-Neuberg-Straße 1, D-30625 Hannover, Germany*
[c]*Division of Hematology/Oncology, The Hospital for Sick Children, 555 University Avenue,
Toronto, ON M5G 1X8, Canada*
[d]*Developmental and Stem Cell Biology, The Hospital for Sick Children Research Institute,
University of Toronto, Toronto, ON M5G 1X8, Canada*
[e]*Medical Research Council Molecular Haematology Unit, John Radcliffe Hospital and the
Weatherall Institute of Molecular Medicine, University of Oxford, Oxford OX3 9DS, UK*

Childhood leukemias often originate from a premalignant clone, a generally asymptomatic condition that can only be detected by demonstrating leukemia-specific genetic changes in peripheral blood, including that obtained from Guthrie cards or in cord-blood [1]. Subsequently, secondary genetic events cause outgrowth of this dormant clone and result in frank leukemia. However, the likelihood of developing leukemia in children who carry premalignant clones, harboring genetic aberrations such as TEL-AML or AML1-ETO is low. Because of the very low transformation into frank leukemia, prevention strategies are generally considered not feasible.

Children with Down syndrome (DS) (for a review on DS, see Roizen and Patterson in [2]) have an increased risk of developing leukemias, which was already recognized in the 1950s [3], although their risk of cancer in general is not increased because of a reduced propensity for solid tumors [3,4]. This increased risk of leukemia includes both acute lymphoblastic leukemia as well as myeloid leukemia. Approximately 10% of newborns with DS

None of the authors have direct financial interests to disclose. P. Vyas receives research support from the Leukemia Research Fund; M. Zwaan receives research support from Stichting Kinderen Kankervrij.
    * Corresponding address.
    E-mail address: c.m.zwaan@erasmusmc.nl (M.C. Zwaan).

0031-3955/08/$ - see front matter © 2008 Elsevier Inc. All rights reserved.
doi:10.1016/j.pcl.2007.11.001

develop a preleukemic clone, originating from myeloid progenitors in the fetal liver that are characterized by a somatic mutation in the gene encoding for the hematopoietic transcription factor GATA1, which is localized on the X-chromosome. Mutations in this transcription factor lead to a truncated mutant protein GATA1short or GATA1s [5,6]. This preleukemia is referred to as transient leukemia (TL), transient myeloproliferative disease (TMD), or transient abnormal myelopoiesis (TAM).

Transient leukemia is associated with a variable clinical presentation, ranging from a-symptomatic to severe complications, which may even be fatal [7,8]. As TL originates in the liver, peripheral blood blast counts are usually higher than the bone marrow blast count. Subsequently, approximately 20% of children who have been diagnosed with TL develop myeloid leukemia of Down syndrome (ML DS; this term has been introduced to refer to the unique subtype of AML that develops in children with DS, as explained later in this article), usually with an onset before the age of 5 years [7]. Studying TL and ML DS may contribute significantly to our understanding of the stepwise process of leukemogeneis [9]. However, so far the genetic factors that drive this progression are unknown. Mutations in the GATA1 gene are present both in both TL and ML DS, and are therefore not sufficient to explain this progression [10].

Of interest, children with DS are also predisposed to develop acute lymphoblastic leukemia (ALL), which is not associated with an overt preleukemic phase. Both ML and ALL in patients with DS are biologically distinct when compared with their non-DS counterparts, and are characterized by a different clinical behavior [11–14]. For children with DS who develop ALL, this does not lead to improved outcome, as is observed for children with DS who develop ML. This article reviews the current knowledge and research questions regarding TL and the DS-associated acute leukemias.

Hematologic abnormalities in children with Down syndrome

Tunstall-Pedoe and colleagues [15] studied hematopoiesis in fetal bood, bone marrow, and liver cells from 16 fetuses with DS with a gestational age of 15 to 37 weeks. GATA1 mutations were not detected in the hematopoietic cells of these fetuses, although minor clones may have been missed, as explained later in this article. A marked increase in the megakaryocyte-erythrocyte progenitors in the fetal liver was found, as well as dysmegakaryopoiesis and dyserythropoiesis in the peripheral blood, but not in the bone marrow, when compared with non-DS fetuses. The investigators conclude that trisomy 21 by itself affects fetal hematopoiesis, and that the expansion of fetal liver progenitors creates a cellular substrate for GATA1 mutations to occur, which subsequently gives rise to TL (see later in this article and Fig. 1).

In DS newborns (n = 158), peripheral blood abnormalities in the first week of life included neutrophilia in 80% of children, thrombocytopenia in 66% (6% had platelets less than $50 \times 10^9/l$) and polycythemia in 33%

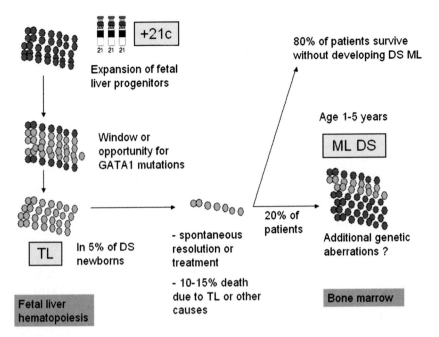

Fig. 1. Stepwise development of ML DS following TL. Transient leukemia arises from expanded fetal liver progenitors as a result of constitutional trisomy 21, providing a window of opportunity for the occurrence of acquired mutations in the hematopoietic transcription factor GATA1. In most cases TL spontaneously disappears, but some children may need treatment because of severe TL-related symptoms. Approximately 20% of children with TL subsequently develop ML DS, which requires additional hits.

[16]. Anemia, neutropenia, and thrombocytosis were present in less than 1% of DS newborns. In 6% of children, TL was diagnosed. Widness and colleagues [17] suggested that the observed polycythemia may be caused by increased erythopoietin levels when compared with non-DS newborns.

After the first week of life, the main peripheral blood abnormalities consist of red blood cell macrocytosis and thrombocytosis, although this study was limited to DS children who were younger than 1 year of age [18].

De Hingh and colleagues [19] have studied T- and B-lymphocyte counts in children with DS and compared these to children without trisomy 21. Over time, the T-lymphocyte subpopulation gradually reached normal levels, but the B-lymphocyte population appeared severely decreased (88% of values were below the tenth percentile, and 61% below the fifth percentile of normal). These abnormalities may at least in part explain the increased susceptibility to infections, which children with DS may experience.

How frequent is transient leukemia in Down syndrome children?

The frequency of TL is estimated to be around 10% in DS children, although this was studied in a selected (hospitalized) population [18]. Most investigators assume that the true frequency is higher, but recent data suggest that his may not be the case. In The Netherlands, children with DS are registered in different nation-wide registries (the Dutch Pediatric Surveillance Unit and the National Dutch Neonatal and Obstetrical Registry), which provide population-based data. After matching these databases, it was assessed that 322 children (95% confidence interval 303–341) with DS were born in 2003, resulting in a prevalence of 16 out of 10,000 live-born babies [20]. To date, five children with DS who were born in 2002 and 2003 have been diagnosed with myeloid leukemia (by the Dutch Childhood Oncology Group, E.R. van Wering, personal communication, 2007). As ML in patients with DS typically occurs before the age of 5 years, with a median age of approximately 2 years, and the frequency for progression from TL to ML DS is well established at 20%, these data suggest that the true frequency of TL is in the 3% to 5% range.

This is further supported by a recent study from Pine and colleagues [21], who screened Guthrie cards from 590 infants with DS for mutations in the GATA1 gene and found a mutation in 3.8% of children. However, GATA1 mutations may have been missed in those patients with minor preleukemic clones, subclonal mutations, low numbers of cells on Guthrie cards, or extramedullary TL without circulating blasts. In addition, one has to consider that some fetuses with DS may die in utero from causes that may include TL [22]. Prospective population-based studies regarding the incidence of TL are currently underway in The Netherlands.

Down syndrome transient leukemia: clinical presentation

Massey and colleagues [7] recently published the clinical data of a Children's Oncology Group (COG) retrospective study in which 48 neonates with TL were enrolled. The median age at diagnosis of TL was 7 days (range 1–65 days). Approximately 25% of patients were a-symptomatic, although this study may have been biased toward registration of symptomatic patients. Hepatosplenomagaly (in 56% of cases), effusions (in 21%), and bleeding or petechiae (in 25%) were the most common findings in symptomatic infants. In terms of outcome, 9 out of 47 (19.1%) patients developed ML DS at a mean of 20 months (range 9–38 months). The development of subsequent leukemia was associated with cytogenetic abnormalities other than the constitutional +21, although there were no clear recurrent abnormalities. Eight out of 47 (17%) patients died early at a mean of 90 days. These eight children all had signs of liver failure and diffuse intravascular coagulation, as well as effusions (including pericardial, pleural, and ascitic effusions). Four patients had liver biopsies showing liver fibrosis, cholestasis, and infiltration with leukemic cells. None of the eight children had normalized their blood counts before death, although in three the blasts had disappeared completely from the peripheral blood. Overall, in 42 out of 47 (89%) patients the blasts disappeared after a mean of 58 days (range

2–194 days). Of these 42 children, four developed subsequent leukemia and three died early because of complications. The other 35 children did not have detectable hematologic abnormalities at follow-up, and normalized their blood counts at a mean of 84 days (range 2–201 days). See Fig. 2A for an example of a blood smear of a TL patient.

The study from Massey and colleagues was recently confirmed by two other series, one from Japan and one from the AML-Berlin Frankfurt Münster Study Group (AML-BFM SG). The Japanese study evaluated 70 children with TL, and reported an early death rate of 23% and development of ML DS in 17% of surviving children [23]. The AML-BFM SG registered 148 children with TMD between 1993 and 2006, mainly consisting of children with symptomatic TL (D. Reinhardt, unpublished data, 2007). Median white blood cell count at diagnosis was 40.3×10^9 per liter. Complete remission was achieved spontaneously in 66% of children; 19% of children were

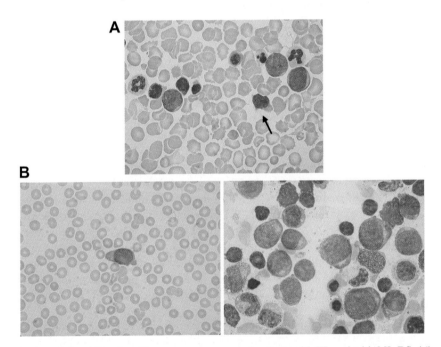

Fig. 2. Peripheral blood and bone marrow smears of patients with TL and with ML DS. (*A*) Peripheral blood smear (63×, May-Grünwald-Giemsa staining), from a baby with DS admitted at the neonatal intensive care for meconium aspiration. A high white blood cell count (56×10^9/l, after correction for normoblasts) was found. The smear shows transient leukemia, with four identifiable blasts, one with typical blebs (*arrow*), among several other normal blood cells. (*B*) Peripheral blood (*left panel*) and bone marrow (*right panel*) smear (63×, May-Grünwald-Giemsa staining), from a child that was diagnosed previously with TL (white blood cell count at birth 88×10^9/l with 37% blasts, which normalized within 3 months) and developed thrombocytopenia at the age of 1.5 years. Peripheral blood showed 3% blasts. Bone marrow examination showed 24% blasts, and was morphologically classified as French-American-British (FAB) M0.

treated with low-dose cytarabine to relieve symptoms and achieved remission. Two children progressed to ML DS after 9 and 13 months of follow-up, without clearing their peripheral blood TL cells in the meantime. In total, 24 children died, including 21 in the first 23 months of life. Death was attributed to TL in 13 of these children, including seven cases with liver fibrosis. In most children (85%) blasts were cleared from the peripheral blood after 4 weeks. Of the 124 surviving children, 29 developed ML DS (23.4%) after a median remission of 1.5 years (0.5–3.0 years).

One of the most relevant questions unanswered to date is whether the development of ML DS following TL can be inhibited by treating children for TL. The AML BFM SG and the Dutch COG are currently performing a study to prospectively investigate this.

Clinical features of Down syndrome leukemias

Myeloid leukemia of Down syndrome: clinical characteristics and classification

According to the World Health Organization (WHO) classification, AML requires the presence of at least 20% blasts in the bone marrow or peripheral blood [24]. However, the pediatric literature suggests that this 20% threshold does not apply to ML in patients with DS [25]. Overt leukemia in these children is preceded in 20% to 60% of cases by an indolent prephase of myelodysplasia (MDS), characterized by thrombocytopenia and dysplastic changes in the bone marrow, often with accompanying marrow fibrosis [26,27]. This MDS may last several months or even years before progressing to overt leukemia. In contrast to MDS in non-DS children, which requires stem-cell transplantation for cure, MDS in children with DS shows a highly favorable response to chemotherapy alone [26–28]. Therefore, Hasle and colleagues [25] suggested that all cases of MDS and overt myeloid leukemia in DS, children should be classified as one disease entity, and referred to as "myeloid leukemia of Down syndrome" or ML DS. As this is a unique disease, it should be classified separately from other cases of AML in the WHO-classification.

The presenting characteristics of DS patients with ML differ from those with non-DS AML [14,26,27,29]. In general, patients with ML DS are younger than 5 years of age at diagnosis, have a low diagnostic white blood cell count, and do not show meningeal involvement. Roughly two-thirds of cases are classified as acute megakaryoblastic leukemia (FAB M7), with the other patients being classified as FAB M0, M2, and M6 (see Fig. 2B). Cytogenetic abnormalities, such as t(8;21) or inv(16), which can frequently be found in the blasts of non-DS AML patients, typically do not occur in patients with DS who develop ML. In contrast, somatic mutations of GATA1 are specific for ML DS. Additional copies of chromosome 8 and 21 (in addition to the constitutional trisomy 21) are the most frequently occurring cytogenetic abnormalities, and are found in approximately 10% to 15% each. Cytogenetic findings associated with a high rate of relapse in non-DS AML, such as monosomy 7 and $-5/5q-$ also occur in DS patients (together in approximately 10%–20% of cases), but do not seem to have a negative impact on prognosis, although numbers are small [14,30].

Myeloid leukemia in Down syndrome: treatment outcome

DS children with ML have a superior outcome when compared with children without DS who develop AML. This was first recognized by investigators from the Pediatric Oncology Group (POG) [31], and the Nordic Society for Pediatric Hematology and Oncology (NOPHO) [32]. However, to obtain excellent outcome rates it is crucial that high intensity treatment, which is required for cure of non-DS AML, is avoided, as this results in unacceptable high induction and treatment-related mortality rates in children with DS [14,27,33]. This observation has led to specific treatment guidelines for children with DS who develop ML, mostly with reduced treatment intensity regimens [13,14,29]. Recent results from several collaborative groups confirm the favorable outcome for this patient population. The 10-year overall survival (OS) for 61 patients treated according to the NOPHO between 1984 and 2001 was 74% [29]. Similarly, the 5-year OS for 161 patients treated according to the Children's Cancer Group study CCG 2891 between 1989 and 1999 was 79% [14]. Finally, the 3-year OS for 67 children treated between 1998 and 2003, according to the AML-BFM 98 study, was 91% [13]. Together, these data confirm a fairly favorable outcome for DS patients who develop myeloid leukemia.

Based on the excellent results in the AML-BFM 98 study, a prospective European treatment protocol was recently opened. DS patients with ML will receive the standard BFM chemotherapy regimen, with significant dose-reductions for cytarabine (28 g/m^2 versus 41 g/m^2 –47 g/m^2 for non-DS patients) and anthracyclines (230 mg/m^2 versus 320 mg/m^2–450 mg/m^2 for non-DS patients). Moreover, DS patients will not receive maintenance therapy, nor cranial radiation, nor stem-cell transplantation [13,34]. The COG has chosen a different approach in their 2971A trial, in which several drugs (etoposide and dexamethasone), as well as the 3-month maintenance period, were eliminated from the standard chemotherapy schedule used in the 2891 AML trial. In contrast to the European approach, there are no dose-reductions of the remaining drugs in the COG study, and the cumulative anthracycline and cytarabine dosages will be 320 mg/m^2 and 44 g/m^2, respectively [30]. Preliminary analysis shows outcome data (3-year probability of OS 84%) which are comparable to the CCG 2891 standard timing arm [28].

The potential for reduced treatment intensity is based on the unique hypersensitivity of myeloid leukemia cells of DS patients to chemotherapy, when compared with AML cells from non-DS individuals, as demonstrated by various investigators [35–38]. This increased sensitivity to chemotherapy extends to agents with different mechanisms of action. Zwaan and colleagues [35] have reported that myeloid blasts were significantly more sensitive to cytarabine (median, 12-fold), anthracyclines (2- to 7-fold), mitoxantrone (9-fold), amsacrine (16-fold), etoposide (20-fold), 6-thioguanine (3-fold), busulfan (5-fold) and vincristine (23-fold), than non-DS AML cells. Taub and colleagues have provided evidence for specific mechanisms to explain the observed differences in drug sensitivity, and linked sensitivity to a gene-dosage effect of chromosome 21 localized genes [39,40]. For instance, cytarabine sensitivity may be caused by increased expression levels of the cystathionine-beta-synthase gene, which is located on chromosome 21 [41,42]. Other studies from this group have shown the impact of GATA1s on cytidine deaminase levels and cytarabine sensitivity [43]. However, the fact that enhanced in-vitro sensitivity was described for drugs that exert therapeutic effect by different mechanisms of action may suggest a more general mechanism of enhanced chemotherapy susceptibility, such as a propensity to undergo apoptosis [35]. Interestingly, ALL cells from DS patients do not differ in drug sensitivity when compared with those of patients without constitutional trisomy 21. This further supports the notion that ML in DS is a unique disease, and that sensitivity is cell-lineage specific rather than associated with a gene-dosage effect of genes located on chromosome 21 [35,37].

It is currently unknown to what extent treatment intensity can be reduced in DS children with ML. In a small case series, a 77% overall survival in a selected group of patients (n=18) was reported with a regimen consisting of cytarabine 10 mg/m^2 per dose subcutaneously, twice daily for 7 days every 2 weeks; vincristine 1 mg/m^2 intravenously every 2 weeks; and retinylpalmitate 250,000 units/m^2 per day orally [44]. The NOPHO reported that approximately half of the patients included in their AML-93 protocol had dose-reductions of 75% and 67% of anthracyclines and cytarabine, respectively, which did not influence the relapse rate in those patients [45]. These data suggest that further treatment reduction may be possible, at least in some patients. However, most studies have also reported resistant or relapsed cases of ML DS. Therefore, it would be helpful if investigators could identify subgroups of patients with ML DS, at low risk of resistant or relapsed disease, for whom further dose-reduction of treatment intensity is feasible.

So far, such prognostic subgroups have not been described, and most published series lack the statistical power to identify prognostic factors because of small patient numbers [30]. Gamis and colleagues reported that children older than 4 years of age with ML DS had a poorer outcome than younger children. The older children, however, may have suffered from non-DS AML rather than typical DS associated ML, which occurs almost invariably in children younger than 5 years of age [14,33]. Indeed, Hasle and colleagues [46] have shown that only 2 out of 12 DS children over 4 years of age, with myeloid leukemia, had a GATA1 mutation. Hence, the authors suggest that ML occurring in children with DS may be classified based on GATA1 mutations as its unique molecular genetic basis. Cases lacking this mutation may benefit from treatment according to a protocol developed for non-DS AML, rather than treatment according to the less dose-intensive protocols developed for GATA1-mutation positive ML DS. It is still unclear whether real-time quantitative polymerase chain reaction (PCR) analysis for mutated GATA1 will be able to successfully measure minimal residual disease (MRD) levels, and therefore could be used for further risk stratification of ML in DS patients [47]. The disadvantage of this assay is that it is laborious, given that GATA1 mutations are private. Alternative methods for MRD-detection that could be employed include flowcytometry or reverse transcription-PCR for the Wilms tumor gene WT1 [48].

Acute lymphoblastic leukemia in patients with Down syndrome

In contrast to children with ML DS, children with ALL do not have a superior outcome when compared with their non-DS counterparts [11,12,29,49–52]. Whitlock and colleagues [11], summarizing the CCG data on ALL in patients with DS treated between 1983 and 1995, reported that DS patients stratified to the standard risk ALL arm had a poorer outcome than those who did not have DS, while this difference was not present for those treated according to the high-risk ALL arm. This suggests that DS children with ALL may be under-treated when stratified in a standard risk arm, based on classical National Cancer Institute risk criteria (age 1–9 years and white blood cell count less than or equal to $50 \times 10^9/l$). This was confirmed in the CCG 1952 study, which enrolled patients between 1996 and 2000 [12]. Another possible explanation for this observation could be that physicians may have dose-reduced DS children with ALL in fear of enhanced toxicity (see later in this article). This may also have contributed to the observed higher relapse rate in these reports, although details on dose intensity were not provided. In the BFM 2000 study, which used MRD-based stratification using T-cell receptor and immunoglobulin gene rearrangements, there were no significant differences between DS and non-DS ALL patients in MRD-based risk-group assignment, nor in day-15 marrow response or in antileukemic efficacy between DS and non-DS ALL [50]. However, there was an increased rate of toxic deaths in the DS patients. At 5-years of follow-up, probability for event free survival was equivalent with 82% (standard error 5%) for DS children and 82% (standard error 1%) for non-DS children.

Despite a similar distribution over MRD-subgroups in the BFM study, there are clear biologic differences between DS and non-DS ALL cases [12]. When considering favorable prognostic factors, the frequency of hyperdiploid (more than 50 chromosomes) ALL is lower in DS patients [11,12,29,49,50]. The prognostically favorable trisomies, such as trisomy of chromosome 4, 10, and 17, are considerably less frequent in DS patients with ALL [12]. Several [12,50,53], but not all [54] investigators report a lower frequency of TEL-AML1 rearranged ALL in children with DS. Considering the unfavorable prognostic factors, there are neither cases of infant ALL with DS, nor CD10-negative pro-B ALL cases, while the frequency of T-cell ALL is lower in children with DS. In addition, unfavorable cytogenetic abnormalities, such as t(1;19), the Philadelphia chromosome, or MLL-gene rearrangements occur less frequently in DS ALL [11,12,29,51], although this was not confirmed by all groups [50]. It needs to be stressed however, that the definitions for favorable and unfavorable characteristics in all these studies were based on ALL in non-DS patients. It is unknown whether these abnormalities have the same impact in the context of constitutional trisomy 21.

Similar to ML treatment, an optimal balance between antileukemic efficacy and treatment-related toxicity needs to be established for children with DS and ALL, who lack the typical enhanced chemotherapy sensitivity that characterizes the myeloid blasts in DS patients. There are two studies describing in vitro cellular drug resistance profiles of ALL lymphoblasts in DS, and both studies did not report enhanced sensitivity of DS lymphoblasts when compared with non-DS lymphoblasts [35,37]. However, the data in these studies were not corrected for the differences in genetic make-up of DS and non-DS ALL, and therefore need to be interpreted with caution. Dördelmann and colleagues [49] reported a tendency for ALL to have a better initial steroid response in DS patients. However this was not confirmed in the BFM 2000 study, which showed a nonsignificant difference of 5.8% nonresponders in non-DS ALL, and 3.2% in DS ALL cases [50].

Increased risk for toxicity in children with Down syndrome

In children with DS, there is a delicate balance between the antileukemic efficacy of intensive chemotherapy and the increased toxic morbidity and mortality rates with which chemotherapy in these vulnerable children is associated [12–14,29,30]. Given the enhanced sensitivity of myeloid leukemic cells in these patients, dose-reductions in ML regimens for DS patients are easier accepted than for ALL regimens. For instance, in the CCG 2891 AML study, excessive toxicity resulted in poor prognosis and subsequent exclusion of children with ML and DS from the intensively timed induction regimen and stem cell transplantation [14]. Moreover, the excellent results of study AML BFM-98 were in part achieved by a significant reduction of induction mortality (the early death rate in the AML-BFM 93 study was 11%, in the subsequent AML-BFM 98-study, 0%) [13]. Similarly, in the ALL 2000 study, children with DS experienced life-threatening adverse events in 23% of subjects, versus 6% in non-DS children [50]. The main side effects include mucositis, and an increased susceptibility to infections [14,30,50,55,56]. Mucositis is mainly associated with high-dose methotrexate (MTX), and probably caused by altered MTX pharmacokinetics in children with DS [55]. It needs to be mentioned, however, that many of these studies only comprised small numbers of patients, and were performed in an era preceding modern supportive care with well-established leucovorin rescue regimens. In addition, the reduced folate carrier (RFC), which is responsible for MTX transport into the cell, is localized on chromosome 21, and may be involved in an enhanced sensitivity for MTX, including gastrointestinal toxicity, although RFC transcript levels were not increased in the DS myeloblasts that were studied by Taub and colleagues [39,41]. Unfortunately, a consensus regarding MTX-dosing in children with DS and ALL is currently lacking.

An important aspect in treating children with DS is whether they have an increased risk of long-term cardiotoxicity following anthracycline exposure, given the fact that a significant proportion of DS children may have a compromised cardiac function because of congenital abnormalities to begin with. O'Brien and colleagues report on 57 DS patients treated on POG 9421, of whom 33% had a structural cardiac abnormality at inclusion [57,58]. One patient with an uncorrected tetralogy of Fallot died early because of a cardiac event as a consequence of fatal hypoxia during septicemia. Of the 54 patients in first complete remission, one patient with an atrioventricular canal was taken off study for congestive heart failure (CHF), and another patient died from CHF. At later follow-up, 21% of patients had documented CHF, requiring diuretics or inotropes. The cumulative anthracycline dose in this study was 135 mg/m^2 of daunorubicin and 80 mg/m^2 of mitoxantrone (cumulative dose of 535 mg/m^2 daunorubicin equivalents when assuming a ratio of 1:5). Creutzig and colleagues [59] describe the cardiotoxicity in DS patients (n=121) treated according to protocol AML BFM 93 and -98, and report early cardiac toxicity in 4% and late cardiac toxicity in 5% of the subjects. In this study, there was no increased cardiotoxicity in DS children, but these children were treated with reduced dosages of anthracyclines (approximately 200 mg/m^2 –300 mg/m^2 daunorubicin dose equivalents).

GATA1 mutations

GATA1 is a double zinc finger DNA-binding transcription factor that has a critical role in promoting specification and terminal maturation of myeloid progenitor cells to red cells and megakaryocytes, that has been conserved through evolution [60]. Acquired mutations in the hemopoietic transcription factor GATA1 in ML DS were initially described by Wechsler and colleagues [61], and subsequently by a number of groups. Three studies have studied the function of N-terminal region of GATA1 in murine megakaryopoiesis [6,62,63]. Expression of the mutated GATA1 protein GATA1s in embryonic and fetal megakaryocyte progenitors results in excessive megakaryocyte proliferation, and to a lesser extent abnormal differentiation of megakaryocytes into platelets [6,62,63].

GATA1 mutations occur both in TL and ML in DS, as well as in blood and fetal liver samples from DS neonates [64–71]. GATA1 mutations are disease specific, as they are not detectable in remission samples. As GATA1 is encoded on the X-chromosome, the mutant clone expresses only the mutant allele in both males and females (because of X-inactivation). Over 100 different somatic genomic GATA1 mutations have been reported, which uniformly result in the expression of the amino-terminal truncated mutated GATA1 protein GATA1s (Fig. 3). Reports of newborns with multiple oligoclonal GATA1 mutations suggest that GATA1 mutations are a frequent event in hematopoietic cells of DS children [69]. Given the high frequency of GATA1 mutations in fetal blood cells trisomic for chromosome 21, and the fact that DS children are not prone to cancer in general, it has been suggested that GATA1 mutations impart a selective advantage, rather than trisomy 21 being a mutator phenotype [69]. The mutations occur principally in the 5' end of the gene, in exon 2, and less commonly in exon 3. Most are small insertions, duplications, deletions, or point mutations, though rare cases of large deletions have been reported. Given this, most mutations can be detected by PCR amplification of GATA1 exons 2 and 3, followed by direct sequencing or analysis by direct high pressure liquid chromatography (DHPLC). The ability to detect mutations depends on the proportion of mutant cells in the sample. In general, for direct sequencing, approximately 20% of the sample has to contain mutant cells. The sensitivity of DHPLC is higher, at approximately 2% to 5%. Once a mutation has been identified, mutation-specific probes and primers for mutation detection by real-time PCR can be designed that allow for more sensitive detection of mutant cells, which may be indicted for MRD detection [47].

Expression profile analysis of GATA1s and the full-length GATA1-expressing murine fetal megakaryocytes showed that GATA1s fails to repress a number of transcription factor genes (GATA2, Ikaros, MYB and MYC), that have a proproliferative effect on hemopoietic cell growth [6,63].

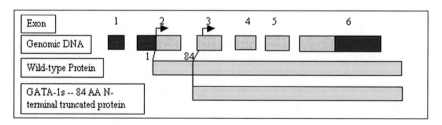

Fig. 3. Mutations in GATA1 in ML DS and TL. The GATA1 gene is composed of six exons with noncoding (blue) and coding (brown) regions. Two translational start sites (*arrows*) are present, one in exon 2, the other in exon 3. Protein translated from the second ATG, GATA1s, lacks the first 84 amino acids. Mutations in TL and ML DS are principally in exons 2 and 3 and introduce stop codons in the first 84 amino acids, or abrogate splicing of exon 2 to 3.

Cooperating genetic events involved in progression from transient leukemia to myeloid leukemia of Down syndrome

AML is hypothesized to result from at least two types of cooperating genetic events, including growth promoting mutations (referred to as type 1 genetic aberrations) in, for example, receptor tyrosine kinases (such as FLT3 or KIT) or the RAS-oncogene, as well as translocations—such as t(8;21) or t(15;17)—that mainly impair differentiation (type 2 abnormalities) [72]. In agreement with this hypothesis, recent studies have shown that GATA1s is insufficient to induce leukemia without other cooperating events [6,73].

Little is known about the proliferation-enhancing type 1 mutations that are frequently encountered in non-DS AMLs, and their role in TL and ML DS. However, several articles have recently reported a potential role for mutations in the gene encoding for the non-receptor tyrosine kinase family of Janus kinases, (ie, JAK2 and JAK3) [74–79]. These mutations were first identified in cell-lines using a proteomic approach [77,79]. So far, JAK2 gene mutations have not been found in the 38 primary samples from children with DS and TL or ML studied to date [75,78]. JAK3 mutations, however, were found in 13 out of 68 (19%) samples studied, suggesting a role in TL and ML in DS [74–78]. Given the fact that mutations were detected both in TL and ML DS, it is suggested that they are not sufficient for disease progression. Moreover, their contribution to DS malignancies still needs to be proven. No mutations in the gene encoding for well-known tyrosine kinases involved in non-DS AML, such as FLT3 or KIT, the RAS oncogene, or the gene encoding for the thrombopoietin receptor c-MPL were identified in any TL or ML samples from DS patients [75,76,78].

Expression profiles from whole bone marrow or peripheral blood samples obtained from DS patients with ML showed that they have a quite distinct expression signature from other myeloid malignancies, including increased expression of GATA2, MYC (as in the mouse studies above), KIT and GATA1 itself [80]. Moreover, the chromosome 21 encoded transcription factor BACH1, which has been implicated as a repressor of megakaryocyte differentiation, was overexpressed, as well as SON, a gene with homology to the MYC family [80]. In contrast, expression of the chromosome 21 encoded transcription factor RUNX1, the most commonly mutated gene in non-DS AML, was reduced. This is an intriguing finding, as in most human AML cases reduced RUNX1 function is leukemogenic. ETS2 and ERG were not differentially expressed, despite their localization on chromosome 21. These genes are involved in megakaryocytic differentiation, and ERG-overexpression can frequently be found in AML cells from non-DS individuals, in particular in normal karyotype AML [81,82]. Whether ERG contributes to the development of TL awaits further study [83].

These findings suggest a complex network of deregulated expression of key genes controlling the cell fate of megakaryocyte-erythroid lineage cells. A major caveat in attributing an oncogenic effect to these deregulated genes is that these gene expression profiles are not compared with relevant nonmalignant cell populations. Thus, it is impossible to assess if the observed gene expression profiles reflect the arrested differentiation of the leukemic cell population or in fact contribute to leukemogenesis.

Summary

Constitutional trisomy 21 results in an enhanced risk of developing leukemias, both ALL as well as ML DS. TL and ML DS offer a unique model to obtain insight into the stepwise progression of leukemia, and of gene dosage effects mediated by aneuploidy. TL arises from expanded fetal liver progenitors as a result of constitutional trisomy 21, providing a window of opportunity for the occurrence of acquired mutations in the hematopoietic transcription factor GATA1. Many questions, however, remain unanswered. These include the true frequency of TL among infants with DS, the events involved in the subsequent development of ML in 20% of children diagnosed with TL, and the mechanisms underlying the spontaneous remission of TL. From a clinical point of view, studies assessing whether timely initiated cytarabine treatment may reduce the number of children dying early from TL-related complications (such as effusions, hydrops, or liver fibrosis), and whether the subsequent development of ML can be prevented by treating TL, are underway. Specific treatment protocols for children with ML DS have been designed, and show that treatment can safely be reduced, probably related to the unique hypersensitivity to chemotherapy of ML blasts in children with DS. Prospective studies need to identify to which extent and for which subgroups treatment can be further reduced, without an increase in recurrent disease. Recent attention has focused on ALL in patients with DS, which may be biologically distinct from non-DS ALL. ALL in DS is not characterized by increased sensitivity to chemotherapy. Given the enhanced sensitivity of DS children to the side effects of intensive chemotherapy, the development of new treatment modalities that confer less toxic side effects needs to be prioritized, and the recent discovery of mutations in JAK3 may be an example of a leukemia-specific target. Meanwhile, investigators will have to carefully assess the balance between the antileukemic efficacy and treatment-related mortality of current chemotherapy regimens. Several studies are currently in progress that will answer some of the questions raised above.

References

[1] Greaves M. In utero origins of childhood leukaemia. Early Hum Dev 2005;81(1):123–9.
[2] Roizen NJ, Patterson D. Down's syndrome. Lancet 2003;361(9365):1281–9.
[3] Krivit W, Good RA. The simultaneous occurrence of leukemia and mongolism; report of four cases. AMA J Dis Child 1956;91(3):218–22.
[4] Hasle H, Clemmensen IH, Mikkelsen M. Risks of leukaemia and solid tumours in individuals with Down's syndrome. Lancet 2000;355:165–9.
[5] Hitzler JK, Zipursky A. Origins of leukaemia in children with Down syndrome. Nat Rev Cancer 2005;5(1):11–20.

[6] Li Z, Godinho FJ, Klusmann JH, et al. Developmental stage-selective effect of somatically mutated leukemogenic transcription factor GATA1. Nat Genet 2005;37(6):613–9.

[7] Massey GV, Zipursky A, Chang MN, et al. A prospective study of the natural history of transient leukemia (TL) in neonates with Down syndrome (DS): a Children's Oncology Group (COG) study POG-9481. Blood 2006;107:4606–13.

[8] Al Kasim F, Doyle JJ, Massey GV, et al. Incidence and treatment of potentially lethal diseases in transient leukemia of Down syndrome: Pediatric Oncology Group Study. J Pediatr Hematol Oncol 2002;24(1):9–13.

[9] Vyas P, Roberts I. Down myeloid disorders: a paradigm for childhood preleukaemia and leukaemia and insights into normal megakaryopoiesis. Early Hum Dev 2006;82(12):767–73.

[10] Vyas P, Crispino JD. Molecular insights into Down syndrome-associated leukemia. Curr Opin Pediatr 2007;19(1):9–14.

[11] Whitlock JA, Sather HN, Gaynon P, et al. Clinical characteristics and outcome of children with down syndrome and acute lymphoblastic leukemia: a Children's Cancer Group study. Blood 2005;106:4043–9.

[12] Bassal M, La MK, Whitlock JA, et al. Lymphoblast biology and outcome among children with Down syndrome and ALL treated on CCG-1952. Pediatr Blood Cancer 2005;44: 21–8.

[13] Creutzig U, Reinhardt D, Diekamp S, et al. AML patients with Down syndrome have a high cure rate with AML-BFM therapy with reduced dose intensity. Leukemia 2005;19(8):1355–60.

[14] Gamis AS, Woods WG, Alonzo TA, et al. Increased age at diagnosis has a significantly negative effect on outcome in children with Down syndrome and acute myeloid leukemia: a report from the Children's Cancer Group Study 2891. J Clin Oncol 2003;21(18):3415–22.

[15] Tunstall-Pedoe O, De la Fuente J, Bennet PR. Trisomy 21 expands the megakaryocyte-erytroid progenitor compartment in human fetal liver—implications for Down syndrome AMKL [abstract]. Blood 2006;108(11):170a.

[16] Henry E, Walker D, Wiedmeier SE, et al. Hematological abnormalities during the first week of life among neonates with Down syndrome: data from a multihospital healthcare system. Am J Med Genet A 2007;143(1):42–50.

[17] Widness JA, Pueschel SM, Pezzullo JC, et al. Elevated erythropoietin levels in cord blood of newborns with Down's syndrome. Biol Neonate 1994;66(1):50–5.

[18] Kivivuori SM, Rajantie J, Siimes MA. Peripheral blood cell counts in infants with Down's syndrome. Clin Genet 1996;49(1):15–9.

[19] De Hingh YC, Van der Vossen PW, Gemen EF, et al. Intrinsic abnormalities of lymphocyte counts in children with Down syndrome. J Pediatr 2005;147(6):744–7.

[20] Weijerman ME, Van Furth AM, Vonk-Noordegraaf A, et al. Prevalence, neonatal characteristics and first year mortality of Down syndrome: a national study. J Pediatr, in press.

[21] Pine SR, Guo Q, Yin C, et al. Incidence and clinical implications of GATA1 mutations in newborns with Down syndrome. Blood 2007;110(6):2128–31.

[22] Heald B, Hilden JM, Zbuk K, et al. Severe TMD/AMKL with GATA1 mutation in a stillborn fetus with Down syndrome. Nat Clin Pract Oncol 2007;4(7):433–8.

[23] Muramatsu H, Watanabe N, Matsumoto K, et al. A retrospective analysis of 70 cases of transient leukemia in neonates with Down syndrome [abstract]. Blood 2006;108(11):301b.

[24] Vardiman JW, Harris NL, Brunning RD. The World Health Organization (WHO) classification of the myeloid neoplasms. Blood 2002;100(7):2292–302.

[25] Hasle H, Niemeyer CM, Chessells JM, et al. A pediatric approach to the WHO classification of myelodysplastic and myeloproliferative diseases. Leukemia 2003;17(2):277–82.

[26] Creutzig U, Ritter J, Vormoor J, et al. Myelodysplasia and acute myelogenous leukemia in Down's syndrome. A report of 40 children of the AML-BFM Study Group. Leukemia 1996; 10(11):1677–86.

[27] Lange BJ, Kobrinsky N, Barnard DR, et al. Distinctive demography, biology, and outcome of acute myeloid leukemia and myelodysplastic syndrome in children with Down syndrome: Children's Cancer Group Studies 2861 and 2891. Blood 1998;91(2):608–15.

[28] Gamis AS, Alonzo T, Hiden JM, et al. Outcome of Down syndrome children with acute myeloid leukemia (AML) or myelodysplasia (MDS) treated with a uniform prospective trial—initial report of the COG trial A2971 [abstract]. Blood 2006;108(11):9a.

[29] Zeller B, Gustafsson G, Forestier E, et al. Acute leukaemia in children with Down syndrome: a population-based Nordic study. Br J Haematol 2005;128(6):797–804.

[30] Gamis AS. Acute myeloid leukemia and Down syndrome evolution of modern therapy—state of the art review. Pediatr Blood Cancer 2005;44(1):13–20.

[31] Ravindranath Y, Abella E, Krischer JP, et al. Acute myeloid leukemia (AML) in Down's syndrome is highly responsive to chemotherapy: experience on Pediatric Oncology Group AML Study 8498. Blood 1992;80(9):2210–4.

[32] Lie SO, Jonmundsson G, Mellander L, et al. A population-based study of 272 children with acute myeloid leukaemia treated on two consecutive protocols with different intensity: best outcome in girls, infants, and children with Down's syndrome. Nordic Society of Paediatric Haematology and Oncology (NOPHO). Br J Haematol 1996;94(1):82–8.

[33] Ravindranath Y. Down syndrome and acute myeloid leukemia: the paradox of increased risk for leukemia and heightened sensitivity to chemotherapy. J Clin Oncol 2003;21(18): 3385–7.

[34] Creutzig U, Zimmermann M, Lehrnbecher T, et al. Less toxicity by optimizing chemotherapy, but not by addition of granulocyte colony-stimulating factor in children and adolescents with acute myeloid leukemia: results of AML-BFM 98. J Clin Oncol 2006;24(27):4499–506.

[35] Zwaan CM, Kaspers GJL, Pieters R, et al. Different drug sensitivity profiles of acute myeloid and lymphoblastic leukemia and normal peripheral blood mononuclear cells, in children with and without Down syndrome. Blood 2002;99:245–51.

[36] Taub JW, Stout ML, Buck SA, et al. Myeloblasts from Down syndrome children with acute myeloid leukemia have increased in vitro sensitivity to cytosine arabinoside and daunorubicin. Leukemia 1997;11(9):1594–5.

[37] Frost BM, Gustafsson G, Larsson R, et al. Cellular cytotoxic drug sensitivity in children with acute leukemia and Down's syndrome: an explanation to differences in clinical outcome? [letter] Leukemia 2000;14(5):943–4.

[38] Yamada S, Hongo T, Okada S, et al. Distinctive multidrug sensitivity and outcome of acute erythroblastic and megakaryoblastic leukemia in children with Down syndrome. Int J Hematol 2001;74(4):428–36.

[39] Taub JW, Ge Y. Down syndrome, drug metabolism and chromosome 21. Pediatr Blood Cancer 2005;44(1):33–9.

[40] Taub JW, Matherly LH, Stout ML, et al. Enhanced metabolism of 1-beta-D-arabinofuranosylcytosine in Down syndrome cells: a contributing factor to the superior event free survival of Down syndrome children with acute myeloid leukemia. Blood 1996;87(8):3395–403.

[41] Taub JW, Huang X, Matherly LH, et al. Expression of chromosome 21-localized genes in acute myeloid leukemia: differences between Down syndrome and non-Down syndrome blast cells and relationship to in vitro sensitivity to cytosine arabinoside and daunorubicin. Blood 1999;94(4):1393–400.

[42] Taub JW, Huang X, Ge Y, et al. Cystathionine-beta-synthase cDNA transfection alters the sensitivity and metabolism of 1-beta-D-arabinofuranosylcytosine in CCRF-CEM leukemia cells in vitro and in vivo: a model of leukemia in Down syndrome. Cancer Res 2000;60(22):6421–6.

[43] Ge Y, Jensen TL, Stout ML, et al. The role of cytidine deaminase and GATA1 mutations in the increased cytosine arabinoside sensitivity of Down syndrome myeloblasts and leukemia cell lines. Cancer Res 2004;64(2):728–35.

[44] Al Ahmari A, Shah N, Sung L, et al. Long-term results of an ultra low-dose cytarabine-based regimen for the treatment of acute megakaryoblastic leukaemia in children with Down syndrome. Br J Haematol 2006;133(6):646–8.

[45] Abildgaard L, Ellebaek E, Gustafsson G, et al. Optimal treatment intensity in children with Down syndrome and myeloid leukaemia: data from 56 children treated on NOPHO-AML protocols and a review of the literature. Ann Hematol 2006;85(5):275–80.

[46] Hasle H, Niemeyer C, O'Marcaigh A, et al. Myeloid leukemia in children 4 years or older with Down syndrome. A BFM, DCOG, MRC, NOPHO collaborative study. [abstract]. Presented at the 5th Bi-annual Symposium on Childhood Leukemia. Noordwijkerhout, the Netherlands, April 30–May 2, 2006.

[47] Pine SR, Guo Q, Yin C, et al. GATA1 as a new target to detect minimal residual disease in both transient leukemia and megakaryoblastic leukemia of Down syndrome. Leuk Res 2005; 29(11):1353–6.

[48] Hasle H, Lund B, Nyvold CG, et al. WT1 gene expression in children with Down syndrome and transient myeloproliferative disorder. Leuk Res 2006;30(5):543–6.

[49] Dördelmann M, Schrappe M, Reiter A, et al. Down's syndrome in childhood acute lymphoblastic leukemia: clinical characteristics and treatment outcome in four consecutive BFM trials. Berlin-Frankfurt-Münster Group. Leukemia 1998;12(5):645–51.

[50] Möricke A, Zimmermann M, Schwarz C, et al. Excellent event-free survival despite higher incidence of treatment related toxicity and mortality in Down syndrome patients with ALL as compared to patients without Down syndrome: data from the ALL-BFM 2000 trial [abstract]. Presented at the 5th Bi-annual Symposium on Childhood Leukemia. Noordwijkerhout, the Netherlands, April 30–May 2, 2006.

[51] Pui CH, Raimondi SC, Borowitz MJ, et al. Immunophenotypes and karyotypes of leukemic cells in children with Down syndrome and acute lymphoblastic leukemia. J Clin Oncol 1993; 11(7):1361–7.

[52] Chessells JM, Harrison CJ, Kempski H, et al. Clinical features, cytogenetics and outcome in acute lymphoblastic and myeloid leukaemia of infancy: report from the MRC Childhood Leukaemia Working Party. Leukemia 2002;16(5):776–84.

[53] Lanza C, Volpe G, Basso G, et al. The common TEL/AML1 rearrangement does not represent a frequent event in acute lymphoblastic leukaemia occuring in children with Down syndrome. Leukemia 1997;11(6):820–1.

[54] Steiner M, Attarbaschi A, Konig M, et al. Equal frequency of TEL/AML1 rearrangements in children with acute lymphoblastic leukemia with and without Down syndrome. Pediatr Hematol Oncol 2005;22(3):229–34.

[55] Garré ML, Relling MV, Kalwinsky D, et al. Pharmacokinetics and toxicity of methotrexate in children with Down syndrome and acute lymphocytic leukemia. J Pediatr 1987;111(4):606–12.

[56] Whitlock JA. Down syndrome and acute lymphoblastic leukaemia. Br J Haematol 2006; 135(5):595–602.

[57] Becton D, Dahl GV, Ravindranath Y, et al. Randomized use of Cyclosporin A (CSA) to modulate P-glycoprotein in children with AML in remission: Pediatric Oncology Group study 9421. Blood 2006;107:1315–24.

[58] O'Brien M, Taub J, Stine K, et al. Excessive cardiotxocity despite excellent leukemia-free survival for pediatric patients with Down syndrome and acute myeloid leukemia: results from POG (Pediatric Oncology Group) protocol 9421 [abstract]. Blood 2006;108(11):168a–9a.

[59] Creutzig U, Diekamp S, Zimmermann M, et al. Longitudinal evaluation of early and late anthracycline cardiotoxicity in children with AML. Pediatr Blood Cancer 2007;48(7):651–62.

[60] Cantor AB. GATA transcription factors in hematologic disease. Int J Hematol 2005;81(5): 378–84.

[61] Wechsler J, Greene M, McDevitt MA, et al. Acquired mutations in GATA1 in the megakaryoblastic leukemia of Down syndrome. Nat Genet 2002;32(1):148–52.

[62] Kuhl C, Atzberger A, Iborra F, et al. GATA1-mediated megakaryocyte differentiation and growth control can be uncoupled and mapped to different domains in GATA1. Mol Cell Biol 2005;25(19):8592–606.

[63] Muntean AG, Crispino JD. Differential requirements for the activation domain and FOG-interaction surface of GATA-1 in megakaryocyte gene expression and development. Blood 2005;106(4):1223–31.

[64] Hitzler JK, Cheung J, Li Y, et al. GATA1 mutations in transient leukemia and acute megakaryoblastic leukemia of Down syndrome. Blood 2003;101(11):4301–4.

[65] Mundschau G, Gurbuxani S, Gamis AS, et al. Mutagenesis of GATA1 is an initiating event in Down syndrome leukemogenesis. Blood 2003;101(11):4298–300.

[66] Rainis L, Bercovich D, Strehl S, et al. Mutations in exon 2 of GATA1 are early events in megakaryocytic malignancies associated with trisomy 21. Blood 2003;102:981–6.

[67] Groet J, McElwaine S, Spinelli M, et al. Acquired mutations in GATA1 in neonates with Down's syndrome with transient myeloid disorder. Lancet 2003;361(9369):1617–20.

[68] Xu G, Nagano M, Kanezaki R, et al. Frequent mutations in the GATA-1 gene in the transient myeloproliferative disorder of Down syndrome. Blood 2003;102(8):2960–8.

[69] Ahmed M, Sternberg A, Hall G, et al. Natural history of GATA1 mutations in Down syndrome. Blood 2004;103(7):2480–9.

[70] Shimada A, Xu G, Toki T, et al. Fetal origin of the GATA1 mutation in identical twins with transient myeloproliferative disorder and acute megakaryoblastic leukemia accompanying Down syndrome [letter]. Blood 2004;103(1):366.

[71] Taub JW, Mundschau G, Ge Y, et al. Prenatal origin of GATA1 mutations may be an initiating step in the development of megakaryocytic leukemia in Down syndrome. Blood 2004; 104(5):1588–9.

[72] Deguchi K, Gilliland DG. Cooperativity between mutations in tyrosine kinases and in hematopoietic transcription factors in AML. Leukemia 2002;16(4):740–4.

[73] Hollanda LM, Lima CS, Cunha AF, et al. An inherited mutation leading to production of only the short isoform of GATA-1 is associated with impaired erythropoiesis. Nat Genet 2006;38(7):807–12.

[74] De Vita S, Mulligan C, McElwaine S, et al. Loss-of-function JAK3 mutations in TMD and AMKL of Down syndrome. Br J Haematol 2007;137(4):337–41.

[75] Klusmann JH, Reinhardt D, Hasle H, et al. Janus kinase mutations in the development of acute megakaryoblastic leukemia in children with and without Down's syndrome. Leukemia 2007;21(7):1584–7.

[76] Kiyoi H, Yamaji S, Kojima S, et al. JAK3 mutations occur in acute megakaryoblastic leukemia both in Down syndrome children and non-Down syndrome adults. Leukemia 2007; 21(3):574–6.

[77] Walters DK, Mercher T, Gu TL, et al. Activating alleles of JAK3 in acute megakaryoblastic leukemia. Cancer Cell 2006;10(1):65–75.

[78] Norton A, Fisher C, Liu H, et al. Analysis of JAK3, JAK2, and C-MPL mutations in transient myeloproliferative disorder and myeloid leukemia of Down syndrome blasts in children with Down syndrome. Blood 2007;110(3):1077–9.

[79] Mercher T, Wernig G, Moore SA, et al. JAK2T875N is a novel activating mutation that results in myeloproliferative disease with features of megakaryoblastic leukemia in a murine bone marrow transplantation model. Blood 2006;108(8):2770–9.

[80] Bourquin JP, Subramanian A, Langebrake C, et al. Identification of distinct molecular phenotypes in acute megakaryoblastic leukemia by gene expression profiling. Proc Natl Acad Sci USA 2006;103:3339–44.

[81] Marcucci G, Baldus CD, Ruppert AS, et al. Overexpression of the ETS-related gene, ERG, predicts a worse outcome in acute myeloid leukemia with normal karyotype: a Cancer and Leukemia Group B study. J Clin Oncol 2005;23(36):9234–42.

[82] Rainis L, Toki T, Pimanda JE, et al. The proto-oncogene ERG in megakaryoblastic leukemias. Cancer Res 2005;65(17):7596–602.

[83] Izraeli S, Rainis L, Hertzberg L, et al. Trisomy of chromosome 21 in leukemogenesis. Blood Cells Mol Dis 2007;39(2):156–9.

Indications and Donor Selections for Allogeneic Stem Cell Transplantation in Children with Hematologic Malignancies

Rupert Handgretinger, MD[a],*,
Joanne Kurtzberg, MD[b], R. Maarten Egeler, MD, PhD[c]

[a]*Department of Hematology/Oncology and General Pediatrics,
Children's University Hospital, Hoppe-Seyler-Strasse 1, 72076 Tuebingen, Germany*
[b]*Pediatric Bone Marrow and Stem Cell Transplant Program,
Duke University Medical Center, Box 3350 Durham, NC 27710, USA*
[c]*Department of Pediatrics, Leiden University Medical Center,
Albinusdreef 2, 2300 RC Leiden, the Netherlands*

Acute lymphoblastic leukemia

Pediatric acute lymphoblastic leukemia (ALL) is the most common malignant disease in childhood. International studies of childhood ALL, in developed countries between 1986 and 1998, have achieved 5-year event-free (EFS) survival rates, ranging from 63% to 83% [1] or even higher [2]. However, despite these impressive improvements in therapy and survival of patients with ALL, there are still a significant number of patients who will experience a relapse after initial treatment. Stem cell transplantation (SCT) may be the only curative approach in these patients. The goal of most therapeutic ALL studies is to identify patients at risk of relapse as early as possible during initial treatment, and then proceed with intensified chemotherapy. Subgroups of these patients with high-risk features of relapse will proceed to an allogeneic SCT while in first complete remission (CR1).

Although the strategy described above helps decrease the incidence of relapse after first-line therapy, a considerable number of children will still relapse. Relapsed ALL is the fourth most common malignant disease of childhood, with a higher incidence than many newly diagnosed pediatric malignancies [3].

---

* Corresponding author.
E-mail address: rupert.handgretinger@med.uni-tuebingen.de (R. Handgretinger).

0031-3955/08/$ - see front matter © 2008 Elsevier Inc. All rights reserved.
doi:10.1016/j.pcl.2007.10.013

Various treatment strategies for patients with relapsed ALL are under study, including intensified chemotherapy and SCT. Because outcomes of SCT are best if performed in CR1 or second complete remission (CR2), the best strategy would be to identify patients in CR2 who would best benefit from allogeneic SCT, and in whom the risks of the procedure are justified.

Patients in third complete remission (CR3) and beyond have an extremely poor prognosis with conventional therapy alone, and can only be cured with SCT. However, the success of SCT in these patients with more advanced disease is not as favorable when compared with patients with earlier stage disease. This article discusses the indications for SCT in patients with ALL in CR1, CR2, and beyond.

Indications for stem cell transplantation in patients with high-risk features of acute lymphoblastic leukemia in first complete remission

The identification of patients at risk of relapse after CR1 is one of the major goals in most therapeutic studies. Patients identified with high-risk features require additional therapy after achieving CR1. High-risk features include the presence of chromosomal translocations such as t(4;11) or 11q23 (MLL)[4], Philadelphia chromosome t (9;22), hypodiploidy (fewer than 44 chromosomes) [5,6], and poor response to induction, such as induction failure (5% or more leukemic cells) or the presence of minimal residual disease (MRD) of more than 1% after 4 to 6 weeks of first-line therapy. Early clearance of blasts, as measured by morphology [7] or by flow cytometry [8], seems to be an important favorable prognostic factor. Once patients have been identified as being at high risk of relapse in CR1, optimal treatment might include an allogeneic SCT in CR1.

A recent study collecting data from 10 study groups of patients with Philadelphia chromosome-positive ALL, showed that SCT in CR1 with bone marrow from human leukocyte antigen (HLA)-matched related donors was associated with a significantly better outcome than with chemotherapy alone [9].

In another prospective study conducted in seven countries, the outcome of patients with very high risk ALL in CR1 was investigated. Subjects were either allocated to chemotherapy alone or chemotherapy followed by SCT, depending on the availability of a compatible related donor [10]. High risk features were defined by the presence of at least one of the following criteria: (1) failure to achieve complete remission after the first four-drug induction phase, (2) the presence of t(9;22) or t(4;11) clonal abnormalities, and (3) poor response to prednisone associated with T-immunophenotype, white blood count of greater than 100 times 10^9/L, or both. The 5-year disease-free survival was 40.6% in children allocated to chemotherapy only, and 56.7% in those assigned to SCT ($P = .02$). In another study, the role of SCT versus chemotherapy alone was investigated in high-risk T-cell leukemia [11]. Very high-risk features were consistent with the presence T-cell immunophenotype and a poor in vivo response to initial treatment (prednisone-poor response or nonresponse at day 33). The 5-year disease-free survival was 67% for 36 subjects who received SCT in CR1, and 42% for the 120 subjects treated with chemotherapy alone. The overall survival at 5 years was 67% for the SCT group and 47% for subjects receiving chemotherapy alone ($P = .01$). The Children's Cancer Study group (CCG-1921) investigated the role of SCT from HLA-matched family donors in patients with ultra-high risk features of ALL in CR1 [12]. Twenty-nine patients proceeded to SCT. The 5-year EFS was 58.6% for all patients, and 77.8% for patients without cytogenetic abnormalities. Patients with Philadelphia chromosome-positive ALL had a 5-year EFS of 66.7%.

Because the role of allogeneic SCT in patients with high-risk features in ALL is not yet clearly defined, the Berlin-Frankfurt-Münster (BFM) study group, the International BFM (IBFM) study group, and the Pediatric Disease Working Party of the European Group for Blood and Marrow Transplantation (EBMT) (PD-WP-EBMT) initiated a multicenter prospective trial enrolling patients with ALL in first, second, or subsequent remission, with a high risk of relapse as defined by cytogenetics, the response to the induction chemotherapy, and the time and site of relapse, respectively [13]. In addition, the levels of MRD at certain time points of the first-line therapy are used for risk stratification. In Table 1, the indications and type of transplants in patients with high risk ALL and CR1 according to the BFM criteria are shown. While all patients with the depicted high-risk features will receive a transplant from an available HLA-matched sibling donor, only subgroups of high-risk patients will proceed to an allogeneic

Table 1
List of indications for allogeneic stem cell transplantation in acute lymphoblastic leukemia in first complete remission according to the Berlin-Frankfurt-Munster criteria

Indication	Criteria	MSD	MD	MMD
Poor prednisone response	t(9;22)	+	+	+
	t(4;11)	+	+	−
	Pro-B-ALL	+	−	−
	M3 marrow d15	+	−	−
	WBC ≥ 10 000	+	−	−
Good prednisone response	t(9;22)	+	+	−
	t(4;11)	+	−	−
MRD level	R2 ≥ 10^{-2}	+	+	+
	R2 = 10^{-3}	+	+	−
Remission	NR d + 33	+	+	+

Abbreviations: MD, matched donor; MMD, mismatched donor; MSD, matched sibling donor; R2 MRD level at time point 2 of induction; WBC, white blood cell count; + recommended; − not recommended.

Data from Peters C, Schrauder A, Schrappe M, et al. Allogeneic haematopoietic stem cell transplantation in children with acute lymphoblastic leukaemia: the BFM/IBFM/EBMT concepts. Bone Marrow Transplant 2005;35 (Suppl 1):S9–11.

SCT from an HLA-matched unrelated donor or an HLA-mismatched donor. The results of this study will hopefully help to better define the role of allogeneic SCT in patients with high risk ALL in CR1.

Indications for stem cell transplantation in patients with relapsed acute lymphoblastic leukemia, second complete remission and beyond

The most common reason for treatment failure in children with ALL is relapse. Although the disease-free survival with conventional chemotherapy has increased considerably over the decades [2,14], approximately 20% to 25% of children suffer a relapse following initial therapy. Relapsed ALL is as common as most pediatric tumors and more common than newly diagnosed acute myeloid leukemia (AML) [15]. In a retrospective analysis of the outcome of 505 patients with relapsed ALL in a single institution, 74% of the relapses occurred within 3 years from diagnosis, and most relapses involved the bone marrow alone or in combination with overt extramedullary involvement [16]. Early relapse, that is, relapse within 3 years after initial diagnosis, was more common in children with T-lineage ALL and in those with unfavorable cytogenetics. The German BFM relapse score (standard, intermediate, and high risk), which takes into account the time of relapse, site of relapse, and subsequent immunophenotype [17], was applied to these patients and was highly predictive of outcome. A retrospective comparison between patients treated with SCT and those that received chemotherapy only showed no difference in EFS for those assigned to the intermediate-risk group, but a possible advantage in the highest risk group [16].

A retrospective analysis of the United Kingdom ALL R2 protocol analyzed 150 children, of whom 139 achieved a CR2. Using the BFM risk score, the overall survival (OS) and EFS for standard, intermediate, and high-risk groups was 92% and 92%, 64% and 51%, and 14% and 15%, respectively [18]. In this study, children with a very early (ie, within 18 months after initial diagnosis) isolated extramedullary relapse were at higher risk for subsequent relapse.

In another study, the long-term outcome in children with relapsed ALL after risk-stratified salvage therapy was analyzed [19]. Of 207 registered patients, 183 were stratified into three groups: (A) early bone marrow relapse (relapse occurring on therapy or up to 6 months after cessation of front-line treatment), (B) late bone marrow relapse, and (C) isolated extra-medullary relapse. The probability of EFS and OS of all registered patients at 15 years was 0.30 and 0.37, respectively. The differences of the probability of EFS between the groups were 0.18 and 0.20 for group A, 0.44 and 0.52 for group B, and 0.35 and 0.42 for group C. In a uni- and multivariate analysis, an early time point of relapse and T-lineage imunophenotype were significant predictors of inferior EFS.

The St. Jude group reported the clinical outcome of 106 children who developed a bone marrow recurrence as the first event after contemporary intensified therapy [20]. Bone marrow relapses were isolated in 79 patients, and combined with extramedullary sites in 27 patients. The 5-year survival among all patients was 24.2%. On multivariate analysis, time to first disease recurrence and blast cell lineage were found to be independent predictors of a second EFS. The 5-year EFS estimate in patients with an initial disease remission of greater than or equal to 36 months was 42.6%, and only 12.5% for children with a short duration of remission (less than 36 months).

In a nonrandomized retrospective analysis, the outcome of patients with B-precursor ALL in CR2 was analyzed. Outcome was compared in 188 patients enrolled in chemotherapy trials and 186 HLA-matched sibling transplants [21]. For children with early first relapse (less than 36 months after diagnosis), the risk of a second relapse was significantly lower after a total body irradiation (TBI)-containing conditioning regimen than after chemotherapy regimens. In contrast, for children with late relapse (greater than or equal to 36 months after diagnosis), the risk of second relapse was similar after TBI-containing SCT and chemotherapy alone. These data support HLA-matched sibling SCT, using a TBI-containing preparative regimen in children with early relapse and those in CR2 or beyond.

In a Children's Oncology Group study (CCG-1941), the outcome for children with early first bone marrow relapse (within 12 months after completion of primary therapy) after matched sibling SCT, alternative donor bone marrow transplantation (BMT), and chemotherapy alone was compared [22]. In this study, 214 subjects received multiagent induction therapy, and 163 subjects with fewer than 25% marrow blasts and count recovery at the end of induction (CR2) were allocated by donor availability. Fifty subjects with sibling donors proceeded to SCT, and 72 subjects were randomly assigned to alternative donor SCT or chemotherapy, while 41 subjects refused allocation. The 3-year EFS from study entry was 19%. Thirty-two of the 50 subjects with a matched sibling donor and 19 of 37 subjects allocated to alternative donor SCT proceeded to SCT in CR2, with a 3-year disease-free survival (DFS) of 42% and 29%, respectively. The 3-year DFS for subjects allocated to matched sibling, alternative donor SCT, and chemotherapy was 29%, 21%, and 27%, respectively. More than half of the subjects died, failed reinduction, or relapsed again before 3 months after achieving CR2, which was the median time to BMT. Therefore, these investigators concluded that SCT is indisputably life-saving for some children, but not the whole answer to curing patients with ALL and early marrow relapse.

In a retrospective matched-pair analysis of the BFM-relapse group, matched unrelated SCT was compared with chemotherapy alone in patients with ALL in second remission and without an HLA-matched family donor [17]. Altogether, 81 pairs could be matched exactly for site of relapse and immunophenotype, and as closely as possible for duration of first remission, age, diagnosis date, and peripheral blast count at relapse. No significant difference in the probability of EFS between SCT and chemotherapy was seen in 28 pairs with an intermediate risk (0.39 versus 0.49, $P = .105$), whereas the probability of the EFS was significantly different in the 53 pairs of the high-risk group, with an EFS of 0.44 for the SCT group and 0.00 for the chemotherapy-alone group. In another study, the impact of allogeneic SCT was investigated in 117 subjects who experienced relapse from ALL. CR2 was attained in 90 subjects, and 30 are in remission with an EFS of 25.1% [23]. The significant prognostic factors in a multivariate analysis were time of relapse and the treatment after relapse. Subjects proceeding to SCT had an EFS of 60.2%, as compared with 25.7% in the subjects receiving chemotherapy alone.

The outcome of children with very late relapse of ALL was investigated in patients who relapsed greater than or equal to 60 months after attainment of CR1 [24]. In this study, 93 children had a first relapse at a median time of 6.1 years (range 5.8–13.7 years) after initial diagnosis. After a median follow-up, the 5-year EFS and OS was 39.5% and 55.6%, respectively. In a multivariate analysis, the site of relapse was the only significant predictor of duration of the CR2, as patients with isolated bone marrow relapse fared worse (5-year EFS 24.5%) than those with combined or isolated extrame-dullary relapse (5-year EFS 68.4%). All of the seven children who received SCT from a matched-related donor following a late relapse are alive in CR2. SCT should therefore be considered for subgroups of patients.

Another prognostic feature in patients with relapsed ALL is their MRD status after initiation of relapse chemotherapy. In a retrospective study of 30 children, all of whom were treated according to the relapsed ALL BFM trials, the MRD status during the first stages of treatment was monitored [25]. In subjects with MRD less than 10^{-3} at day 36, the probability of event-free survival was 0.86 (or 86%), whereas none of the patients with MRD of greater than or equal to 10^{-3} survived. In another study, similar results were obtained in 41 subjects using flow cytometry techniques for determination of MRD levels at the end of remission reinduction [26]. Thirty-five subjects were in morphologic remission. Of these 35 subjects, 19 had MRD greater than or equal to 0.01% with a 2-year cumulative incidence of second relapse of 70.2%, whereas it was only 27.9% for subjects with negative MRD. The time of relapse and MRD status were the only two significant predictors of outcome in a multivariate analysis.

To decide which patients in CR2 would benefit most from SCT, the BFM study group, IBFM study group, and the PD-WP-EBMT initiated a prospective cooperative multicenter trial to better define risk groups according to time to relapse, site of relapse, immunophenotype, and MRD status [13]. In this study, patients with relapsed ALL are subdivided into risk groups according to the parameters mentioned above. High-risk group patients (early isolated or very early isolated combined bone marrow relapse of a B-cell precursor ALL, and any bone marrow involving relapse of a T-lineage ALL) will proceed to a transplant with any allogeneic donor. Intermediate-risk patients (early or late combined bone marrow relapse, late isolated bone marrow relapse of B-cell precursor ALL) and patients with a MRD level greater than or equal to 10^{-3} will proceed to a matched sibling or matched unrelated donor SCT, and patients with intermediate-risk features and MRD less than 10^{-3} will receive SCT only if a matched sibling donor is available (Table 2).

The MRD status before SCT has also been shown an important prognostic factor for assessing which patients might be at risk of relapse after SCT. Patients with high MRD burden before transplant had a significant poorer outcome when compared with MRD-negative subgroups [27–30]. These data were challenged by another study, which found no correlation between the pretransplant MRD burden and the posttransplant relapse [31]. In a more recent study, detectable levels of MRD before SCT predicted an extremely poor prognosis because of the high rate of relapses in the MRD-positive group [32]. Further prospective studies will hopefully lead to better use of MRD detection for risk-adapted stratification and treatment.

Patients with CR3 and beyond have a very high risk for subsequent relapse with chemotherapy alone, and allogeneic SCT from any donor source might offer the only chance of cure.

The role of allogeneic SCT in infant ALL is controversial. Most infants have rearrangements of the MLL gene on chromosome 11q23, which is associated with a poor outcome [33]. SCT with matched sibling donors does not seem to improve the prognosis for this patient group [34]. Clinical studies are needed to further evaluate innovative strategies in this disease [35].

Acute myeloid leukemia

As in ALL, the prognosis of childhood AML has improved over the decades [36]. With current aggressive induction chemotherapy protocols, approximately 80% to 90% of children with AML achieve remission and

Table 2
Indication for allogeneic stem cell transplantation according to Berlin-Frankfurt-Munster criteria for patients after first relapse

Risk status	Donor selection		
High risk T-lineage: any BM involvement	MSD	MD	MMD
BCP-ALL: very early BM involving relapse, early isolated BM relapse ($>$ CR 2: according to risk for TRM)	MSD	MD	MMD
Intermediate-risk, MRD $\geq 10^{-3}$ after 2nd induction BCP-ALL: early combined BM MSD relapse, late BM involving relapse (all t(9;22) with IR feature)	MSD	MD	
Intermediate-risk, MRD $< 10^{-3}$ after 2nd induction BCP-ALL: early combined BM relapse	MSD		

Groups are defined by immunophenotype, site of relapse and time point of relapse (very early, $<$ 18 months after primary diagnosis; early, $\geq$ 18 months after primary diagnosis and $<$ 6 months of cessation of front-line therapy; late, $\geq$ 6 months after cessation of front-line therapy).

Abbreviations: BCP, B-cell precurser; BM, bone marrow; IR feature, intermediate risk feature; TRM, transplant-related mortality.

Data from Peters C, Schrauder A, Schrappe M, et al. Allogeneic haematopoietic stem cell transplantation in children with acute lymphoblastic leukaemia: the BFM/IBFM/EBMT concepts. Bone Marrow Transplant 2005;35 (Suppl 1):S9–11.

nearly 50% remain in remission and are long-term survivors [37,38]. Given the improvements of survival with chemotherapy alone, the role of SCT—especially in patients in CR1—has not yet been clearly defined by prospective randomized trials. The survival of patients with relapsed AML in CR2 or beyond and patients with refractory AML is poor, and allogeneic SCT is for most patients the only change for long-term cure.

Indications for stem cell transplantation in patients with acute myeloid leukemia in first complete remission

The best therapy for patients with AML in first remission remains controversial. The definition of risk factors for subsequent therapy failure might help to decide which patients should proceed to SCT in CR1. Patients with AML associated with the t(8;21), t(15;17), or inv(16) have a favorable prognosis, whereas those with complex karyotypes, such as -5, del(5q), -7, or 3q abnormalities might benefit from SCT [39]. Hyperleucocytosis indicates a high risk, especially for early failure. Multivariate analysis showed a high correlation of hyperleucocytosis with other parameters, such as blast cell count greater than or equal to 5% in the bone marrow on day 15 of induction chemotherapy [40]. Favorable or low-risk groups can be defined by morphologic and response criteria or cytogenetic and molecular findings. Morphology includes French-American-British (FAB) subtypes with granulocytic differentiation (FAB M1 to M4) and additional features, such as Auer rods or eosinophils with a blast cell reduction in the bone marrow at day 15 [40]. Favourable cytogenetic features [41] correlate with the FAB types M1 and M2 with Auer rods, M3, and M4eo [40,42,43].

While the North American study groups seem to favor SCT from a matched related family donor (MSD-SCT) in all patients in CR1 [44], European groups take a more conservative approach, and MSD-SCT is limited in some European studies to patients at high risk of relapse [45]. The North Americans derive their preference from results obtained in studies that compared allogeneic with autologous SCT [36,46–49]. Because these studies all show fewer relapses in the allogeneic groups, this approach is supported in the United States and Canada. Moreover, studies have shown a role for graft-versus-leukemia in the maintenance of disease-free survival in AML patients [50].

In a large analysis of the postremission outcome of 1,464 children under 21 years old, enrolled between 1979 and 1996 in five consecutive Children's Cancer Group AML trials, 373 children were allocated to SCT in CR1 if a matched family donor was available [51]. The remaining children were assigned to chemotherapy (n = 688), autologous purged SCT (n = 217), withdrawn from the study without assignment, or had unknown data (n = 186). The overall and disease-free survival was superior for children assigned to allogeneic SCT. In this analysis, a high diagnostic white blood cell (WBC) count (greater than 50,000 $\times$ 10^9/l) was prognostic for inferior outcome, whereas the FAB subtypes were not. Benefit from allogeneic SCT was evident in most children, including those with high or low diagnostic WBC count, each FAB subtype, and the presence of t(8;21). The benefit was not seen in patients with inv(16). Because the North American studies have demonstrated that the best relapse-free and OS for pediatric patients with AML is achieved in those receiving family donor SCT, MSD-SCT is routinely performed in patients in CR1, except for patients with inv(16).

The reasoning for the more conservative European approach is that several cooperative groups, including the Medical Research Council and BFM, have shown that patients with good-risk AML can be effectively treated with chemotherapy alone, and that SCT can therefore be reserved for patients who relapse [45,52]. While most of the European study groups recommend SCT from a matched family donor in patients with high-risk AML in CR1, the German cooperative AML-BFM study group has completely abandoned SCT in CR1 following their 2006 amendment, independent of the risk features and even if a matched family donor is available (Ursula Creutzig, MD, Hannover, Germany, personal communication, August 2007). In the current AML-BFM trial, allogeneic SCT is reserved for patients with de-novo refractory AML (persistent blasts after second induction or continuous aplasia after 6 weeks after second induction).

One of the main reasons leading the German investigators to abandon SCT in all patients with AML in CR1, besides long-term effects, is the high treatment-related mortality (TRM) associated with this approach. However, similar to the more aggressive chemotherapeutic regimens, the improved supportive care of patients undergoing SCT and the optimization of conditioning regimens, has significantly decreased TRM in matched sibling, matched unrelated, and even in haploidentical transplantation [53]. The enormous advances in the field of allogeneic SCT with a decrease of TRM, improved prevention and treatment of graft-versus-host disease (GVHD), and increase of overall survival must be taken into account, and the benefit might outweigh the reduced risk with better supportive care.

A low TRM of 6% was reported in a recent study in children receiving allogeneic transplantation from a matched sibling donor for acute leukemia [54]. In this study, 55 subjects with AML in CR1 received allogeneic SCT. The 5-year OS was 74%. Relapse was not seen in subjects with AML developing acute GVHD, thus corroborating the previously published graft-versus-leukemia affect in AML. In a recent update of the Children's Cancer group (CCG 2891), the clinical outcome of those patients with no available HLA-matched family donor was reported. Patients were randomized to receive either an autologous SCT or consolidation chemotherapy [55]. DFS, relapse-free-survival, and OS at 8 years were 47%, 50%, and 55%, respectively, thus confirming previous studies that autologous SCT might be an effective post remission therapy for patients with AML in first remission.

The definition of patients at risk of relapse will remain a major goal for future research, and it remains to be seen whether, similar to patients with ALL, the determination of minimal residual disease and MRD-directed therapy will improve the outcome of patients with AML [56]. Further clinical prospective and ideally randomized trials in patients with AML in CR1 will be necessary to define the best therapy for these patients.

Indications for stem cell transplantation in patients with acute myeloid leukemia in second complete remission and beyond

While with contemporary treatment, 80% to 90% of patients achieve remission, 30% to 40% of these patients subsequently suffer recurrence. After recurrence, the likelihood of survival is poor, ranging from 21% to 33% [57–61]. In these studies, the length of first remission was the best predictor of survival.

Allogeneic SCT in CR2 is associated with improved outcome after relapse. The survival of 64 children undergoing SCT as part of their relapse therapy was 62% [62]. In another retrospective analysis, the outcome in 58 children with advanced AML after allogeneic SCT was analyzed. At time of SCT, 12 children were in CR2, 11 in untreated first relapse, and 35 had refractory disease. Estimates of 5-year DFS for patients in CR2, untreated first relapse, and refractory disease were 58%, 36%, and 9%, respectively [63]. In this analysis, advanced disease phase and cytogenetic abnormalities at time of transplantation were each associated with decreased EFS and increased risk of relapse. The survival of children transplanted in CR2 or untreated first relapse in this study was higher than previously reported [64]. In another study, survival for 25 patients who relapsed after autologous SCT (n = 11) or allogeneic SCT (n = 14) was analyzed in patients who then underwent a second allogeneic SCT from either a matched related, mismatched related, or unrelated donor [65]. Patients who received their second transplant less than or equal to 6 months after the first transplantation were at higher risk of relapse. The disease-free survival at 10 years was 44%.

Outcome of patients with relapsed AML has been shown to be dependent on the length of initial remission, and those patients with CR1 longer than 12 months had a better survival than patients with CR1 less than 12 months [59]. In contrast to patients in CR1, there is less controversy over the indication for SCT in patients with AML in CR2 or with refractory disease (less than 20% bone marrow blasts). In patients with a short CR1, SCT is the only chance for long-term cure.

Myelodysplastic syndromes

The prognosis of most children with a myelodysplastic syndrome (MDS) is poor. SCT is currently the therapy of choice for most of these patients. MDS can be divided into refractory cytopenia, high-grade MDS, and secondary MDS.

Stem cell transplantation in patients with refractory cytopenias

Patients with lesser risk of life-threatening complications secondary to cytopenias, or lesser risk of progression to leukemia, will respond best to allogeneic transplantation [66]. This group includes patients with refractory anemia, refractory anemia with ringed sideroblasts, and those with normal cytogenetics. In the patients with refractory cytopenia, the karyotype is the most important factor for progression to high grade MDS and survival. Patients with trisomy 8 or chromosomal abnormalities other than monosomy 7 may experience a longer stable course of the disease [67]. Patients with monosomy 7, 7q-, or complex karyotypes should proceed to SCT as soon as the diagnosis has been established and a donor has been identified. In patients with all other karyotypes, an absolute neutrophil count (ANC) greater than 1,000/μl, and no need for transfusions, a watch-and-wait strategy can be adopted. In patients with a karyotype other than monosomy 7 and in the absence of complex karyotype abnormalities, who have an ANC less than 1,000/μl, or those that are transfusion-dependent, SCT from a matched related or unrelated donor is indicated. More recently, immunosuppressive therapy in selected patients, with hypoplastic refractory cytopenia and normal karyotype or trisomy 8, has been shown to induce complete or partial remissions [68].

The role of conditioning, that is, myeloablative versus reduced-intensity conditioning (RIC), still needs to be established in clinical trials. In a pilot trial of the European Working Group (EWOG) study, 19 patients with hypocellular refractory cytopenia and normal karyotypes were transplanted from a matched (n = 14) or mismatched (n = 5) unrelated donor using a RIC regimen consisting of thiotepa, fludarabine, and antithymocyte globuline. The Kaplan-Meier estimate for EFS and OS at 3 years was 74% and 84%, respectively [69].

High-grade myelodysplastic syndrome

MDS with increased blast counts comprises the MDS subtype refractory anemia with excess blasts (RAEB) and refractory anemia with excess blasts in transformation (RAEB-t). The distinction between high-grade MDS and de novo AML is difficult and important, because de novo AML is chemosensitive, while MDS is resistant to chemotherapy. Patients with cytogenetic abnormalities normally associated with AML should be treated as de novo AML independent of the blast count [70]. Myelodysplasia-related AML (MDR-AML) is associated with MDS progressing to disease, with bone marrow blasts greater than 30%. It is currently not clear whether MDS with monosomy 7 and progression to MDR-AML is biologically the same as de novo AML with monosomy 7. Patients diagnosed with AML and monosomy 7 have a poorer outcome when compared with patients with AML without monosomy 7 [71–73].

There is no controversy at all that allogeneic SCT is the treatment of choice for patients with high-grade MDS. The children who will most likely benefit from SCT are those with RAEB, RAEB-t, an age younger than 2 years, and a hemoglobin F level of 10% or higher [74,75]. Because of the rarity of these diseases in children, international studies by cooperative groups, such as the EWOG of MDS in Childhood, are required to find out the best treatment strategies.

There is controversy, however, whether or not intensive chemotherapy before SCT should routinely be performed. Patients with RAEB-t might have a high relapse rate if transplanted without preceding chemotherapy, whereas those with less than 5% blasts do better with SCT performed in the absence of induction chemotherapy [76,77]. A large prospective study of children with MDS found that patients with RAEB-t often do as well as those with AML when treated with AML therapy at diagnosis, including SCT when an HLA-matched sibling is available [72]. On the other hand, children with refractory anemia or RAEB do very poorly with standard AML therapy, and should be considered for SCT without preceding chemotherapy [78,79].

Juvenile myelomonocytic leukemia

The optimal treatment for juvenile myelomonocytic leukemia (JMML) is not clearly established, but there are no drugs known to be curative in the absence of SCT. Pretransplant therapy might be useful to control tumor burden [80]. Other approaches, such as isoretinoin, have shown nonconclusive results [81,82]. In a recent European Working Group MDS/EBMT trial, intensive chemotherapy before SCT had no influence on the outcome [83]. The survival of patients with JMML is very poor without SCT [84], and SCT offers the greatest likelihood for cure [80,84–86]. In the analysis of the EWOG-MDS/EBMT trial of 100 patients with JMML, the 5-year EFS was 52%, and there was no difference in the EFS of patients receiving a transplant from a matched related or matched unrelated donor [83]. In this study, age greater than 4 years and female sex predicted a poorer outcome, whereas cytogenetic abnormalities were not associated with a worse prognosis. Another study reported that monosomy 7 was associated with an outcome comparable to or even better that of patients with normal karyotypes [87].

The role of GVHD on the rate of relapse is not clear. One study showed that chronic GVHD was associated with a lower risk of relapse and better survival, and acute GVHD (greater than or equal to grade III) with a poor survival [88]. The success of SCT is limited primarily by the tendency of this disease to relapse, generally within the first year after transplant [89]. Therefore, additional posttransplant interventions, such as alpha-interferon, biologic differentiation agents, such as retinoic acids or farnesyltransferase inhibitors, are under investigation [90]. Following relapse, a substantial number of patients might still be cured by a second SCT [91].

Therapy-related myelodysplastic syndrome and acute myeloid leukemia

Therapy-related MDS (t-MDS) and AML (t-AML) are defined as clonal malignant disorders that arise after exposure to cytoxic agents. While many of the clinical and biologic features of t-MDS and t-AML are similar to those of de novo disorders, patients with t-MDS and t-AML often have a rapidly progressive disease, and their neoplastic clones usually have distinct chromosomal abnormalities [92]. Most likely as a result of the high frequency of poor prognostic factors, including unfavorable cytogenetic abnormalities characteristic of secondary disorders, chemotherapy yields fewer and shorter complete remissions [93]. Patients with favorable karyotypes, such as the t(8;21), inv(16) or t(15;17) translocations might be treated as any other case of de novo AML [92]. SCT seems to be a potential curative treatment, especially for patients who lack poor-risk cytogenetic features [94], and might be the only curative option for a small number of patients with primary refractory disease [95]. However, outcome in these children is negatively impacted by high TRM rates [96].

Chronic myeloid leukemia

Allogeneic transplantation from an MSD or matched unrelated donor offers long-term disease-free survival in patients with chronic phase, and is the only proven curative approach [97]. The survival in children after SCT ranges from 70% to 80% with matched related donors to 40% to 60% with unrelated donors [98–101]. A shorter time between diagnosis and transplantation resulted in a better outcome [102]. One study comparing the use of peripheral blood SCT with bone marrow as a stem cell source found the former method to have a significant survival advantage (1,000-day overall survival of 94% versus 66%) [103]. Conversely, a retrospective analysis by the Center for International Blood and Marrow Transplant Research (CIBMTR) showed a significantly poorer EFS for children transplanted with peripheral blood precursor cells, as compared with bone marrow [104]. In children, a 3-year OS of 65% after matched unrelated donor transplants with a myeloablative conditioning regimen has been described [98]. In this study, however, 55% of the matched unrelated donor transplants were performed 1 year after diagnosis and were associated with a higher TRM (31% in chronic phase 1 and 46% in advanced phase). Relapse rates were higher in advanced phase patients, especially after MSD transplants. The outcomes for patients in advanced phase were 3-year OS of 46% for MSD, and 39% for matched unrelated donor transplants. In an early pediatric study, the 12-year OS for patients transplanted within 3 years of diagnosis with MSD and matched unrelated donors was 62% [105]. In all of these studies, TRM has limited the success rate, especially after SCT from unrelated donors. In a study including pediatric patients, however, it was indicated that comparable survival after related and unrelated SCT can be obtained [106].

The use of RIC conditioning regimens and the known sensitivity of chronic myelogenous leukemia (CML) to immunologic approaches, like donor lymphocyte infusions, might decrease TRM and long-term side effects of SCT [107] and increase long-term survival [108,109]. However, the efficacy of RIC needs to be confirmed in larger pediatric studies comparing RIC and myeloablative approaches.

There is no broad consensus on the use of imatinib mesylate as front-line therapy in children with CML [110]. While imatinib might be chosen as primary therapy to bridge the time until a suitable donor has been identified, it should be kept in mind that the delay of transplant more than 1 year after diagnosis was associated in the pre-imatinib era with a higher TRM, especially after SCT from unrelated donors. It must be anticipated that patients treated with imatinib and not proceeding to transplant before developing accelerated phase or blast phase, will have a poor outcome with transplant [111]. Because the goal of therapy in children is cure rather than palliation, all new nontransplant approaches must aim for long-term cure. The risk of the gradual emergence of resistance in patients continuing imatinib [112] should be kept in mind when abandoning SCT, and only carefully planned, controlled clinical studies comparing these different approaches should be performed, especially when the transplantation is delayed beyond 1 year after diagnosis.

Together, the information available suggests that pediatric patients with chronic phase 1 or advanced phase, who have an MSD or a matched unrelated donor, should proceed to an allogeneic SCT after initial therapy with imatinib.

Preparative regimens

The most commonly used preparative regimes before allogeneic transplantation for leukemia include various doses (12 gray–15.75 gray) of fractionated total-body irradiation (TBI) and cyclophosphamide or melphalan, with or without the addition of etoposide, cytarabine, thiotepa, or fludarabine. Non-TBI-based regimens with busulfan or cyclophosphamide, with or without additional cytotoxic drugs such as melphalan, etoposide, thiotepa, and fludarabine, are also used, but no conclusive studies to support either TBI- or non-TBI-based regimens have been reported for children. The preparative regimen should have a cytotoxic antileukemic effect, but should also provide adequate immunosuppression to ensure engraftment. Other non-TBI-based myeloablative regimens based on melphalan, fludarabine, and thiotepa have been reported to facilitate safe engraftment in three-loci mismatched haploidentical transplants with low TRM [53]. For patients with ALL, the use of TBI-containing regimens was associated with better survival, compared with busulfan-containing regimens [113,114]. From these data, TBI-based regimens should be recommended for preparative regimens in patients with ALL undergoing matched sibling or matched unrelated donor transplantation.

Less aggressive so-called nonmyeloablative SCT regimens are attracting increasing interest, especially for patients who otherwise cannot tolerate a conventional myeloablative regimen. Such regimens range from minimal, to facilitate engraftment (fludarabine plus low-dose TBI) [115], to more intensive but still not myeloablative (reduced intensity conditioning), such as reduced doses of fludarabine plus busulfan [116]. The rationale behind nonmyeloablative stem cell transplantation is to induce an optimal graft-versus-leukemia effect by donor-alloreactive effector cells [117]. While this form of transplantation is mostly applied in adult and elderly patients, the data in children with leukemia remains insufficient to conclude that the reduced cytotoxic antileukemic effect of the preparative regimen is counter-balanced by an increased antileukemic effect of the allograft. Furthermore, children have a healthier immune system and a greater capacity to reject grafts in the setting of reduced intensity conditioning; hence, these regimens should be used only in the context of controlled clinical trials.

Donor selection for stem cell transplantation

There are several types of allogeneic donors for SCT in children. These include related or unrelated donors, cells from bone marrow, umbilical cord blood or mobilized peripheral blood, unmanipulated or T-cell depleted, or CD34 or CD133 selected grafts. Donor selection is influenced by donor availability, the size and age of the patient, and the underlying diagnosis and risk for relapse.

In case of the rather unlikely availability of more than one HLA-matched related donor, additional selection criteria will include the donor's cytomeg-alovirus (CMV) status (negative preferred), donor age (younger preferred), and donor health or social issues. If more than one adult unrelated donor is available, the age of the donor (younger), donor sex (male preferred), and donor CMV status (negative preferred) are factored into the selection of the optimal donor.

The most important selection factor in donor selection is HLA matching. Identification of an HLA-matched donor at the DNA level is prioritized. DNA typing for HLA antigens has identified disparities between patients and serologically matched donors [118], and high resolution HLA matching at one or more alleles is associated with decreased mortality after SCT from unrelated donors [119]. While the role of high resolution matching at HLA-A, HLA-B, and HLA-DRB1 is clearly established, the significance of the other loci, including HLA-C, HLA-DQ, HLA-DRB3 and DRB5, and HLA-DPB1 is less clear and under current investigation. It has been shown that HLA-C mismatching is associated with increased rejection and strong adverse effects on transplantation outcome [120].

Some transplant centers consider 6 out of 6 matched (A, B, DR) donor-recipient pair a match, others require 8 out of 8 (A, B, C, DR), whereas the majority of centers would consider a 10 out of 10 (HLA-A, -B, -C, -DRB1, and -DQB1) recipient-donor pair as best match for adult donors [121–123]. For most centers, a single allele-mismatch (9 out of 10) would be acceptable.

A low mortality was reported in children after SCT from 7 out of 10 or 8 out of 10 HLA allele-matched unrelated donors with the use of antithymocyte globulin [124]. Therefore, the decision to proceed with a mismatch unrelated transplant needs to be made in the context of the experience of the preparative regimens, the use of in vivo or in vitro T-cell depletion strategies, GVHD prophylaxis regimens, the probability to identify a better matched donor within a reasonable time, and the availability of alternative transplant strategies. If there are more than one HLA-matched donor, other non-HLA donor characteristics have to be taken into account, such as CMV status, donor age, donor gender, parity for female donors, and ABO blood group.

In a large retrospective analysis, the influence of various donor characteristics on the overall and disease-free survival was analyzed [125]. In this analysis, age was the only donor trait significantly associated with overall and disease-free survival. The 5-year overall survival rates for recipients were 33%, 29%, and 25%, respectively, with donors aged 18 to 30 years, 31 to 45 years, and more than 45 years ($P = .0002$). A similar effect was observed among HLA-mismatched cases. Patients with older donors had a higher incidence of acute GVHD, and recipients with female donors who had undergone multiple pregnancies had a higher rate of chronic GVHD. Therefore, the use of younger, male donors may lower the incidence of GVHD and improve survival. In this analysis, the donor serologic CMV status did not affect the survival of either seropositive or seronegative recipients, and a race mismatch also did not affect the outcome. Other studies have demonstrated a distinct survival advantage when the donor is CMV seronegative [126,127]. If there is a choice among several matched donors, a CMV-negative donor would be preferred for a CMV-negative patient. The most optimal donor would be a young male who shares he same blood type with the patient and is HLA-matched at 10 out of 10 loci.

With the higher degree of HLA-matching of unrelated donors and improved supportive care strategies, the differences in the outcome between matched sibling donors and matched unrelated donors have become small, and comparable outcomes after unrelated and HLA-matched sibling SCTs have been reported [128,129].

Despite the availability of matched sibling donor or a 10 out of 10 allele-matched unrelated donor, transplant-related complications, especially GVHD, can still be observed, and further research will be necessary to determine factors that influence the outcome after transplantation. Such factors might be minor histocompatiblity antigens [130], genetic single nucleotide polymorphisms within the promoter regulatory regions of non-HLA encoded genes, such as those for cytokines and cytokines receptors [131,132], or killer immunoglobulin-like receptor polymorphisms of the donors [133]. Additional research will be necessary to determine the influence of these factors on the overall outcome after allogeneic SCT.

Given the improvements of HLA typing and matching, and the further evaluation of the role on non-HLA donor characteristics, it is questionable whether it is beneficial to a patient to proceed to SCT only if an HLA-matched sibling is available, and not to proceed to allogeneic transplant even if a 10 out of 10 allele-matched donor would be available. In fact, the incidence of posttransplant leukemic relapse might be lower in patients undergoing unrelated donor transplantation, as compared with those transplanted with matched siblings. The promising outcome after matched unrelated donor SCT does not support such an approach, and further clinical studies are needed to demonstrate whether transplantations from matched sibling donors can continue to be considered as the gold standard superior to all other transplant approaches.

The time to identify an HLA-matched unrelated donor negatively influences the outcome. Because of the lack of prospective "intend-to-transplant" studies, the number of patients progressing and succumbing from disease during donor search is not clear, but up to 50% of the patients might progress during donor search before transplantation [134]. Therefore, this factor has to be taken into account in each individual patient for whom a donor search is initiated. Probability estimates to identify a 10 out of 10 allele-matched donor might be helpful to decide the best treatment strategy for patients [135], so that alternative strategies can be planned. The chance of survival in patients who are at high risk for rapid progression might be better if they proceed with a lesser matched unrelated donor transplant or with an alternative transplant strategy, such as matched or mismatched umbilical cord blood (UCB) or haploidentical SCT before disease progression.

Alternative transplantations: umbilical cord blood and haploidentical transplantation

A distinct advantage of unrelated donor UCB or haploidentical related donors is their rapid availability. Promising results have been reported with matched and mismatched unrelated UCB transplants from a single donor [136], or from two partially HLA-matched donors [137]. Important predictors of success after UCB transplant are the number of cells in the UCB graft and the degree of HLA disparity [138]. In a recent pediatric study, patients who received a cell dose of less than 3 times 10^7/kg had a much lower survival when compared with patients who received more than 3 times 10^7/kg [139]. Other studies have also reported promising results in children [140,141], and transplantation with UCB might be a reasonable option for children lacking a matched related donor. A recent review of outcomes data reported to the CIBMTR showed a hierarchy of success, with the best survival in recipients of fully matched (6 out of 6) UCB donors. Outcomes using 5 out of 6 matched UCB donors were equivalent to those with matched bone marrow [136].

Initial experiences with haploidentical transplantation using bone marrow and less effective T-cell depletion methods resulted in a higher rate of GVHD [142]. However, newer, more efficient methods for T-cell depletion, using CD34+ positive selection from mobilized peripheral stem cells, has allowed for successful haploidentical transplantation without GVHD in adults [143] and children [144], with comparable outcomes as compared with matched unrelated donor transplantation [145]. More recent developed T-cell depletion techniques and the use of less intensive conditioning regimens were associated with a very low TRM and improved immune reconstitution [53]. Because of the further availability of haploidentical donors posttransplant, adoptive transfer of additional cells, such as stem cell boosts [146], virus-specific T-cells [147], or natural killer [35,148] cells can be systematically investigated in clinical protocols.

For each patient, an individual risk-benefit analysis based on the disease status, the risk of progression, patient age and the likelihood to identify an HLA-suitable donor within a reasonable time (less than or equal to 3–4 months) has to be performed to determine the best treatment options. With the inclusion of matched or partially matched UCBs and haploidentical donors into the donor pool, almost every child with a high-risk hematologic malignancy should be able to find a suitable donor and can proceed to an allogeneic transplantation, if the benefit outweighs the risk.

References

[1] Pui CH, Campana D, Evans WE. Childhood acute lymphoblastic leukaemia—current status and future perspectives. Lancet Oncol 2001;2:597–607.

[2] Pui CH, Evans WE. Treatment of acute lymphoblastic leukemia. N Engl J Med 2006;354: 166–78.

[3] Gaynon PS, Qu RP, Chappell RJ, et al. Survival after relapse in childhood acute lymphoblastic leukemia: impact of site and time to first relapse—the Children's Cancer Group Experience. Cancer 1998;82:1387–95.

[4] Johansson B, Moorman AV, Haas OA, et al. Hematologic malignancies with t(4;11) (q21;q23)—a cytogenetic, morphologic, immunophenotypic and clinical study of 183 cases. European 11q23 Workshop participants. Leukemia 1998;12:779–87.

[5] Heerema NA, Nachman JB, Sather HN, et al. Hypodiploidy with less than 45 chromosomes confers adverse risk in childhood acute lymphoblastic leukemia: a report from the Children's Cancer Group. Blood 1999;94:4036–45.

[6] Nachman JB, Heerema NA, Sather H, et al. Outcome of treatment in children with hypodiploid acute lymphoblastic leukemia. Blood 2007;110:1112–5.

[7] Sandlund JT, Harrison PL, Rivera G, et al. Persistence of lymphoblasts in bone marrow on day 15 and days 22 to 25 of remission induction predicts a dismal treatment outcome in children with acute lymphoblastic leukemia. Blood 2002;100:43–7.

[8] Coustan-Smith E, Sancho J, Behm FG, et al. Prognostic importance of measuring early clearance of leukemic cells by flow cytometry in childhood acute lymphoblastic leukemia. Blood 2002;100:52–8.

[9] Arico M, Valsecchi MG, Camitta B, et al. Outcome of treatment in children with Philadelphia chromosome-positive acute lymphoblastic leukemia. N Engl J Med 2000;342: 998–1006.

[10] Balduzzi A, Valsecchi MG, Uderzo C, et al. Chemotherapy versus allogeneic transplantation for very-high-risk childhood acute lymphoblastic leukaemia in first complete remission: comparison by genetic randomisation in an international prospective study. Lancet 2005;366:635–42.

[11] Schrauder A, Reiter A, Gadner H, et al. Superiority of allogeneic hematopoietic stem-cell transplantation compared with chemotherapy alone in high-risk childhood T-cell acute lymphoblastic leukemia: results from ALL-BFM 90 and 95. J Clin Oncol 2006;24:5742–9.

[12] Satwani P, Sather H, Ozkaynak F, et al. Allogeneic bone marrow transplantation in first remission for children with ultra-high-risk features of acute lymphoblastic leukemia: a Children's Oncology Group study report. Biol Blood Marrow Transplant 2007;13:218–27.

[13] Peters C, Schrauder A, Schrappe M, et al. Allogeneic haematopoietic stem cell transplantation in children with acute lymphoblastic leukaemia: the BFM/IBFM/EBMT concepts. Bone Marrow Transplant 2005;35(Suppl 1):S9–11.

[14] Schrappe M, Reiter A, Zimmermann M, et al. Long-term results of four consecutive trials in childhood ALL performed by the ALL-BFM study group from 1981 to 1995. Berlin-Frankfurt-Münster. Leukemia 2000;14:2205–22.

[15] Chessells JM. Relapsed lymphoblastic leukaemia in children: a continuing challenge. Br J Haematol 1998;102:423–38.

[16] Chessells JM, Veys P, Kempski H, et al. Long-term follow-up of relapsed childhood acute lymphoblastic leukaemia. Br J Haematol 2003;123:396–405.

[17] Borgmann A, von SA, Hartmann R, et al. Unrelated donor stem cell transplantation compared with chemotherapy for children with acute lymphoblastic leukemia in a second remission: a matched-pair analysis. Blood 2003;101:3835–9.

[18] Roy A, Cargill A, Love S, et al. Outcome after first relapse in childhood acute lymphoblastic leukaemia - lessons from the United Kingdom R2 trial. Br J Haematol 2005;130:67–75.

[19] Einsiedel HG, von SA, Hartmann R, et al. Long-term outcome in children with relapsed ALL by risk-stratified salvage therapy: results of trial acute lymphoblastic leukemia-relapse study of the Berlin-Frankfurt-Münster Group 87. J Clin Oncol 2005;23:7942–50.

[20] Rivera GK, Zhou Y, Hancock ML, et al. Bone marrow recurrence after initial intensive treatment for childhood acute lymphoblastic leukemia. Cancer 2005;103:368–76.

[21] Eapen M, Raetz E, Zhang MJ, et al. Outcomes after HLA-matched sibling transplantation or chemotherapy in children with B-precursor acute lymphoblastic leukemia in a second remission: a collaborative study of the Children's Oncology Group and the Center for International Blood and Marrow Transplant Research. Blood 2006;107:4961–7.

[22] Gaynon PS, Harris RE, Altman AJ, et al. Bone marrow transplantation versus prolonged intensive chemotherapy for children with acute lymphoblastic leukemia and an initial bone marrow relapse within 12 months of the completion of primary therapy: Children's Oncology Group study CCG-1941. J Clin Oncol 2006;24:3150–6.

[23] Matsuzaki A, Nagatoshi Y, Inada H, et al. Prognostic factors for relapsed childhood acute lymphoblastic leukemia: impact of allogeneic stem cell transplantation—a report from the Kyushu-Yamaguchi Children's Cancer Study Group. Pediatr Blood Cancer 2005;45: 111–20.

[24] Rizzari C, Valsecchi MG, Arico M, et al. Outcome of very late relapse in children with acute lymphoblastic leukemia. Haematologica 2004;89:427–34.

[25] Eckert C, Biondi A, Seeger K, et al. Prognostic value of minimal residual disease in relapsed childhood acute lymphoblastic leukaemia. Lancet 2001;358:1239–41.

[26] Coustan-Smith E, Gajjar A, Hijiya N, et al. Clinical significance of minimal residual disease in childhood acute lymphoblastic leukemia after first relapse. Leukemia 2004;18:499–504.

[27] Knechtli CJ, Goulden NJ, Hancock JP, et al. Minimal residual disease status before allogeneic bone marrow transplantation is an important determinant of successful outcome for children and adolescents with acute lymphoblastic leukemia. Blood 1998;92:4072–9.

[28] Bader P, Hancock J, Kreyenberg H, et al. Minimal residual disease (MRD) status prior to allogeneic stem cell transplantation is a powerful predictor for post-transplant outcome in children with ALL. Leukemia 2002;16:1668–72.

[29] van der Velden VH, Joosten SA, Willemse MJ, et al. Real-time quantitative PCR for detection of minimal residual disease before allogeneic stem cell transplantation predicts outcome in children with acute lymphoblastic leukemia. Leukemia 2001;15:1485–7.

[30] Krejci O, van der Velden VH, Bader P, et al. Level of minimal residual disease prior to haematopoietic stem cell transplantation predicts prognosis in paediatric patients with acute lymphoblastic leukaemia: a report of the Pre-BMT MRD Study Group. Bone Marrow Transplant 2003;32:849–51.

[31] Imashuku S, Terui K, Matsuyama T, et al. Lack of clinical utility of minimal residual disease detection in allogeneic stem cell recipients with childhood acute lymphoblastic leukemia: multi-institutional collaborative study in Japan. Bone Marrow Transplant 2003;31:1127–35.

[32] Sramkova L, Muzikova K, Fronkova E, et al. Detectable minimal residual disease before allogeneic hematopoietic stem cell transplantation predicts extremely poor prognosis in children with acute lymphoblastic leukemia. Pediatr Blood Cancer 2007;48:93–100.

[33] Pui CH, Behm FG, Downing JR, et al. 11q23/MLL rearrangement confers a poor prognosis in infants with acute lymphoblastic leukemia. J Clin Oncol 1994;12:909–15.

[34] Pui CH, Gaynon PS, Boyett JM, et al. Outcome of treatment in childhood acute lymphoblastic leukaemia with rearrangements of the 11q23 chromosomal region. Lancet 2002;359: 1909–15.

[35] Triplett B, Handgretinger R, Pui CH, et al. KIR-incompatible hematopoietic-cell transplantation for poor prognosis infant acute lymphoblastic leukemia. Blood 2006;107: 1238–9.

[36] Stevens RF, Hann IM, Wheatley K, et al. Marked improvements in outcome with chemotherapy alone in paediatric acute myeloid leukemia: results of the United Kingdom Medical Research Council's 10th AML trial. MRC Childhood Leukaemia Working Party. Br J Haematol 1998;101:130–40.

[37] Creutzig U, Ritter J, Zimmermann M, et al. Improved treatment results in high-risk pediatric acute myeloid leukemia patients after intensification with high-dose cytarabine and mitoxantrone: results of Study Acute Myeloid Leukemia-Berlin-Frankfurt-Münster 93. J Clin Oncol 2001;19:2705–13.

[38] Krance RA, Hurwitz CA, Head DR, et al. Experience with 2-chlorodeoxyadenosine in previously untreated children with newly diagnosed acute myeloid leukemia and myelodysplastic diseases. J Clin Oncol 2001;19:2804–11.

[39] Wells RJ, Arthur DC, Srivastava A, et al. Prognostic variables in newly diagnosed children and adolescents with acute myeloid leukemia: Children's Cancer Group Study 213. Leukemia 2002;16:601–7.

[40] Creutzig U, Zimmermann M, Ritter J, et al. Definition of a standard-risk group in children with AML. Br J Haematol 1999;104:630–9.

[41] Wheatley K, Burnett AK, Goldstone AH, et al. A simple, robust, validated and highly predictive index for the determination of risk-directed therapy in acute myeloid leukaemia derived from the MRC AML 10 trial. United Kingdom Medical Research Council's Adult and Childhood Leukaemia Working Parties. Br J Haematol 1999;107:69–79.

[42] Dastugue N, Payen C, Lafage-Pochitaloff M, et al. Prognostic significance of karyotype in de novo adult acute myeloid leukemia. The BGMT group. Leukemia 1995;9:1491–8.

[43] Raimondi SC, Chang MN, Ravindranath Y, et al. Chromosomal abnormalities in 478 children with acute myeloid leukemia: clinical characteristics and treatment outcome in a Cooperative Pediatric Oncology Group study-POG 8821. Blood 1999;94:3707–16.

[44] Chen AR, Alonzo TA, Woods WG, et al. Current controversies: which patients with acute myeloid leukaemia should receive a bone marrow transplantation?—an American view. Br J Haematol 2002;118:378–84.

[45] Creutzig U, Reinhardt D. Current controversies: which patients with acute myeloid leukaemia should receive a bone marrow transplantation?—a European view. Br J Haematol 2002;118:365–77.

[46] Amadori S, Testi AM, Arico M, et al. Prospective comparative study of bone marrow transplantation and postremission chemotherapy for childhood acute myelogenous leukemia. The Associazione Italiana Ematologia ed Oncologia Pediatrica Cooperative Group. J Clin Oncol 1993;11:1046–54.

[47] Nesbit ME Jr, Buckley JD, Feig SA, et al. Chemotherapy for induction of remission of childhood acute myeloid leukemia followed by marrow transplantation or multiagent chemotherapy: a report from the Children's Cancer Group. J Clin Oncol 1994;12:127–35.

[48] Ravindranath Y, Yeager AM, Chang MN, et al. Autologous bone marrow transplantation versus intensive consolidation chemotherapy for acute myeloid leukemia in childhood. Pediatric Oncology Group. N Engl J Med 1996;334:1428–34.

[49] Woods WG, Neudorf S, Gold S, et al. A comparison of allogeneic bone marrow transplantation, autologous bone marrow transplantation, and aggressive chemotherapy in children with acute myeloid leukemia in remission. Blood 2001;97:56–62.

[50] Neudorf S, Sanders J, Kobrinsky N, et al. Allogeneic bone marrow transplantation for children with acute myelocytic leukemia in first remission demonstrates a role for graft versus leukemia in the maintenance of disease-free survival. Blood 2004;103.3655 61.

[51] Alonzo TA, Wells RJ, Woods WG, et al. Postremission therapy for children with acute myeloid leukemia: the Children's Cancer Group experience in the transplant era. Leukemia 2005;19:965–70.

[52] Burnett AK, Wheatley K, Goldstone AH, et al. The value of allogeneic bone marrow transplant in patients with acute myeloid leukaemia at differing risk of relapse: results of the UK MRC AML 10 trial. Br J Haematol 2002;118:385–400.

[53] Handgretinger R, Chen X, Pfeiffer M, et al. Feasibility and outcome of reduced-intensity conditioning in haploidentical transplantation. Ann N Y Acad Sci 2007;1106:279–89, Epub 2007 Apr 18.

[54] Willemze AJ, Geskus RB, Noordijk EM, et al. HLA-identical haematopoietic stem cell transplantation for acute leukaemia in children: less relapse with higher biologically effective dose of TBI. Bone Marrow Transplant 2007;40:319–27.

[55] Neudorf S, Sanders J, Kobrinsky N, et al. Autologous bone marrow transplantation for children with AML in first remission. Bone Marrow Transplant 2007;40:313–8.

[56] Goulden N, Virgo P, Grimwade D. Minimal residual disease directed therapy for childhood acute myeloid leukaemia: the time is now. Br J Haematol 2006;134:273–82.

[57] Webb DK, Wheatley K, Harrison G, et al. Outcome for children with relapsed acute myeloid leukaemia following initial therapy in the Medical Research Council (MRC) AML 10 trial. MRC Childhood Leukaemia Working Party. Leukemia 1999;13:25–31.

[58] Stahnke K, Boos J, der-Gotze C, et al. Duration of first remission predicts remission rates and long-term survival in children with relapsed acute myelogenous leukemia. Leukemia 1998;12:1534–8.

[59] Aladjidi N, Auvrignon A, Leblanc T, et al. Outcome in children with relapsed acute myeloid leukemia after initial treatment with the French Leucemie Aique Myeloide Enfant (LAME) 89/91 protocol of the French Society of Pediatric Hematology and Immunology. J Clin Oncol 2003;21:4377–85.

[60] Wells RJ, Adams MT, Alonzo TA, et al. Mitoxantrone and cytarabine induction, high-dose cytarabine, and etoposide intensification for pediatric patients with relapsed or refractory acute myeloid leukemia: Children's Cancer Group Study 2951. J Clin Oncol 2003;21:2940–7.

[61] Johnston DL, Alonzo TA, Gerbing RB, et al. Risk factors and therapy for isolated central nervous system relapse of pediatric acute myeloid leukemia. J Clin Oncol 2005;23:9172–8.

[62] Abrahamsson J, Clausen N, Gustafsson G, et al. Improved outcome after relapse in children with acute myeloid leukaemia. Br J Haematol 2007;136:229–36.

[63] Nemecek ER, Gooley TA, Woolfrey AE, et al. Outcome of allogeneic bone marrow transplantation for children with advanced acute myeloid leukemia. Bone Marrow Transplant 2004;34:799–806.

[64] Webb DK. Management of relapsed acute myeloid leukaemia. Br J Haematol 1999;106: 851–9.

[65] Meshinchi S, Leisenring WM, Carpenter PA, et al. Survival after second hematopoietic stem cell transplantation for recurrent pediatric acute myeloid leukemia. Biol Blood Marrow Transplant 2003;9:706–13.

[66] Luger S, Sacks N. Bone marrow transplantation for myelodysplastic syndrome—who? when? and which? Bone Marrow Transplant 2002;30:199–206.

[67] Kardos G, Baumann I, Passmore SJ, et al. Refractory anemia in childhood: a retrospective analysis of 67 patients with particular reference to monosomy 7. Blood 2003;102: 1997–2003.

[68] Yoshimi A, Baumann I, Fuhrer M, et al. Immunosuppressive therapy with anti-thymocyte globulin and cyclosporine A in selected children with hypoplastic refractory cytopenia. Haematologica 2007;92:397–400.

[69] Strahm B, Locatelli F, Bader P, et al. Reduced intensity conditioning in unrelated donor transplantation for refractory cytopenia in childhood. Bone Marrow Transplant 2007;40: 329–33.

[70] Chan GC, Wang WC, Raimondi SC, et al. Myelodysplastic syndrome in children: differentiation from acute myeloid leukemia with a low blast count. Leukemia 1997;11:206–11.

[71] Hasle H, Arico M, Basso G, et al. Myelodysplastic syndrome, juvenile myelomonocytic leukemia, and acute myeloid leukemia associated with complete or partial monosomy 7. European Working Group on MDS in Childhood (EWOG-MDS). Leukemia 1999;13: 376–85.

[72] Woods WG, Barnard DR, Alonzo TA, et al. Prospective study of 90 children requiring treatment for juvenile myelomonocytic leukemia or myelodysplastic syndrome: a report from the Children's Cancer Group. J Clin Oncol 2002;20:434–40.

[73] Hasle H, Alonzo TA, Auvrignon A, et al. Monosomy 7 and deletion 7q in children and adolescents with acute myeloid leukemia: an international retrospective study. Blood 2007; 109:4641–7.

[74] Passmore SJ, Hann IM, Stiller CA, et al. Pediatric myelodysplasia: a study of 68 children and a new prognostic scoring system. Blood 1995;85:1742–50.

[75] Heaney ML, Golde DW. Myelodysplasia. N Engl J Med 1999;340:1649–60.

[76] Anderson JE, Appelbaum FR, Storb R. An update on allogeneic marrow transplantation for myelodysplastic syndrome. Leuk Lymphoma 1995;17:95–9.

[77] Sutton L, Chastang C, Ribaud P, et al. Factors influencing outcome in de novo myelodysplastic syndromes treated by allogeneic bone marrow transplantation: a long-term study of 71 patients Societe Francaise de Greffe de Moelle. Blood 1996;88:358–65.

[78] Davies SM, Wagner JE, Defor T, et al. Unrelated donor bone marrow transplantation for children and adolescents with aplastic anaemia or myelodysplasia. Br J Haematol 1997;96: 749–56.

[79] Anderson JE, Anasetti C, Appelbaum FR, et al. Unrelated donor marrow transplantation for myelodysplasia (MDS) and MDS-related acute myeloid leukaemia. Br J Haematol 1996;93:59–67.

[80] Lutz P, Zix-Kieffer I, Souillet G, et al. Juvenile myelomonocytic leukemia: analyses of treatment results in the EORTC Children's Leukemia Cooperative Group (CLCG). Bone Marrow Transplant 1996;18:1111–6.

[81] Castleberry RP, Emanuel PD, Zuckerman KS, et al. A pilot study of isotretinoin in the treatment of juvenile chronic myelogenous leukemia. N Engl J Med 1994;331:1680–4.

[82] Pui CH, Arico M. Isotretinoin for juvenile chronic myelogenous leukemia. N Engl J Med 1995;332:1520–1.

[83] Locatelli F, Nollke P, Zecca M, et al. Hematopoietic stem cell transplantation (HSCT) in children with juvenile myelomonocytic leukemia (JMML): results of the EWOG-MDS/ EBMT trial. Blood 2005;105:410–9.

[84] Niemeyer CM, Arico M, Basso G, et al. Chronic myelomonocytic leukemia in childhood: a retrospective analysis of 110 cases. European Working Group on Myelodysplastic Syndromes in Childhood (EWOG-MDS). Blood 1997;89:3534–43.

[85] Locatelli F, Giorgiani G, Comoli P. Allogeneic transplantation of haematopoietic progenitors for myelodysplastic syndromes and myeloproliferative disorders. Bone Marrow Transplant 1998;21(Suppl 2):S17–20.

[86] Manabe A, Okamura J, Yumura-Yagi K, et al. Allogeneic hematopoietic stem cell transplantation for 27 children with juvenile myelomonocytic leukemia diagnosed based on the criteria of the International JMML Working Group. Leukemia 2002;16:645–9.

[87] Passmore SJ, Chessells JM, Kempski H, et al. Paediatric myelodysplastic syndromes and juvenile myelomonocytic leukaemia in the UK: a population-based study of incidence and survival. Br J Haematol 2003;121:758–67.

[88] Smith FO, King R, Nelson G, et al. Unrelated donor bone marrow transplantation for children with juvenile myelomonocytic leukaemia. Br J Haematol 2002;116:716–24.

[89] MacMillan ML, Davies SM, Orchard PJ, et al. Haemopoietic cell transplantation in children with juvenile myelomonocytic leukaemia. Br J Haematol 1998;103:552–8.

[90] Emanuel PD, Snyder RC, Wiley T, et al. Inhibition of juvenile myelomonocytic leukemia cell growth in vitro by farnesyltransferase inhibitors. Blood 2000;95:639–45.

[91] Yoshimi A, Mohamed M, Bierings M, et al. Second allogeneic hematopoietic stem cell transplantation (HSCT) results in outcome similar to that of first HSCT for patients with juvenile myelomonocytic leukemia. Leukemia 2007;21:556–60.

[92] Dann EJ, Rowe JM. Biology and therapy of secondary leukaemias. Best Pract Res Clin Haematol 2001;14:119–37.

[93] Ballen KK, Antin JH. Treatment of therapy-related acute myelogenous leukemia and myelodysplastic syndromes. Hematol Oncol Clin North Am 1993;7:477–93.

[94] Yakoub-Agha I, de La SP, Ribaud P, et al. Allogeneic bone marrow transplantation for therapy-related myelodysplastic syndrome and acute myeloid leukemia: a long-term study of 70 patients-report of the French Society of Bone Marrow Transplantation. J Clin Oncol 2000;18:963–71.

[95] Barnard DR, Lange B, Alonzo TA, et al. Acute myeloid leukemia and myelodysplastic syndrome in children treated for cancer: comparison with primary presentation. Blood 2002;100:427–34.

[96] Woodard P, Barfield R, Hale G, et al. Outcome of hematopoietic stem cell transplantation for pediatric patients with therapy-related acute myeloid leukemia or myelodysplastic syndrome. Pediatr Blood Cancer 2006;47:931–5.

[97] Clift RA, Appelbaum FR, Thomas ED. Treatment of chronic myeloid leukemia by marrow transplantation. Blood 1993;82:1954–6.

[98] Cwynarski K, Roberts IA, Iacobelli S, et al. Stem cell transplantation for chronic myeloid leukemia in children. Blood 2003;102:1224–31.

[99] Dini G, Rondelli R, Miano M, et al. Unrelated-donor bone marrow transplantation for Philadelphia chromosome-positive chronic myelogenous leukemia in children: experience of eight European countries. The EBMT Paediatric Diseases Working Party. Bone Marrow Transplant 1996;18(Suppl 2):80–5.

[100] Gamis AS, Haake R, McGlave P, et al. Unrelated-donor bone marrow transplantation for Philadelphia chromosome-positive chronic myelogenous leukemia in children. J Clin Oncol 1993;11:834–8.

[101] Millot F, Esperou H, Bordigoni P, et al. Allogeneic bone marrow transplantation for chronic myeloid leukemia in childhood: a report from the Societe Francaise de Greffe de Moelle et de Therapie Cellulaire (SFGM-TC). Bone Marrow Transplant 2003;32:993–9.

[102] van RF, Szydlo RM, Hermans J, et al. Long-term results after allogeneic bone marrow transplantation for chronic myelogenous leukemia in chronic phase: a report from the Chronic Leukemia Working Party of the European Group for Blood and Marrow Transplantation. Bone Marrow Transplant 1997;20:553–60.

[103] Elmaagacli AH, Basoglu S, Peceny R, et al. Improved disease-free-survival after transplantation of peripheral blood stem cells as compared with bone marrow from HLA-identical unrelated donors in patients with first chronic phase chronic myeloid leukemia. Blood 2002;99:1130–5.

[104] Eapen M, Horowitz MM, Klein JP, et al. Higher mortality after allogeneic peripheral-blood transplantation compared with bone marrow in children and adolescents: the

Histocompatibility and Alternate Stem Cell Source Working Committee of the International Bone Marrow Transplant Registry. J Clin Oncol 2004;22:4872–80.

[105] Creutzig U, Ritter J, Zimmermann M, et al. Prognosis of children with chronic myeloid leukemia: a retrospective analysis of 75 patients. Klin Padiatr 1996;208:236–41 [in German].

[106] Davies SM, DeFor TE, McGlave PB, et al. Equivalent outcomes in patients with chronic myelogenous leukemia after early transplantation of phenotypically matched bone marrow from related or unrelated donors. Am J Med 2001;110:339–46.

[107] Barta A, Denes R, Masszi T, et al. Remarkably reduced transplant-related complications by dibromomannitol non-myeloablative conditioning before allogeneic bone marrow transplantation in chronic myeloid leukemia. Acta Haematol 2001;105:64–70.

[108] Chakraverty R, Peggs K, Chopra R, et al. Limiting transplantation-related mortality following unrelated donor stem cell transplantation by using a nonmyeloablative conditioning regimen. Blood 2002;99:1071–8.

[109] Kolb HJ, Mittermuller J, Clemm C, et al. Donor leukocyte transfusions for treatment of recurrent chronic myelogenous leukemia in marrow transplant patients. Blood 1990;76: 2462–5.

[110] Thornley I, Perentesis JP, Davies SM, et al. Treating children with chronic myeloid leukemia in the imatinib era: a therapeutic dilemma? Med Pediatr Oncol 2003;41:115–7.

[111] Pulsipher MA. Treatment of CML in pediatric patients: should imatinib mesylate (STI-571, Gleevec) or allogeneic hematopoietic cell transplant be front-line therapy? Pediatr Blood Cancer 2004;43:523–33.

[112] Walz C, Sattler M. Novel targeted therapies to overcome imatinib mesylate resistance in chronic myeloid leukemia (CML). Crit Rev Oncol Hematol 2006;57:145–64.

[113] Bunin N, Aplenc R, Kamani N, et al. Randomized trial of busulfan vs total body irradiation containing conditioning regimens for children with acute lymphoblastic leukemia: a Pediatric Blood and Marrow Transplant Consortium study. Bone Marrow Transplant 2003;32:543–8.

[114] Davies SM, Ramsay NK, Klein JP, et al. Comparison of preparative regimens in transplants for children with acute lymphoblastic leukemia. J Clin Oncol 2000;18:340–7.

[115] Niederwieser D, Maris M, Shizuru JA, et al. Low-dose total body irradiation (TBI) and fludarabine followed by hematopoietic cell transplantation (HCT) from HLA-matched or mismatched unrelated donors and postgrafting immunosuppression with cyclosporine and mycophenolate mofetil (MMF) can induce durable complete chimerism and sustained remissions in patients with hematological diseases. Blood 2003;101:1620–9.

[116] Or R, Shapira MY, Resnick I, et al. Nonmyeloablative allogeneic stem cell transplantation for the treatment of chronic myeloid leukemia in first chronic phase. Blood 2003;101(2): 441–5.

[117] Giralt S, Estey E, Albitar M, et al. Engraftment of allogeneic hematopoietic progenitor cells with purine analog-containing chemotherapy: harnessing graft-versus-leukemia without myeloablative therapy. Blood 1997;89:4531–6.

[118] Prasad VK, Kernan NA, Heller G, et al. DNA typing for HLA-A and HLA-B identifies disparities between patients and unrelated donors matched by HLA-A and HLA-B serology and HLA-DRB1. Blood 1999;93:399–409.

[119] Speiser DE, Tiercy JM, Rufer N, et al. High resolution HLA matching associated with decreased mortality after unrelated bone marrow transplantation. Blood 1996;87:4455–62.

[120] Flomenberg N, Baxter-Lowe LA, Confer D, et al. Impact of HLA class I and class II high-resolution matching on outcomes of unrelated donor bone marrow transplantation: HLA-C mismatching is associated with a strong adverse effect on transplantation outcome. Blood 2004;104:1923–30.

[121] Chalandon Y, Tiercy JM, Schanz U, et al. Impact of high-resolution matching in allogeneic unrelated donor stem cell transplantation in Switzerland. Bone Marrow Transplant 2006; 37:909–16.

[122] Yakoub-Agha I, Mesnil F, Kuentz M, et al. Allogeneic marrow stem-cell transplantation from human leukocyte antigen-identical siblings versus human leukocyte antigen-allelic-matched unrelated donors (10/10) in patients with standard-risk hematologic malignancy: a prospective study from the French Society of Bone Marrow Transplantation and Cell Therapy. J Clin Oncol 2006;24:5695–702.

[123] Petersdorf EW. HLA matching in allogeneic stem cell transplantation. Curr Opin Hematol 2004;11:386–91.

[124] Sedlacek P, Formankova R, Keslova P, et al. Low mortality of children undergoing hematopoietic stem cell transplantation from 7 to 8/10 human leukocyte antigen allele-matched unrelated donors with the use of antithymocyte globulin. Bone Marrow Transplant 2006; 38:745–50.

[125] Kollman C, Howe CW, Anasetti C, et al. Donor characteristics as risk factors in recipients after transplantation of bone marrow from unrelated donors: the effect of donor age. Blood 2001;98:2043–51.

[126] Ljungman P, Brand R, Einsele H, et al. Donor CMV serologic status and outcome of CMV-seropositive recipients after unrelated donor stem cell transplantation: an EBMT megafile analysis. Blood 2003;102:4255–60.

[127] Ljungman P, Perez-Bercoff L, Jonsson J, et al. Risk factors for the development of cytomegalovirus disease after allogeneic stem cell transplantation. Haematologica 2006;91:78–83.

[128] Eapen M, Rubinstein P, Zhang MJ, et al. Comparable long-term survival after unrelated and HLA-matched sibling donor hematopoietic stem cell transplantations for acute leukemia in children younger than 18 months. J Clin Oncol 2006;24:145–51.

[129] Dahlke J, Kroger N, Zabelina T, et al. Comparable results in patients with acute lymphoblastic leukemia after related and unrelated stem cell transplantation. Bone Marrow Transplant 2006;37:155–63.

[130] Hambach L, Spierings E, Goulmy E. Risk assessment in haematopoietic stem cell transplantation: minor histocompatibility antigens. Best Pract Res Clin Haematol 2007;20: 171–87.

[131] Bettens F, Passweg J, Gratwohl A, et al. Association of TNFd and IL-10 polymorphisms with mortality in unrelated hematopoietic stem cell transplantation. Transplantation 2006;81:1261–7.

[132] Dickinson AM, Middleton PG. Beyond the HLA typing age: genetic polymorphisms predicting transplant outcome. Blood Rev 2005;19:333–40.

[133] Mulligan CG, Petersdorf EW. Genomic polymorphism and allogeneic hematopoietic transplantation outcome. Biol Blood Marrow Transplant 2006;12:19–27.

[134] Souillet G, Rey S, Bertrand Y, et al. Outcome of unrelated bone marrow donor searches in 174 children resulting in 45 patients transplanted in the HLA-matched and -mismatched situation. Bone Marrow Transplant 2000;26:31–43.

[135] Tiercy JM, Nicoloso G, Passweg J, et al. The probability of identifying a 10/10 HLA allele-matched unrelated donor is highly predictable. Bone Marrow Transplant 2007;40:515–22.

[136] Eapen M, Rubinstein P, Zhang MJ, et al. Outcomes of transplantation of unrelated donor umbilical cord blood and bone marrow in children with acute leukaemia: a comparison study. Lancet 2007;369:1947–54.

[137] Barker JN, Weisdorf DJ, DeFor TE, et al. Transplantation of 2 partially HLA-matched umbilical cord blood units to enhance engraftment in adults with hematologic malignancy. Blood 2005;105:1343–7.

[138] Gluckman E, Rocha V, Arcese W, et al. Factors associated with outcomes of unrelated cord blood transplant: guidelines for donor choice. Exp Hematol 2004;32:397–407.

[139] Sawczyn KK, Quinones R, Malcolm J, et al. Cord blood transplant in childhood ALL. Pediatr Blood Cancer 2005;45:964–70.

[140] Rocha V, Cornish J, Sievers EL, et al. Comparison of outcomes of unrelated bone marrow and umbilical cord blood transplants in children with acute leukemia. Blood 2001;97: 2962–71.

[141] Wall DA, Carter SL, Kernan NA, et al. Busulfan/melphalan/antithymocyte globulin followed by unrelated donor cord blood transplantation for treatment of infant leukemia and leukemia in young children: the Cord Blood Transplantation study (COBLT) experience. Biol Blood Marrow Transplant 2005;11:637–46.

[142] Henslee-Downey PJ, Abhyankar SH, Parrish RS, et al. Use of partially mismatched related donors extends access to allogeneic marrow transplant. Blood 1997;89:3864–72.

[143] Aversa F, Terenzi A, Tabilio A, et al. Full haplotype-mismatched hematopoietic stem-cell transplantation: a phase II study in patients with acute leukemia at high risk of relapse. J Clin Oncol 2005;23:3447–54.

[144] Handgretinger R, Klingebiel T, Lang P, et al. Megadose transplantation of purified peripheral blood CD34(+) progenitor cells from HLA-mismatched parental donors in children. Bone Marrow Transplant 2001;27:777–83.

[145] Klingebiel T, Lang P, Schumm M, et al. Experiences with haploidentical stem cell transplantation in children with acute lymphoblastic leukemia. Pathol Biol (Paris) 2005;53:159–61.

[146] Larocca A, Piaggio G, Podesta M, et al. Boost of CD34+-selected peripheral blood cells without further conditioning in patients with poor graft function following allogeneic stem cell transplantation. Haematologica 2006;91:935–40.

[147] Feuchtinger T, Matthes-Martin S, Richard C, et al. Safe adoptive transfer of virus-specific T-cell immunity for the treatment of systemic adenovirus infection after allogeneic stem cell transplantation. Br J Haematol 2006;134:64–76.

[148] Passweg JR, Koehl U, Uharek L, et al. Natural-killer-cell-based treatment in haematopoietic stem-cell transplantation. Best Pract Res Clin Haematol 2006;19:811–24.

ELSEVIER
SAUNDERS

PEDIATRIC CLINICS
OF NORTH AMERICA

Pediatr Clin N Am 55 (2008) 97–120

Neuroblastoma: Biology, Prognosis, and Treatment

Julie R. Park, MD[a],*, Angelika Eggert, MD[b],
Huib Caron, MD, PhD[c]

[a]*Division of Hematology and Oncology, University of Washington School of Medicine
and Children's Hospital and Regional Medical Center, 4800 Sand Pt. Way NE,
MS: B6553, Seattle, WA 98105-0371, USA*
[b]*Department of Hematology/Oncology, University Children's Hospital Essen,
Hufelandstr. 55, 45122 Essen, Germany*
[c]*Department of Pediatric Oncology and Hematology, Emma Children's Hospital AMC,
EKZ/AMC, P.O. Box 22700, 1100 DE, Amsterdam, the Netherlands*

Neuroblastoma, a neoplasm of the sympathetic nervous system, is the second most common extracranial malignant tumor of childhood and the most common solid tumor of infancy. Neuroblastoma is a heterogeneous malignancy with prognosis ranging from near uniform survival to high risk for fatal demise. Neuroblastoma serves as a paradigm for the prognostic utility of biologic and clinical data and the potential to tailor therapy for patient cohorts at low, intermediate, and high risk for recurrence. Overall survival is excellent for patients who have low- and intermediate-risk neuroblastoma with a general trend toward minimization of therapy. In contrast, a marked intensification of therapy has led to only incremental improvement in survival for high-risk disease because less than 40% of high-risk patients survive. Chemotherapy and radiotherapy resistance remain the hallmark of failure. This article summarizes our understanding of neuroblastoma biology and prognostic features and discusses their impact on current and proposed risk stratification schemas, risk-based therapeutic approaches, and the development of novel therapies for patients at high risk for failure.

Epidemiology and cause

The incidence of neuroblastoma per year is 10.5 per million children less than 15 years of age [1]. Neuroblastoma accounts for 8% to 10% of all

---

* Corresponding author.
E-mail address: julie.park@seattlechildrens.org (J.R. Park).

0031-3955/08/$ - see front matter © 2008 Elsevier Inc. All rights reserved.
doi:10.1016/j.pcl.2007.10.014

childhood cancers and for approximately 15% of cancer deaths in children. There seems to be no significant geographical variation in the incidence between North America and Europe, and there are no differences between races. Neuroblastoma occurs slightly more frequently in boys than girls (ratio 1.2:1). The incidence peaks at age 0 to 4 years, with a median age of 23 months. Forty percent of patients who present with clinical symptoms at diagnosis are under 1 year of age, and less than 5% with clinical symptoms are over the age of 10 years. Cases of familial neuroblastoma have been reported [2]. Environmental factors are implicated in the development of neuroblastoma (eg, paternal exposure to electromagnetic fields or prenatal exposure to alcohol, pesticides, or phenobarbital). A potential relationship with assisted pregnancies has also been made. None of these environmental factors has been confirmed in independent studies [3,4].

Screening for neuroblastoma was pioneered by Japanese investigators who demonstrated that asymptomatic tumors could be detected in infants by measurement of urinary catecholamine metabolites. The implementation of infant screening for neuroblastoma resulted in a doubling of neuroblastoma incidence to 20.1 per million children [5], and the tumors detected possessed favorable biological characteristics [6]. Although the outcome for the children with the detected tumors was excellent, these studies were not population based and did not demonstrate a resultant reduction in neuroblastoma mortality rates. The Quebec Neuroblastoma Screening Project and the German Neuroblastoma Screening Study were designed to identify whether screening a large cohort of infants for neuroblastoma at the ages of 3 weeks, 6 months, and 12 months could reduce the population-based incidence of advanced disease and mortality. These studies demonstrate that screening for neuroblastoma at or under the age of 1 year identifies tumors with a good prognosis and molecular pathology, doubles the incidence, and fails to detect the poor-prognosis disease that presents clinically at an older age [7,8].

Genetic predisposition

Neuroblastoma can occur in patients affected with other neural crest disorders or malignancies, such as Hirschsprung disease, neurofibromatosis type 1, and congenital central hypoventilation syndrome [9–11]. Genomic linkage studies have not found evidence of a link between Hirschsprung disease and neuroblastoma development. The co-occurrence of neuroblastoma and von Recklinghausen disease is of interest because both disorders are deviations of normal neural-crest cell development in the embryo. An analysis of the reported coincidence of neuroblastoma and neurofibromatosis indicates that most of these cases can probably be accounted for by chance [12]. The *PHOX2B* gene is the major disease gene for the congenital central hypoventilation disorder, and constitutional *PHOX2B* mutations have been identified in familial neuroblastoma cases [13] and in 2.3% of patients who have sporadic neuroblastoma [14].

Several cases of constitutional chromosome abnormalities have been reported in individuals who have neuroblastoma, but no consistent pattern has emerged [12]. Constitutional abnormalities involving the short arm of chromosome 1 have been reported for three neuroblastoma cases, possibly implicating chromosome 1 p loci in neuroblastoma predisposition. A report that familial neuroblastoma is not linked to 1p36 indicates that the predisposition locus for familial cases lies elsewhere.

Familial forms of neuroblastoma are rare, accounting for about 1% of all cases. There are few reported pedigrees of familial neuroblastoma [15]. In those families, the median age at diagnosis is 9 months, as opposed to 2 to 3 years in sporadic cases. An increased incidence of multiple primary tumors is also apparent. Analysis of the pedigree structures suggests a dominant mode of inheritance with low penetrance [15]. The limited number of families available for linkage studies has hindered the ability to map neuroblastoma-predisposing genes. Linkage studies aimed at chromosomal regions involved in neuroblastoma and candidate genes have not demonstrated convincing evidence of linkage [16,17]. Linkage of neuroblastoma predisposition to the chromosomal region 16p12-p13 was demonstrated in North American families [18]. In studies of European pedigrees, linkage to chromosome 12 p and 2 p was found [15]. No constitutional mutations in candidate genes in those regions have been reported.

Pathology

Cell of origin and cancer stem cell hypothesis

The peripheral neuroblastic tumors (pNTs), including neuroblastoma, belong to the "small blue round cell" neoplasms of childhood [19]. They are derived from progenitor cells of the sympathetic nervous system: the sympathogonia of the sympathoadrenal lineage. After migrating from the neural crest, these pluripotent sympathogonia form the sympathetic ganglia, the chromaffin cells of the adrenal medulla, and the paraganglia, reflecting the typical localizations of neuroblastic tumors.

The mechanisms causing persistence of embryonal cells that later give rise to pNTs are mainly unknown. Defects in embryonic genes controlling neural crest development are likely to underlie the unbalanced proliferation and disturbed differentiation of neuroblastoma [13,14,20]. These defects cause a disruption of the normal genetic differentiation program, resulting in an early or late differentiation block. The classic histopathologic pNT subtypes of neuroblastoma, ganglioneuroblastoma, and ganglioneuroma reflect a spectrum of maturation ranging from tumors with predominant undifferentiated neuroblasts to those largely consisting of fully differentiated neurons surrounded by a dense stroma of Schwann cells.

A hallmark of neuroblastoma is cellular heterogeneity. Although the presence of phenotypically diverse cells could be explained by ongoing mutagenesis, the cancer stem cell hypothesis has provided an intriguing alternative explanation for neuroblastoma heterogeneity. This hypothesis suggests that rare multipotent stem cells with indefinite potential for self-renewal drive the onset and growth of tumors. Although the existence of cancer stem cells in leukemia and some solid tumors has been established [21–23], neuroblastoma stem cells have not been clearly identified. Developmental programs controlling self-renewal in neuronal stem cells, including the Notch, Sonic hedgehog, and Wnt/β-catenin pathways, have been implicated in embryonal tumorigenesis [24–26]. It is conceivable that neuroblastoma stem cells arise from normal neural crest stem cells, partly preserving and partly dysregulating these pathways. The identification and characterization of cancer stem cells in neuroblastoma should permit a targeted approach to more effective treatment.

Histopathologic assessment

Primary, pretreatment tumor specimens obtained by open biopsy are optimal material for histologic examination and prognostic evaluation. The typical neuroblastoma is composed of small, uniformly sized cells containing dense hyperchromatic nuclei and scant cytoplasm. The Homer-Wright pseudorosette composed of neuroblasts surrounding areas of eosinophilic neuropil is seen in up to 50% of cases [27]. Distinguishing pNTs from other "small blue round cell" tumors often requires techniques beyond hematoxylin-eosin staining and light microscopy. In the immunohistochemical diagnosis of pNTs, positive staining for neural markers, including neuron-specific enolase, synaptophysin, neurofilament protein, ganglioside GD2, chromogranin A, and tyrosine hydroxylase, combined with negative staining for markers of other small-round-cell tumors should be considered. Electron microscopy typically demonstrates dense core, membrane-bound neurosecretory granules, microfilaments, and parallel arrays of microtubules within neuritic processes (neuropil) [19].

As early as 1963, Beckwith and Perrin suggested a natural history of pNTs that might include involution (regression) and maturation [28]. This hypothesis was based on their observation of "in situ neuroblastoma," an adrenal lesion of microscopic size that is cytologically identical to typical neuroblastoma and is detected in infants with a frequency of 50 times the expected incidence of primary adrenal neuroblastoma. The concept of Beckwith and Perrin has been adopted and incorporated in the International Neuroblastoma Pathology Classification (INPC) [29]. The INPC was established in 1999 by adopting the original system proposed by Shimada in 1984 [30]. The INPC was revised in 2003 [31]. The INPC distinguishes a favorable histology group from an unfavorable histology group of pNTs by applying the concept of age-dependent normal ranges of morphologic features, such as Schwannian stromal development, grade of neuroblastic differentiation, and mitosis-karyorrexis index (Fig. 1).

According to the INPC, the pNTs are assigned to one of the following four basic morphologic categories.

Neuroblastoma (Schwannian-stroma poor)

A neuroblastoma is a tumor composed of neuroblastic cells forming groups or nests separated by stromal septa with none to limited Schwannian proliferation. This category consists of the three subtypes: (1) undifferentiated, (2) poorly differentiated (background of recognizable neuropil and <5% of cells showing differentiation), and (3) differentiating (abundant neuropil and >5% cells showing differentiation toward ganglion cells).

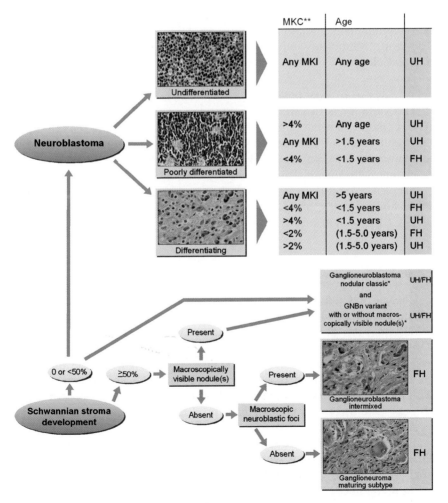

Fig. 1. International Neuroblastoma Pathology Classification.

Ganglioneuroblastoma, intermixed (Schwannian stroma-rich)

An intermixed ganglioneuroblastoma is a tumor containing well-defined microscopic nests of neuroblastic cells intermixed or randomly distributed in the ganglioneuromatous stroma. The nests are composed of a mixture of neuroblastic cells in various stages of differentiation, usually dominated by differentiating neuroblasts and maturing ganglion cells in a background of neuropil.

Ganglioneuroblastoma, nodular (composite Schwannian stroma-rich/stroma dominant and stroma-poor)

A nodular ganglioneuroblastoma is characterized by the presence of grossly visible, usually hemorrhagic neuroblastic nodules (stoma-poor component, representing an aggressive clone) co-existing with ganglioneuroblastoma, intermixed (stroma-rich component) or with ganglioneuroma (stroma-dominant component), both representing a nonaggressive clone. The term "composite" implies that the tumor is composed of biologically different clones.

Ganglioneuroma (Schwannian-stroma-dominant)

This variant has two subtypes: maturing and mature. The maturing subtype is composed predominantly of ganglioneuromatous stroma with scattered collections of differentiating neuroblasts or maturing ganglion cells in addition to fully mature ganglion cells. The mature subtype is composed of mature Schwannian stroma and ganglion cells.

There is a significant correlation between morphologic features of the INPC and biological properties of the pNTS, such as *MYCN* amplification or *TrkA* Expression.

Clinical presentation, diagnosis, and staging

Clinical presentation of neuroblastoma is dependent upon site of tumor origin, disease extent, and the presence of paraneoplastic syndromes. Neuroblastoma can arise anywhere along the sympathetic nervous system. The majority of tumors (65%) arise in the abdomen, with over half of these arising in the adrenal gland. Additional sites of origin include the neck, chest, and pelvis. There is a concordance with age and site of disease, with infants more likely to present with thoracic and cervical primary sites (Fig. 2). One percent of patients have no detectable primary tumor.

Approximately 50% of patients present with localized or regional disease, and approximately 35% of patients have regional lymph node spread at the time of diagnosis. Patients who have localized disease are often asymptomatic, with disease coincidently diagnosed after testing for unassociated medical conditions. Alternatively, mass or abdominal distension and pain are present. Patients who have localized cervical disease arising from the

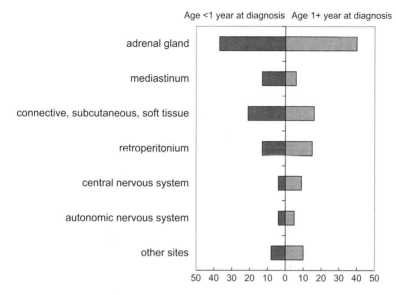

Fig. 2. Percent distribution of neuroblastomas by primary site and age; SEER 1975–1995. (*Data from* Ries LA, Smith MA, Gurney JG, et al. Cancer incidence and survival among children and adolescents: United States SEER Program 1975–1995. NIH Pub. No. 99-4649. Bethesda (MD): NIH; 1999.)

superior cervical ganglion may present with Horner syndrome. Epidural or intradural extension of tumor occurs in approximately 5% to 15% of patients diagnosed with neuroblastoma and may be accompanied by neurologic impairments [32,33]. Well-documented paraneoplastic or clinical syndromes can be present at diagnosis and are summarized in Table 1.

Disease dissemination occurs through lymphatic and hematogenous routes. Bone, bone marrow, and liver are the most common sites of hematogenous spread, with particular predilection for metaphyseal, skull, and orbital bone sites. In contrast to the frequent lack of symptoms with locoregional disease, patients who have widespread disease are often ill appearing with fever, pain, and irritability. A classic presentation of periorbital swelling and ecchymoses ("raccoon eyes") is seen in children who have disease spread to periorbital region. Rarely, infants can present with respiratory compromise secondary to diffuse tumor involvement in the liver and massive hepatomegaly [34].

The current criteria for diagnosis and staging of neuroblastoma are based upon the International Neuroblastoma Staging System (INSS) criteria initially formulated in 1986 and revised in 1988 [35,36]. Neuroblastoma diagnosis is defined by pathologic confirmation from tumor tissue or by pathologic confirmation of neuroblastoma tumor cells in a bone marrow sample in the setting of increased urine or serum catecholamines or catecholamine metabolites (dopamine, vanillylmandelic acid, and homovanillic

Table 1
Syndromes associated with neuroblastoma

Eponym	Syndrome features
Pepper syndrome	Massive involvement of the liver with metastatic disease with or without respiratory distress.
Horner syndrome	Unilateral ptosis, myosis, and anhydrosis associated with a thoracic or cervical primary tumor. Symptoms do not resolve with tumor resection.
Hutchinson syndrome	Limping and irritability in young child associated with bone and bone marrow metastases.
Opsoclonus Mycoclonus Ataxia syndrome	Myoclonic jerking and random eye movement with or without cerebellar ataxia. Often associated with a biologically favorable and differentiated tumor. The condition is likely immune mediated, may not resolve with tumor removal, and often exhibits progressive neuropsychologic sequelae [118–120].
Kerner-Morrison syndrome	Intractable secretory diarrhea due to tumor secretion of vasointestinal peptides. Tumors are generally biologically favorable [121–122].
Neurocristopathy syndrome	Neuroblastoma associated with other neural crest disorders, including congenital hypoventilation syndrome or Hirshprung disease. Germline mutations in the paired homeobox gene PHOX2B have been identified in a subset of such patients [13,20].

Adapted from Castleberry RP. Biology and treatment of neuroblastoma. Pediatr Clin North Am 1997;44:919–37; with permission.

acid). Initial diagnostic testing should include CT or MRI to evaluate primary tumor size and regional extent and to assess for distant spread to neck, thorax, abdomen, or pelvic sites. Brain imaging is recommended only if clinically indicated by examination or neurologic symptoms. Bilateral posterior iliac crest marrow aspirates and core biopsies are required to exclude marrow involvement. Metaiodobenzylguanidine, a norepinephrine analog, is concentrated selectively in sympathetic nervous tissue and, when labeled with radioactive iodine (I^{131} or I^{123}), is an integral component of neuroblastoma staging and response evaluation [37]. A technetium bone scan should be considered for detection of cortical bone disease, especially in patients who have a negative metaiodobenzylguanidine scan.

The INSS definitions for neuroblastoma stage are listed in Table 2. Resectability implies tumor removal without removal of vital organs, compromise of major vessels, or patient disfigurement. Completely resected tumors are classified as stage 1, and partially resected regional tumors with or without regional nodal involvement are classified as stages 2 and 3 dependent upon amount of tumor resection, local invasion, and regional lymph node involvement. Stage 4 disease is defined as distant nodal or hematogenous spread of disease. A unique pattern of dissemination limited to liver, skin, and minimal bone marrow involvement has been described in infants (stage 4s), which has a potential for spontaneous regression in marked contrast to

Table 2
International Neuroblastoma Staging System

Stage 1	Localized tumor with complete gross excision with or without microscopic residual disease; representative ipsilateral lymph nodes negative for tumor microscopically (nodes attached to and removed with the primary tumor may be positive)
Stage 2A	Localized tumor with incomplete gross resection; representative ipsilateral nonadherent lymph nodes negative for tumor microscopically
Stage 2B	Localized tumor with or without complete gross excision with ipsilateral nonadherent lymph nodes positive for tumor; enlarged contralateral lymph nodes must be negative microscopically
Stage 3	Unresectable unilateral tumor infiltrating across the midline[a] with or without regional lymph node involvement, localized unilateral tumor with contralateral regional lymph node involvement, or midline tumor with bilateral extension by infiltration (unresectable) or by lymph node involvement[b]
Stage 4	Any primary tumor with dissemination to distant lymph nodes, bone, bone marrow, liver, skin, or other organs (except as defined for stage 4S)
Stage 4S	Localized primary tumor (as defined for stage 1, 2A, or 2B) with dissemination limited to skin, liver, or bone marrow[c] (limited to infants < 1 yr of age)

Multifocal primary tumors (eg, bilateral adrenal primary tumors) should be staged according to the greatest extent of disease, as defined in the table, and followed by a subscript "M" (eg, 3_M).

[a] The midline is defined as the vertebral column. Tumors originating on one side and crossing the midline must infiltrate to or beyond the opposite side of the vertebral column.

[b] Proven malignant effusion within the thoracic cavity if it is bilateral or the abdominal cavity upstages the patient to INSS stage 3.

[c] Marrow involvement in stage 4S should be minimal (ie, <10% of total nucleated cells identified as malignant on bone marrow biopsy or marrow aspirate). More extensive marrow involvement would be considered to be stage 4. The metaiodobenzylguanidine scan (if performed) should be negative in the marrow.

Data from Brodeur GM, Pritchard J, Berthold F, et al. Revisions of the international criteria for neuroblastoma diagnosis, staging, and response to treatment. J Clin Oncol 1933;11(8):1466–77.

the disseminated aggressive disease seen in the majority of patients greater than 18 months of age [34].

Tumor biology and prognosis

Numerous clinical and biologic factors have been shown to predict clinical behavior of neuroblastoma. There is international agreement that a combination of clinical and biologic factors best predicts clinical prognosis. The Children's Oncology Group stratifies patients into low-, intermediate-, or high-risk categories based upon age at diagnosis, INSS stage, tumor histopathology, DNA index (ploidy), and *MYCN* amplification status (Table 3), with each group displaying a unique risk for recurrence (Fig. 3). Similar strategies are used internationally; however, several factors outlined below suggest a potential for continued evolution of any classification algorithm.

Table 3
Children's Oncology Group neuroblastoma risk stratification

Risk group	Stage	Age	MYCN Amplification Status	Ploidy	Shimada
Low risk	1	Any	Any	Any	Any
Low risk	2a/2b	Any	Not amplified	Any	Any
High risk	2a/2b	Any	Amplified	Any	Any
Intermediate risk	3	<547 d	Not amplified	Any	any
Intermediate risk	3	≥547 d	Not amplified	Any	FH
High risk	3	Any	Amplified	Any	Any
High risk	3	≥547 d	Not amplified	Any	UH
High risk	4	<365 d	Amplified	Any	Any
Intermediate risk	4	<365 d	Not amp	Any	Any
High risk	4	365 to <547 d	Amplified	Any	Any
High Risk	4	365 to <547 d	Any	DI = 1	Any
High risk	4	365 to <547 d	Any	Any	UH
Intermediate risk	4	365 to <547 d	Not amplified	DI > 1	FH
High risk	4	≥547 d	Any	Any	Any
Low risk	4s	<365 d	Not amplified	DI > 1	FH
Intermediate risk	4s	<365 d	Not amplified	DI = 1	Any
Intermediate risk	4s	<365 d	Not amplified	Any	UH
High risk	4s	<365 d	Amplified	Any	Any

Abbreviations: DI, DNA index; FH, favorable histology; UH, unfavorable histology.
Courtesy of Children's Oncology Group.

Stage and age

Although the prognostic value of classifying patients according to the INSS has been confirmed [38,39], an inherent bias toward complete resection

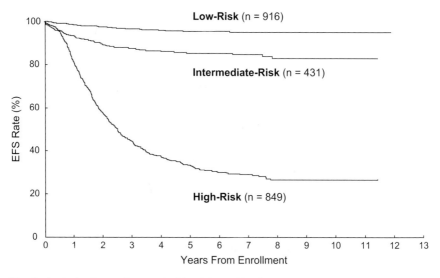

Fig. 3. Analysis of event free survival by risk stratification. (*Courtesy of* W.B. London, PhD, Children's Oncology Group Statistical Office.)

exists. Variation in the surgical approach for resection of locoregional disease has the potential to dramatically alter INSS staging. Such variation has led to considerations of alternative staging approaches. In 1995, the European International Society of Pediatric Oncology Neuroblastoma group demonstrated that radiographic characteristics of the tumor, termed surgical risk factors, were useful in predicting the ability to resect the primary tumor and the risk of developing postoperative complications [40]. This led to proposing an International Risk Group imaging classification system that would use surgical risk factors to more uniformly define extent of disease/staging [41]. The prognostic significance of the International Risk Group classification system will be prospectively validated in ongoing trials within the United States and Europe and, if validated, may replace the current INSS staging.

Age is an important clinical prognostic factor. Patients older than 1 to 2 years have a worse prognosis than those who are younger [42,43], especially for patients who have disseminated disease at diagnosis. Until recently, an age of 365 days has been used as a surrogate for tumor behavior, although alternative ages have been explored. A review of over 3000 neuroblastoma cases confirmed age as a continuous prognostic variable and identified 460 days as the most prognostic age cutoff [44]. Recent reviews demonstrated that patients up to 18 months of age who are diagnosed with biologically favorable INSS stage 3 and 4 neuroblastoma share the same excellent prognosis with those less than 1 year of age [45–47] and suggests that 18 months may be a more clinically relevant predictor of outcome. These outcomes were achieved with dose-intensive chemotherapy regimens, including myeloablative consolidation therapy as compared with the moderately dosed chemotherapy received by the more biologically favorable patient cohorts. The ability to treat children ages 12 to 18 months of age who have metastatic disease or locoregional disease using less aggressive therapy is under investigation.

Pathology

The pathologic characteristics of neuroblastoma have been used to further classify these tumors as outlined previously. Shimada initially proposed a histology-based classification of tumors into "favorable" and "unfavorable" by combining age with extent of tumor differentiation, presence of a Schwannian stromal components, and degree of mitosis and karyorrhexis [30]. The prognostic impacts of the original Shimada classification and the more recently revised INPC have been validated [30,48]. The inclusion of age, which is a strong independent prognostic variable, has led to consideration for examining cellular proliferation and extent of differentiation as independent variables in future multifactorial clinical and biological classification schemas.

Genetic factors

Neuroblastoma can be divided into those with a near-diploid nuclear DNA content ($\approx 45\%$) and near-triploid tumors ($\approx 55\%$). Near-triploid neuroblastomas are characterized by whole chromosome gains and losses without structural genetic aberrations. Clinically, near-triploid tumors are more often localized and show a favorable outcome. Near-diploid neuroblastomas are characterized by the presence of genetic aberrations, such as *MYCN* amplification, 17q gain, and chromosomal losses (reviewed in references [12,49]). For many genetic, molecular, and clinical factors, a prognostic value has been reported. Recently, a systematic review of prognostic tumor markers in neuroblastoma has been published [50]. Riley and coworkers identified 3415 papers with a sensitive literature search for prognostic factors in neuroblastoma, of which 428 were judged to be relevant. In total, 31 prognostic factors were reported, each in five or more papers. Among these 31 prognostic factors, there were six genetic aberrations listed (ploidy, *MYCN* amplification, chromosome 1 p loss, chromosome 17q gain, chromosome14q loss, and loss of chromosome 11q). Meta-analysis of prognostic markers showed that *MYCN* amplification and DNA ploidy had the strongest prognostic impact. The pooled hazard ratio for a bad outcome (measured by overall survival) for *MYCN* amplification was 5.48 (95% confidence interval, 4.30–6.97) and for DNA near-diploidy was 3.23 (95% confidence interval, 2.08–5.00).

Most neuroblastomas have a nuclear DNA content in the diploid range. Tumors from patients who have lower stages of disease can often be hyperdiploid or near-triploid (reviewed in references [12,49]). DNA content is most prognostic in infants who have neuroblastoma. The Children's Oncology Group is the only collaborative group using ploidy of diagnostic tumor specimen for risk stratification (see Table 3).

Allelic gains and amplifications

The *MYCN* oncogene is present in an increased copy number in 25% to 35% of neuroblastomas. *MYCN* amplification is found in 30% to 40% of stage 3 and 4 neuroblastomas and in only 5% of localized or stage 4s neuroblastomas. *MYCN*-amplified neuroblastomas are characterized by a highly aggressive behavior with unfavorable outcome (reviewed in [12,49]). Some discussion remains on the prognostic value of *MYCN* amplification in the rare cases of completely resected localized neuroblastoma. The unfavorable prognostic value also holds in the prognostically favorable group of infants who have stage 4s neuroblastoma. In *MYCN*-amplified neuroblastomas, loss of chromosome 1 p is almost invariably present [49,51].

Allelic gains

Gain of the entire chromosome 17 or gain of parts of chromosome 17q occur in greater than 60% of neuroblastomas. The partial 17q gain most often results from unbalanced translocation of 17q21–25 to another chromosome (eg, chromosome 1). Partial gain of 17q identifies unfavorable neuroblastoma [52]. Obvious candidate genes on 17q are the NM23 and the BIRC5 (survivin) gene.

Tumor suppressor genes

Loss of tumor suppressor regions is reported in neuroblastomas for many chromosomal regions. The most frequently affected regions are chromosome 1 p (30–40%), 4 p (20%), 1lq (25%), and 14q (25%).

Chromosome 1 p loss occurs more frequently in older children who have stage 3 and 4 neuroblastoma and is correlated with increased serum ferritin and serum lactate dehydrogenase. In almost all samples with $MYCN$ amplification, concomitant 1 p loss is demonstrated, but loss of chromosome 1 p also occurs in $MYCN$ single-copy cases [53]. Several studies have shown that 1 p loss is a strong predictor of outcome [12,49,53]. In the meta-analysis of Riley and colleagues [50], $MYCN$ amplification and ploidy were stronger predictors of outcome, indicating that 1 p loss might best be used to identify high-risk patients in $MYCN$ single-copy tumors.

Chromosome 11q loss is demonstrated in approximately 40% of patients (reviewed in [12,49]). Chromosome 11q loss is inversely correlated with $MYCN$ amplification and therefore identifies an additional high-risk subset of patients characterized by advanced stage, older age, and unfavorable pathology. It has recently become clear that "unbalanced" deletion of 11q (deletion of long-arm material with retention or gain of short-arm material) occurs in 15% to 20% of cases but is more clearly associated with high-risk biologic features [54]. Prospective evaluation of 1 p and 11q status is ongoing in several cooperative group trials and is especially aimed at risk stratification of intermediate-risk patients.

Molecular factors

Despite extensive data correlating genomic alterations with disease outcome, no bona fide target genes have been identified for neuroblastoma, with the exception of $MYCN$ [55]. A number of biological pathways regulating cancer seem to be disrupted or affected in neuroblastoma, including tumor differentiation, apoptosis, drug resistance, angiogenesis, and metastasis. Insight into the molecular regulation of these biological pathways will lead to the identification of novel drug targets.

Because neurotrophin signaling has a central role in normal neuronal development and may be involved in differentiation and regression of neuroblastoma there has been interest in alterations of these pathways. The clinical and biological roles of Trk receptors ($NTRK1$, $NTRK2$, and $NTRK3$ encoding TrkA, TrkB, and TrkC, respectively) and their ligands (NGF, BDNF, and NT-3, respectively) have been extensively investigated. Trk-receptors have been identified as important prognostic factors in neuroblastoma [56,57]. High expression of TrkA is present in neuroblastomas, with favorable biological features and correlates with good outome

[58–61]. By contrast, full-length TrkB is highly expressed in biologically un-favorable, *MYCN*-amplified, aggressive neuroblastomas [56,62]. In neuro-blastoma cell culture models, the biological effects of TrkA include neuronal differentiation or apoptosis, depending on the presence or absence of NGF and on inhibition of proliferation and angiogenesis [63,64]. TrkA signaling might also be related to Phox2B- or Delta-Notch–regulated differ-entiation programs. Depending on the microenvironment, NGF/TrkA signaling could provoke differentiation or regression in favorable neuroblas-tomas [14,65]. This would partly explain spontaneous regression as a delayed activation of developmentally programmed cell death resulting from the ab-sence of NGF in the microenvironment.

Activation of TrkB by its ligand BDNF results in enhanced proliferation, migration, angiogenesis, and chemotherapy resistance of neuroblastoma cells [66]. Differential splicing of Trk receptors results in the expression of truncated receptors lacking the kinase domain [67], which may function as dominant negative inhibitors or scavenger receptors sequestering the ligand [68–70]. Truncated TrkB seems to be preferentially expressed in more differ-entiated tumors [62,71]. Recently, a novel NGF-unresponsive TrkA splice variant has been identified, which is predominantly expressed in clinically aggressive neuroblastomas. This splice variant promotes cell survival, xeno-graft tumor growth, and angiogenesis [72]. Thus, the neurotrophins and their receptors govern numerous cellular functions in neuroblastoma, and the complexity of the signaling responses is reflected in the multiplicity of the pathways involved. More detailed insights into the mechanisms regulat-ing differentiation might suggest new options for treatment.

Delayed activation or disruption of normal apoptotic pathways may be an important phenomenon involved in spontaneous regression and therapy resistance of neuroblastoma. Major elements of the apoptotic signaling cas-cade with abnormal expression or activation patterns include the BCL2 fam-ily, survivin, and caspase-8 [73–76]. The latter is mainly affected by inactivation due to epigenetic silencing. CpG-island hypermethylation of gene promoters is a frequent mechanism for functional inactivation of genes. In neuroblastoma, this mode of inactivation has been demonstrated not only for caspase-8 but also for the four TRAIL apoptosis receptors, the caspase-8 inhibitor FLIP, the RASSF1A tumor suppressor, p73, RB1, DAPK, CD44, p14ARF, and p16INK4a [74,77]. Because many of these genes are involved in apoptotic signaling and therapy responsiveness, gene hypermethylation might be a major event leading to resistance. Therefore, the antitumor effects of demethylating agents, including decitabine, are be-ing investigated in preclinical studies.

Acquired resistance to chemotherapeutic agents may be conferred by en-hanced drug efflux due to overexpression of classical multidrug resistance proteins, including multidrug resistance gene 1 and the gene for multidrug resistance-related protein. Their potential clinical significance in neuroblas-toma has been addressed in several studies [78–81], but their interaction with each other and the role of unknown cofactors remains to be elucidated. Several additional factors have been shown to contribute to treatment resistance in neuroblastoma, including expression of oncogenes such as MYCN, TrkB/BDNF signaling, or loss of p53 expression [66,82,83].

Enhanced tumor angiogenesis and high expression of proangiogenic factors such as vascular endothelial growth factor and basic fibroblast growth factor are correlated with an aggressive phenotype in neuroblastoma [64,84], making angiogenesis inhibitors an attractive treatment option that is being evaluated in preclinical studies. Despite the fact that approximately 50% of patients present with disseminated disease at the time of diagnosis, little is known about the biology of invasion and metastases in neuroblastoma. Major molecular players in the regulation of local invasiveness and metastases are metalloproteinases (mainly MMP9), activating matrix-degrading proteolytic enzymes, and molecules regulating tumor cell adhesion and migration, such as CD44 and NM23-H1 [85–88].

Treatment overview

It is imperative that a multidisciplinary approach to diagnosis and therapy be undertaken for all patients. Tumor tissue obtained through surgical tumor biopsy is almost uniformly required to assess tumor genetic and histologic features. The improved understanding of neuroblastoma biology and its impact on prognosis has resulted in successful tailoring of therapy. The requirement for further surgical resection, chemotherapy, or radiotherapy is based upon a patient's risk stratification with general principles of therapy outlined below. When possible, exposure to chemotherapy is limited to patients who have regional or advanced-stage disease, whereas radiotherapy is limited to patients who have advanced disease and unfavorable biologic characteristics.

Low-risk neuroblastoma

Survival rates for patients who have INSS stage 1 disease, regardless of biologic factors, are excellent with surgery alone. Chemotherapy, when necessary, has been an effective salvage therapy for patients who have INSS stage 1 disease who relapse after surgery only [89,90]. Chemotherapy can be omitted for the majority of patients who have biologically favorable but incompletely resected localized tumors (INSS stage 2A and 2B), with a survival rate greater than 95% [90–93]. For patients who have INSS stage 1, 2A, or 2B disease, chemotherapy should be reserved for those who have localized neuroblastoma and experience life- or organ-threatening symptoms at diagnosis or for the minority of patients who experience recurrent or progressive disease.

Stage 4S neuroblastoma without *MYCN* amplification undergoes spontaneous regression in the majority of cases [34,94]. Chemotherapy or low-dose radiotherapy is reserved for patients who have large tumors or massive hepatomegaly causing mechanical obstruction, respiratory insufficiency, or liver dysfunction [95,96].

Intermediate-risk neuroblastoma

The intermediate-risk classification group encompasses a wide spectrum of disease. Surgical resection and moderate–dose, multiagent chemotherapy are the backbone of therapy. The prognosis for patients who have INSS stage 3 disease or infants who have INSS stage 4 disease is highly dependent upon the tumor's histologic and biologic features. Survival after surgical resection and moderate-dose chemotherapy, including cisplatin, doxorubicin, etoposide, and cyclophosphamide, is greater than 95% for children whose tumors exhibit favorable characteristics [97,98]. To reduce acute and long-term toxicity, international groups have successfully reduced the cumulative exposure to chemotherapy and substituted carboplatin for cisplatin while maintaining excellent survival [99]. These promising results have provided the basis for further reduction in therapy for patients who have intermediate-risk disease. Several small series have brought to question whether chemotherapy could be eliminated for patients who have regional disease and favorable biologic characteristics [100,101]. The challenge is to use more recently identified biologic features to identify patients within this heterogeneous intermediate risk group for whom therapy reduction may not be warranted. Prospective clinical trials in the United States and Europe will integrate additional molecular genetic variables (1 p and 11q allelic status) to further refine risk assessment within the intermediate-risk group.

High-risk neuroblastoma

High-risk neuroblastoma is largely chemotherapy responsive, but, despite improvements in complete response rates, only 30% to 40% of patients survive long term [102]. Standard therapy for patients who have high-risk neuroblastoma involves at least four components: induction, local control, consolidation, and treatment of minimal disease with biologic agents. The use of these four components has evolved over the last 20 years based upon work by the Pediatric Oncology Group, the Children's Cancer Group (CCG), international cooperative groups, and smaller cohort studies, with results summarized below.

Induction therapy

There is a direct correlation between achieving complete tumor response after induction therapy and survival [102]. Standard induction chemotherapy consists of a combination of anthracyclines, alkylators, platinum compounds, and topoisomerase II inhibitors. Escalation in chemotherapy dose intensity may improve initial tumor response rates [103]; however, these results have not been reproduced in multicenter trials [104,105]. An alternative induction strategy is to add noncross-resistant cytotoxic agents into this multiagent chemotherapy backbone. The topoisomerase I inhibitor class of agents, including topotecan, has activity in recurrent neuroblastoma [106] and can be safely combined with multiagent induction chemotherapy [107]. The efficacy of this strategy is being studied in a phase III Children's Oncology Group trial for newly diagnosed neuroblastoma.

Local control

Optimal local control is achieved with a combination of aggressive surgical resection and administration of external-beam radiotherapy to the primary tumor site regardless of response to induction chemotherapy. Resection of the primary tumor and bulky metastatic disease is usually necessary to achieve a chance of cure. Delayed surgical resection after initial induction chemotherapy improves resection of the primary tumor, may improve overall survival, and may minimize acute complications of surgical resection [108].

Neuroblastoma is one of the most radiosensitive solid tumors of childhood [109]. Radiation doses of 2160 cGy in daily 180 cGy fractions administered to the primary tumor site, regardless of initial response to chemotherapy, seem to decrease the risk for local recurrence [33,110,111]. The presence of residual tumor at the time of radiation therapy affects risk for recurrence. A single-institution study suggests that patients undergoing an incomplete resection may benefit from a higher radiation dose [112]. Prospective studies are ongoing to assess whether higher-dose radiation to the volume of residual tumor improves local control rates.

Myeloablative consolidation therapy

Over the past decade, several clinical trials have assessed the efficacy of myeloablative consolidation chemotherapy. The CCG-3891 study demonstrated that myeloablative therapy with purged bone marrow transplant improved outcome for patients who had high-risk neuroblastoma [102]. Trials performed in Germany and Europe similarly demonstrate improved outcome after myeloablative therapy compared with maintenance chemotherapy [113] or observation [114]. Taken together, these data indicate that neuroblastoma is one of the few human cancers in which relapse rates are reduced by myeloablative consolidation in first remission and raise the possibility that further intensification of consolidation therapy may improve outcome. George and colleagues have recently published a 3-year, event-free survival of 55% after a rapid sequential tandem transplant consolidation therapy [115], forming the basis for an ongoing randomized trial comparing single- versus tandem transplant consolidation for high-risk neuroblastoma.

Biologic therapy

The CCG-3891 study demonstrated the efficacy of isotretinoin (cis-RA), a synthetic retinoid, in treating minimal residual neuroblastoma and established a standard for the use of noncytotoxic therapy for the treatment of minimal residual disease [102]. Although cis-RA is the standard of care for postremission induction maintenance therapy, monoclonal antibodies directed against neuroblastoma-specific antigens (gangliosidase, GD2) may provide an additional mechanism to kill residual neuroblastoma cells via antibody-dependant cellular cytotoxicity. Preclinical and clinical trials suggest that lymphocyte-, neutrophil-, or natural killer cell–mediated, antibody-dependent cellular cytotoxicity can be enhanced by coadministration of the cytokines granulocyte/macrophage colony-stimulating factor and interleukin-2 [116,117]. Clinical trials are underway to analyze the efficacy of coadministration of soluble cytokines with anti-GD2 (gangliosidase) monoclonal antibodies or the development of fused anti-GD2/cytokine molecules in the setting of minimal residual disease. Alternative retinoid derivatives, including fenretinide, have been tested and show promising response rates in recurrent disease.

Future directions

Neuroblastoma is a heterogenous tumor for which biology dictates clinical behavior. Further advances in our understanding of the molecular biology of neuroblastoma are supported by the use of high-throughput, array-based methods not only with the goal of patient-tailored prognostication but also to identify key targets that can efficiently be exploited therapeutically. We must continue to refine our ability to better identify the rare patients who have apparent low-risk or intermediate-risk disease who are destined to have a poor outcome. For the remaining patients who have low- and intermediate-risk disease, we must minimize the lasting effects of therapy, specifically avoiding organ damage or organ loss from surgery and organ dysfunction or risk for secondary malignancy after chemotherapy. Likewise, it is imperative that we use the mounting knowledge of neuroblastoma tumor biology toward the development of novel therapies for high-risk neuroblastoma. Several rationally chosen biologic agents are in ongoing clinical trials for recurrent neuroblastoma, including histone deacetylase inhibitors, Trk tyrosine kinase inhibitors, and anti-angiogenic agents. If effective, these agents will be moved into front-line therapy and may improve induction response. Alternatively, they may be used to optimize treatment of minimal residual disease.

References

[1] Stiller CA, Parkin DM. International variations in the incidence of neuroblastoma. Int J Cancer 1992;52(4):538–43.

[2] Kushner BH, Gilbert F, Helson L. Familial neuroblastoma: case reports, literature review, and etiologic considerations. Cancer 1986;57(9):1887–93.

[3] Belson M, Kingsley B, Holmes A. Risk factors for acute leukemia in children: a review. Environ Health Perspect 2007;115(1):138–45.

[4] Connelly JM, Malkin MG. Environmental risk factors for brain tumors. Curr Neurol Neurosci Rep May 2007;7(3):208–14.

[5] Yamamoto K, Hayashi Y, Hanada R, et al. Mass screening and age-specific incidence of neuroblastoma in Saitama Prefecture, Japan. J Clin Oncol 1995;13(8):2033–8.

[6] Kaneko Y, Kanda N, Maseki N, et al. Current urinary mass screening for catecholamine metabolites at 6 months of age may be detecting only a small portion of high-risk neuroblastomas: a chromosome and N-myc amplification study. J Clin Oncol 1990;8(12):2005–13.

[7] Schilling FH, Spix C, Berthold F, et al. Neuroblastoma screening at one year of age. N Engl J Med 2002;346(14):1047–53.

[8] Woods WG, Gao RN, Shuster JJ, et al. Screening of infants and mortality due to neuroblastoma. N Engl J Med 2002;346(14):1041–6.

[9] Clausen N, Andersson P, Tommerup N. Familial occurrence of neuroblastoma, von Recklinghausen's neurofibromatosis, Hirschsprung's agangliosis and jaw-winking syndrome. Acta Paediatr Scand 1989;78(5):736–41.

[10] Rohrer T, Trachsel D, Engelcke G, et al. Congenital central hypoventilation syndrome associated with Hirschsprung's disease and neuroblastoma: case of multiple neurocristopathies. Pediatr Pulmonol 2002;33(1):71–6.

[11] Trochet D, O'Brien LM, Gozal D, et al. PHOX2B genotype allows for prediction of tumor risk in congenital central hypoventilation syndrome. Am J Hum Genet 2005;76(3):421–6.

[12] Brodeur GM. Neuroblastoma: biological insights into a clinical enigma. Nat Rev Cancer 2003;3(3):203–16.

[13] Trochet D, Bourdeaut F, Janoueix-Lerosey I, et al. Germline mutations of the paired-like homeobox 2B (PHOX2B) gene in neuroblastoma. Am J Hum Genet 2004;74(4):761–4.

[14] van Limpt V, Schramm A, van Lakeman A, et al. The Phox2B homeobox gene is mutated in sporadic neuroblastomas. Oncogene 2004;23(57):9280–8.

[15] Longo L, Panza E, Schena F, et al. Genetic predisposition to familial neuroblastoma: identification of two novel genomic regions at 2p and 12p. Hum Hered 2007;63(3–4):205–11.

[16] Tonini GP, McConville C, Cusano R, et al. Exclusion of candidate genes and chromosomal regions in familial neuroblastoma. Int J Mol Med 2001;7(1):85–9.

[17] Maris JM, Kyemba SM, Rebbeck TR, et al. Familial predisposition to neuroblastoma does not map to chromosome band 1p36. Cancer Res 1996;56(15):3421–5.

[18] Maris JM, Weiss MJ, Mosse Y, et al. Evidence for a hereditary neuroblastoma predisposition locus at chromosome 16p12-13. Cancer Res 2002;62(22):6651–8.

[19] Triche TJ. Neuroblastoma: biology confronts nosology. Arch Pathol Lab Med 1986;110(11):994–6.

[20] Mosse YP, Laudenslager M, Khazi D, et al. Germline PHOX2B mutation in hereditary neuroblastoma. Am J Hum Genet 2004;75(4):727–30.

[21] O'Brien CA, Pollett A, Gallinger S, et al. A human colon cancer cell capable of initiating tumour growth in immunodeficient mice. Nature 2007;445(7123):106–10.

[22] Singh SK, Hawkins C, Clarke ID, et al. Identification of human brain tumour initiating cells. Nature 2004;432(7015):396–401.

[23] Tirode F, Laud-Duval K, Prieur A, et al. Mesenchymal stem cell features of Ewing tumors. Cancer Cell 2007;11(5):421–9.

[24] Allenspach EJ, Maillard I, Aster JC, et al. Notch signaling in cancer. Cancer Biol Ther 2002;1(5):466–76.

[25] Blanc E, Goldschneider D, Douc-Rasy S, et al. Wnt-5a gene expression in malignant human neuroblasts. Cancer Letters 2005;228(1–2):117–23.

[26] Taipale J, Beachy PA. The Hedgehog and Wnt signalling pathways in cancer. Nature 2001;411(6835):349–54.

[27] Russell D, Rubinstein L. Pathology of tumours of the nervous system. London: Edward Arnold; 1989.

[28] Beckwith J, Perrin E. In situ neuroblastomas: a contribution to the natural history of neural crest tumors. Am J Pathol 1963;43:1089–104.

[29] Shimada H, Ambros IM, Dehner LP, et al. The International Neuroblastoma Pathology Classification (the Shimada system). Cancer 1999;86(2):364–72.

[30] Shimada H, Chatten J, Newton W Jr, et al. Histophatologic prognostic factors in neuroblastic tumors: definition of subtypes of ganglineuroblastoma and an age-linked classification of neuroblastomas. J Natl Cancer Inst 1984;73:405–16.

[31] Peuchmaur M, d'Amore ES, Joshi VV, et al. Revision of the international neuroblastoma pathology classification: confirmation of favorable and unfavorable prognostic subsets in ganglioneuroblastoma, nodular. Cancer 2003;98(10):2274–81.

[32] de Bernardi B, Rogers D, Carli M, et al. Localized neuroblastoma: surgical and pathologic staging. Cancer 1987;60(5):1066–72.

[33] Haas-Kogan DA, Swift PS, Selch M, et al. Impact of radiotherapy for high-risk neuroblastoma: a Children's Cancer Group study. Int J Radiat Oncol Biol Phys 2003;56(1):28–39.

[34] Evans AE, Chatten J, D'Angio GJ, et al. A review of 17 IV-S neuroblastoma patients at the Children's Hospital of Philadelphia. Cancer 1980;45(5):833–9.

[35] Brodeur GM, Pritchard J, Berthold F, et al. Revisions of the international criteria for neuroblastoma diagnosis, staging, and response to treatment. J Clin Oncol 1993;11(8): 1466–77.

[36] Brodeur GM, Seeger RC, Barrett A, et al. International criteria for diagnosis, staging, and response to treatment in patients with neuroblastoma. J Clin Oncol 1988;6(12):1874–81.

[37] Messina JA, Cheng SC, Franc BL, et al. Evaluation of semi-quantitative scoring system for metaiodobenzylguanidine (mIBG) scans in patients with relapsed neuroblastoma. Pediatr Blood Cancer 2006;47(7):865–74.

[38] Castleberry RP, Shuster JJ, Smith EI. The pediatric oncology group experience with the international staging system criteria for neuroblastoma. Member Institutions of the Pediatric Oncology Group. J Clin Oncol 1994;12(11):2378–81.

[39] Haase GM, Atkinson JB, Stram DO, et al. Surgical management and outcome of locoregional neuroblastoma: comparison of the Childrens Cancer Group and the international staging systems. J Pediatr Surg 1995;30(2):289–94 [discussion: 295].

[40] Cecchetto G, Mosseri V, De Bernardi B, et al. Surgical risk factors in primary surgery for localized neuroblastoma: the LNESG1 study of the European International Society of Pediatric Oncology Neuroblastoma Group. J Clin Oncol 2005;23(33):8483–9.

[41] Cohn SL, London W, Monclair T, Matthay KK, Ambros PF, Pearson AD. Update on the development of the international neuroblastoma risk group. Presented at the 43rd Annual Meeting of the American Society of Clinical Oncology. Chicago, June 2–6, 2007.

[42] Breslow N, McCann B. Statistical estimation of prognosis for children with neuroblastoma. Cancer Res 1971;31(12):2098–103.

[43] Evans AE. Staging and treatment of neuroblastoma. Cancer 1980;45(Suppl 7):1799–802.

[44] London WB, Castleberry RP, Matthay KK, et al. Evidence for an age cutoff greater than 365 days for neuroblastoma risk group stratification in the Children's Oncology Group. J Clin Oncol 2005;23(27):6459–65.

[45] George RE, London WB, Cohn SL, et al. Hyperdiploidy plus nonamplified MYCN confers a favorable prognosis in children 12 to 18 months old with disseminated neuroblastoma: a Pediatric Oncology Group study. J Clin Oncol 2005;23(27):6466–73.

[46] Schmidt ML, Lal A, Seeger RC, et al. Favorable prognosis for patients 12 to 18 months of age with stage 4 nonamplified MYCN neuroblastoma: a Children's Cancer Group Study. J Clin Oncol 2005;23(27):6474–80.

[47] Park J, Villablanca J, Seeger R, et al. Favorable outcome of high risk (HR) stage 3 neuroblastoma (NB) with myeloablative therapy and 13-cis-retinoic acid. Presented at the 41st Annual Meeting of American Society of Oncology. Orlando, Florida, May 13–17, 2005.

[48] Shimada H, Stram DO, Chatten J, et al. Identification of subsets of neuroblastomas by combined histopathologic and N-myc analysis. J Natl Cancer Inst 1995;87(19): 1470–6.

[49] Maris JM. The biologic basis for neuroblastoma heterogeneity and risk stratification. Curr Opin Pediatr 2005;17(1):7–13.

[50] Riley RD, Heney D, Jones DR, et al. A systematic review of molecular and biological tumor markers in neuroblastoma. Clin Cancer Res 2004;10(1 Pt 1):4–12.

[51] Westermann F, Schwab M. Genetic parameters of neuroblastomas. Cancer Lett 2002; 184(2):127–47.

[52] Bown N, Cotterill S, Lastowska M, et al. Gain of chromosome arm 17q and adverse outcome in patients with neuroblastoma. N Engl J Med 1999;340(25):1954–61.

[53] Caron H, van Sluis P, de Kraker J, et al. Allelic loss of chromosome 1p as a predictor of unfavorable outcome in patients with neuroblastoma. N Engl J Med 1996;334(4): 225–30.

[54] Attiyeh EF, London WB, Mosse YP, et al. Chromosome 1p and 11q deletions and outcome in neuroblastoma. N Engl J Med 2005;353(21):2243–53.

[55] Maris JM, Hogarty MD, Bagatell R, et al. Neuroblastoma. Lancet 2007;369(9579): 2106–20.

[56] Nakagawara A, Azar CG, Scavarda NJ, et al. Expression and function of Trk-B and BDNF in human neuroblastomas. Mol Cell Biol 1994;14:759–67.

[57] Nakagawara A, Arima-Nakagawara M, Scavarda NJ, et al. Association between high levels of expression of the Trk gene and favorable outcome in human neuroblastomas. N Engl J Med 1993;328:847–54.

[58] Combaret V, Gross N, Lasset C, et al. Clinical relevance of CD44 cell surface expression and MYCN gene amplification in neuroblastoma. Eur J Cancer 1997;33(12):2101–5.

[59] Borrello MG, Bongarzone I, Pierotti MA, et al. TRK and RET protooncogene expression in human neuroblastoma specimens: high frequency of Trk expression in non-advanced stages. Int J Cancer 1993;54:540–5.

[60] Kogner P, Barbany G, Dominici C, et al. Coexpression of messenger RNA for Trk protooncogene and low affinity nerve growth factor receptor in neuroblastomas with favorable prognosis. Cancer Res 1993;53:2044–50.

[61] Suzuki T, Bogenmann E, Shimada H, et al. Lack of high affinity nerve growth factor receptors in aggressive neuroblastomas. J Natl Cancer Inst 1993;85:377–84.

[62] Aoyama M, Asai K, Shishikura T, et al. Human neuroblastomas with unfavorable biologies express high levels of brain-derived neurotrophic factor mRNA and a variety of its variants. Cancer Lett 2001;164(1):51–60.

[63] Eggert A, Grotzer MA, Ikegaki N, et al. Expression of the neurotrophin receptor TrkA down-regulates expression and function of angiogenic stimulators in SH-SY5Y neuroblastoma cells. Cancer Res 2002;62(6):1802–8.

[64] Eggert A, Ikegaki N, Kwiatkowski J, et al. High-level expression of angiogenic factors is associated with advanced tumor stage in human neuroblastomas. Clin Cancer Res 2000; 6:1900–8.

[65] van Limpt V, Chan A, Schramm A, et al. Phox2B mutations and the Delta-Notch pathway in neuroblastoma. Cancer Lett 2005;228(1–2):59–63.

[66] Ho R, Eggert A, Hishiki T, et al. Resistance to chemotherapy mediated by TrkB in neuroblastomas. Cancer Res 2002;62(22):6462–6.

[67] Barbacid M. The trk family of neurotrophin receptors. J Neurobiol 1994;25:1386–403.

[68] Biffo S, Offenhauser N, Carter BD, et al. Selective binding and internalisation by truncated receptors restrict the availability of BDNF during development. Development 1995;121(8): 2461–70.

[69] Eide FF, Vining ER, Eide BL, et al. Naturally occurring truncated trkB receptors have dominant inhibitory effects on brain-derived neurotrophic factor signaling. J Neurosci 1996;16(10):3123–9.

[70] Haapasalo A, Koponen E, Hoppe E, et al. Truncated trkB.T1 is dominant negative inhibitor of trkB.TK+-mediated cell survival. Biochem Biophys Res Commun 2001;280(5): 1352–8.

[71] Brodeur GM, Nakagawara A, Yamashiro D, et al. Expression of TrkA, TrkB and TrkC in human neuroblastomas. J Neurooncol 1997;31:49–55.

[72] Tacconelli A, Farina AR, Cappabianca L, et al. TrkA alternative splicing: a regulated tumor-promoting switch in human neuroblastoma. Cancer Cell 2004;6(4):347–60.

[73] Castle VP, Heidelberger KP, Bromberg J, et al. Expression of the apoptosis-suppressing protein bcl-2, in neuroblastoma is associated with unfavorable histology and N-myc amplification. Am J Pathol 1993;143(6):1543–50.

[74] Eggert A, Grotzer MA, Zuzak TJ, et al. Resistance to tumor necrosis factor-related apoptosis-inducing ligand (TRAIL)-induced apoptosis in neuroblastoma cells correlates with a loss of caspase-8 expression. Cancer Res 2001;61(4):1314–9.

[75] Hopkins-Donaldson S, Bodmer JL, Bourloud KB, et al. Loss of caspase-8 expression in highly malignant human neuroblastoma cells correlates with resistance to tumor necrosis factor-related apoptosis-inducing ligand-induced apoptosis. Cancer Res 2000;60(16): 4315–9.

[76] Teitz T, Wei T, Valentine MB, et al. Caspase 8 is deleted or silenced preferentially in childhood neuroblastomas with amplification of MYCN. Nat Med 2000;6(5):529–35.

[77] van Noesel MM, van Bezouw S, Salomons GS, et al. Tumor-specific down-regulation of the tumor necrosis factor-related apoptosis-inducing ligand decoy receptors DcR1 and DcR2 is associated with dense promoter hypermethylation. Cancer Res 2002;62(7): 2157–61.

[78] Chan HS, Haddad G, Thorner PS, et al. P-glycoprotein expression as a predictor of the outcome of therapy for neuroblastoma. N Engl J Med 1991;325(23):1608–14.

[79] Goldstein LJ, Fojo AT, Ueda K, et al. Expression of the multidrug resistance, MDR1, gene in neuroblastomas. J Clin Oncol 1990;8(1):128–36.

[80] Haber M, Smith J, Bordow SB, et al. Association of high-level MRP1 expression with poor clinical outcome in a large prospective study of primary neuroblastoma. J Clin Oncol 2006; 24(10):1546–53.

[81] Norris MD, Bordow SB, Marshall GM, et al. Expression of the gene for multidrug-resistance-associated protein and outcome in patients with neuroblastoma. N Engl J Med 1996;334(4):231–8.

[82] Jaboin J, Kim CJ, Kaplan DR, et al. Brain-derived neurotrophic factor activation of TrkB protects neuroblastoma cells from chemotherapy-induced apoptosis via phosphatidylinositol 3'-kinase pathway. Cancer Res 2002;62(22):6756–63.

[83] Scala S, Wosikowski K, Giannakakou P, et al. Brain-derived neurotrophic factor protects neuroblastoma cells from vinblastine toxicity. Cancer Res 1996;56:3737–42.

[84] Meitar D, Crawford SE, Rademaker AW, et al. Tumor angiogenesis correlates with metastatic disease, N-myc amplification, and poor outcome in human neuroblastoma. J Clin Oncol 1996;14:405–14.

[85] Almgren MA, Henriksson KC, Fujimoto J, et al. Nucleoside diphosphate kinase A/nm23-H1 promotes metastasis of NB69-derived human neuroblastoma. Mol Cancer Res 2004; 2(7):387–94.

[86] Chantrain CF, Shimada H, Jodele S, et al. Stromal matrix metalloproteinase-9 regulates the vascular architecture in neuroblastoma by promoting pericyte recruitment. Cancer Res 2004;64(5):1675–86.

[87] Gross N, Balmas Bourloud K, Brognara CB. MYCN-related suppression of functional CD44 expression enhances tumorigenic properties of human neuroblastoma cells. Exp Cell Res 2000;260(2):396–403.

[88] Jodele S, Chantrain CF, Blavier L, et al. The contribution of bone marrow-derived cells to the tumor vasculature in neuroblastoma is matrix metalloproteinase-9 dependent. Cancer Res 2005;65(8):3200–8.

[89] Alvarado CS, London WB, Look AT, et al. Natural history and biology of stage A neuroblastoma: a Pediatric Oncology Group Study. J Pediatr Hematol Oncol 2000;22(3): 197–205.

[90] Perez CA, Matthay KK, Atkinson JB, et al. Biologic variables in the outcome of stages I and II neuroblastoma treated with surgery as primary therapy: a children's cancer group study. J Clin Oncol 2000;18(1):18–26.

[91] Simon T, Spitz R, Faldum A, et al. New definition of low-risk neuroblastoma using stage, age, and 1p and MYCN status. J Pediatr Hematol Oncol 2004;26(12):791–6.

[92] Simon T, Spitz R, Hero B, et al. Risk estimation in localized unresectable single copy MYCN neuroblastoma by the status of chromosomes 1p and 11q. Cancer Lett 2006; 237(2):215–22.

[93] Strother DR, London W, Schmidt ML, et al. Surgery alone or followed by chemotherapy for patients with stages 2A and 2B neuroblastoma: results of Children's Oncology Group Study P9641. Presented at the 12th meeting of Advances in Neuroblastoma Research. Los Angeles, May 18–20, 2006.

[94] D'Angio GJ, Evans AE, Koop CE. Special pattern of widespread neuroblastoma with a favourable prognosis. Lancet 1971;1(7708):1046–9.

[95] Nickerson HJ, Matthay KK, Seeger RC, et al. Favorable biology and outcome of stage IV-S neuroblastoma with supportive care or minimal therapy: a Children's Cancer Group study. J Clin Oncol 2000;18(3):477–86.

[96] Katzenstein HM, Bowman LC, Brodeur GM, et al. Prognostic significance of age, MYCN oncogene amplification, tumor cell ploidy, and histology in 110 infants with stage D(S) neuroblastoma: the pediatric oncology group experience–a pediatric oncology group study. J Clin Oncol 1998;16(6):2007–17.

[97] Matthay KK, Perez C, Seeger RC, et al. Successful treatment of stage III neuroblastoma based on prospective biologic staging: a Children's Cancer Group study. J Clin Oncol 1998;16(4):1256–64.

[98] Schmidt ML, Lukens JN, Seeger RC, et al. Biologic factors determine prognosis in infants with stage IV neuroblastoma: a prospective Children's Cancer Group study. J Clin Oncol Mar 2000;18(6):1260–8.

[99] Baker DL, Schmidt ML, Cohn SL, et al. A phase III trial of biologically-based therapy reduction for intermediate risk neuroblastoma. Presented at the 43rd Annual meeting of the American Society of Clinical Oncology. Chicago, June 2–6, 2007.

[100] Kushner BH, Cheung NK, LaQuaglia MP, et al. Survival from locally invasive or widespread neuroblastoma without cytotoxic therapy. J Clin Oncol 1996;14(2):373–81.

[101] Hero B, Thorsten S, Benz-Bohm G, et al. Is a "wait and see" strategy justified in localised neuroblastoma in infancy? Presented at the 12th meeting of Advances in Neuroblastoma Research. Los Angeles, May 18–20, 2006.

[102] Matthay KK, Villablanca JG, Seeger RC, et al. Treatment of high-risk neuroblastoma with intensive chemotherapy, radiotherapy, autologous bone marrow transplantation, and 13-cis-retinoic acid. Children's Cancer Group. N Engl J Med 1999;341(16):1165–73.

[103] Kushner BH, LaQuaglia MP, Bonilla MA, et al. Highly effective induction therapy for stage 4 neuroblastoma in children over 1 year of age. J Clin Oncol 1994;12(12):2607–13.

[104] Valteau-Couanet D, Michon J, Boneu A, et al. Results of induction chemotherapy in children older than 1 year with a stage 4 neuroblastoma treated with the NB 97 French Society of Pediatric Oncology (SFOP) protocol. J Clin Oncol 2005;23(3):532–40.

[105] Kreissman SG, Villablanca JG, Diller L, et al. Response and toxicity to a dose-intensive multi-agent chemotherapy induction regimen for high risk neuroblastoma: a Children's Oncology Group study. Presented at the 43rd Annual meeting of the American Society of Clinical Oncology. Chicago, June 2–6, 2007.

[106] Frantz CN, London WB, Diller L, et al. Recurrent neuroblastoma: randomized treatment with topotecan + cyclophosphamide (T + C) vs. topotecan alone(T). A POG/CCG Intergroup Study. J Clin Oncol 2004;22(14S):8512.

[107] Park JR, Stewart CF, London W, et al. Targeted topotecan during induction therapy of high risk neuroblastoma : A Children's Oncology Group pilot study. Presented at the 42nd annual meeting of the American Society of Clinical Oncology. Atlanta, Georgia, June 2–6, 2006.

[108] Adkins ES, Sawin R, Gerbing RB, et al. Efficacy of complete resection for high-risk neuroblastoma: a Children's Cancer Group study. J Pediatr Surg 2004;39(6):931–6.

[109] Brodeur GM, Maris JM. Neuroblastoma. 4th edition. Philadelphia: Lippincott; 2002.

[110] Kushner BH, Wolden S, LaQuaglia MP, et al. Hyperfractionated low-dose radiotherapy for high-risk neuroblastoma after intensive chemotherapy and surgery. J Clin Oncol 2001;19(11):2821–8.

[111] Bradfield SM, Douglas JG, Hawkins DS, et al. Fractionated low-dose radiotherapy after myeloablative stem cell transplantation for local control in patients with high-risk neuroblastoma. Cancer 2004;100(6):1268–75.

[112] Simon T, Bongartz R, Hero B, et al. Intensified external beam radiation therapy improves the outcome of stage 4 neuroblastoma in children > 1 year with residual local disease [abstract: 314]. Advances in Neuroblastoma Research 2006.

[113] Berthold F, Boos J, Burdach S, et al. Myeloablative megatherapy with autologous stem-cell rescue versus oral maintenance chemotherapy as consolidation treatment in patients with high-risk neuroblastoma: a randomised controlled trial. Lancet Oncol 2005;6(9):649–58.

[114] Pritchard J, Cotterill SJ, Germond SM, et al. High dose melphalan in the treatment of advanced neuroblastoma: results of a randomised trial (ENSG-1) by the European Neuroblastoma Study Group. Pediatr Blood Cancer 2005;44(4):348–57.

[115] George RE, Li S, Medeiros-Nancarrow C, et al. High-risk neuroblastoma treated with tandem autologous peripheral-blood stem cell-supported transplantation: long-term survival update. J Clin Oncol 2006;24(18):2891–6.

[116] Albertini MR, Gan J, Jaeger P, et al. Systemic interleukin-2 modulates the anti-idiotypic response to chimeric anti-GD2 antibody in patients with melanoma. J Immunother Emphasis Tumor Immunol 1996;19(4):278–95.

[117] Hank JA, Surfus J, Gan J, et al. Treatment of neuroblastoma patients with antiganglioside GD2 antibody plus interleukin-2 induces antibody-dependent cellular cytotoxicity against neuroblastoma detected in vitro. J Immunother 1994;15(1):29–37.

[118] Roberts KB. Cerebellar ataxia and "occult neuroblastoma" without opsoclonus. Pediatrics 1975;56(3):464–5.

[119] Altman AJ, Baehner RL. Favorable prognosis for survival in children with coincident opso-myoclonus and neuroblastoma. Cancer 1976;37(2):846–52.

[120] Matthay KK, Blaes F, Hero B, et al. Opsoclonus myoclonus syndrome in neuroblastoma: a report from a workshop on the dancing eyes syndrome at the advances in neuroblastoma meeting in Genoa, Italy. Cancer Lett 2005;228(1–2):275–82.

[121] Scheibel E, Rechnitzer C, Fahrenkrug J, et al. Vasoactive intestinal polypeptide (VIP) in children with neural crest tumours. Acta Paediatr Scand 1982;71(5):721–5.

[122] El Shafie M, Samuel D, Klippel CH, et al. Intractable diarrhea in children with VIP-secreting ganglioneuroblastomas. J Pediatr Surg 1983;18(1):34–6.

ELSEVIER
SAUNDERS

PEDIATRIC CLINICS
OF NORTH AMERICA

Pediatr Clin N Am 55 (2008) 121–145

Central Nervous System Tumors

Roger J. Packer, MD[a,b,c,d,*],
Tobey MacDonald, MD[c,d,e], Gilbert Vezina, MD[c,d,f]

[a]Center for Neuroscience and Behavioral Medicine, Children's National Medical Center,
111 Michigan Avenue, Washington, DC 20010, USA
[b]Division of Neurology, Children's National Medical Center, 111 Michigan Avenue,
Washington, DC 20010, USA
[c]The Brain Tumor Institute, Children's National Medical Center, Children's National
Medical Center, 111 Michigan Avenue, Washington, DC 20010, USA
[d]The George Washington University School of Medicine and Health Sciences,
Washington, DC, USA
[e]Division of Oncology, Center for Cancer and Blood Disorders, Center for Cancer
and Immunology Research, Children's National Medical Center,
111 Michigan Avenue NW, Washington, DC 20010, USA
[f]Department of Radiology, Children's National Medical Center, 111 Michigan Avenue NW,
Washington, DC 20010, USA

Central nervous system (CNS) tumors comprise 15% to 20% of all malignancies occurring in childhood and adolescence [1]. Despite being relatively common, they only occur in between 2500 to 3500 children in the United States each year and may present in a myriad of ways, often delaying diagnosis. Symptoms and signs depend on the growth rate of the tumor, its location in the central nervous system (CNS), and the age of the child. Childhood brain tumors demonstrate greater histological variation, are more likely to be disseminated at the time of diagnosis, and more frequently are embryonal than those arising in adults [1].

The etiology for most childhood brain and spinal cord tumors is unknown. Specific syndromes are associated with a higher incidence of tumors [2]. Patients who have neurofibromatosis type 1 (NF-1) have a higher incidence of low-grade gliomas, including visual pathway gliomas and other types of CNS tumors [3]. Children who have tuberous sclerosis are prone to harbor giant-cell astrocytomas [4], and those who have the Li-Fraumeni syndrome have an increased predisposition to various different tumors including

---

* Corresponding author. Department of Neurology, Children's National Medical Center,
111 Michigan Avenue, NW, Washington, DC 20010.
  E-mail address: rpacker@cnmc.org (R.J. Packer).

0031-3955/08/$ - see front matter © 2008 Elsevier Inc. All rights reserved.
doi:10.1016/j.pcl.2007.10.010   pediatric.theclinics.com

gliomas [5]. Rarer conditions, such as the autosomally dominant inherited nevoid basal cell carcinoma syndrome (Gorlin syndrome) and the recessively inherited Turcot's syndrome (germ line mutation of the adenomatosis polyposis coli gene) are associated with an increased incidence of medulloblastoma [6,7]. Exposure to radiation therapy has been the only environmental factor consistently related to the development of brain tumors [8].

Presentation

Approximately one-half of all childhood brain tumors arise in the posterior fossa (Table 1) [1]. The five major tumor types that arise subtentorially may present with focal neurologic deficits, but those filling the fourth ventricle are as likely to come to clinical attention because of obstruction of cerebrospinal fluid with associated hydrocephalus. The classical triad associated with increased intracranial pressure of morning headaches, nausea, and vomiting, may occur, but nonspecific headaches are more frequent. In infants, cerebrospinal fluid obstruction with dilatation of the third ventricle and the resultant tectal pressure causes paresis of upgaze may result in downward deviation of the eyes, the setting sun sign.

The suprasellar and pineal regions are relatively frequent sites for supratentorial childhood brain tumors [1,9]. Tumors in the suprasellar region, primarily craniopharyngiomas, visual pathway gliomas, and germinomas, may present with complex visual findings including unilateral or bilateral decreased visual acuity and hard to characterize visual field loss, as well as hormonal dysfunction. In the pineal region, various different tumor types may occur in the pediatric years, including germinomas, mixed germ cell tumors, pineoblastomas, and lower-grade pineocytomas. Pineal region lesions characteristically cause compression or destruction of the tectal region of the brain stem, and result in Parinaud's syndrome, manifested by paralysis or paresis of upgaze, retraction or convergence nystagmus, pupils that react better to accommodation than light, and lid retraction. Most cortical childhood tumors are gliomas, usually low-grade, but they are anaplastic in approximately 20% of cases. Other tumor types (supratentorial primitive neuroectodermal tumors and ependymomas) may occur. Unlike the situation in adulthood, pediatric low-grade gliomas do not mutate frequently to higher-grade gliomas during childhood. In younger children, large benign supratentorial lesions, such as diffuse infantile gangliogliomas/gliomas and dysembryoplastic neuroepithelial tumors may be misdiagnosed as more aggressive lesions.

Diagnosis

The diagnosis of pediatric brain and spinal cord tumors has been simplified by advances in neuroimaging [10]. Because of the speed and availability of CT, it is often the first imaging technique obtained for children with

Table 1
Posterior-Fossa tumors of childhood

Tumor	Relative incidence	Presentation	Diagnosis	Prognosis
Medulloblastoma	35% to 40%	2–3 months of headaches, vomiting, truncal ataxia	Heterogeneous or homogeneously enhancing fourth ventricular mass; may be disseminated	65% to 85% survival; dependent on stage/type; poorer (20% to 70%) in infants
Cerebellar astrocytoma	35% to 40%	3–6 months of limb ataxia; secondary headaches, vomiting	Cerebellar hemisphere mass, usually with cystic and solid (mural nodule) components	90% to 100% in totally resected pilocytic type
Brain stem glioma	10% to 15%	1–4 months of double vision, unsteadiness, weakness, and other cranial nerve deficits, facial weakness, swallowing deficits, and other deficits	Diffusely expanded, minimally or partially enhancing mass in 80%; 20% more focal tectal or cervicomedullary lesion	90% + 18-month mortality in diffuse tumors; better in localized
Ependymoma	10% to 15%	2–5 months of unsteadiness, headaches, double vision, and facial asymmetry	Usually enhancing, fourth ventricular mass with cerebellopontine predilection	75% + survival in totally resected lesions
Atypical Teratoid/Rhabdoid	>5 (10% to 15% of infantile malignant tumors)	As in medulloblastoma, but primarily in infants; often associated facial weakness and strabismus	As in medulloblastoma, but often more laterally extended	10% to 20% (or less) survival in infants

suspected intracranial pathology and, if properly done, CT will detect 95% or more of brain tumors. Because of the superior image contrast of MRI, however, it is essential in the diagnosis of brain tumors, and its multiplanar capabilities offer far superior tumor localization. Based on clinical and neuroradiographic findings, brain tumors have characteristic presentations, especially those arising in the posterior fossa (Fig. 1). Other MRI techniques such as magnetic resonance spectroscopy, which supplements anatomic findings with biochemical data and possibly, in the future, diffusion tensor imaging, especially tractography, may aid in characterizing the type of tumor and its anatomic interrelationships.

For the diagnosis of spinal cord tumors or determination of leptomeningeal dissemination of tumors, spinal MRI has supplanted all other techniques, including myelography or CT studies. In attempts to avoid postoperative artifacts, an MRI of the entire neurospinal axis often is undertaken before surgery in patients who have presumed malignant tumors.

In selected cases, positron emission tomography (PET) scanning may provide additional information, but it is usually most useful in supplying baseline diagnostic information, as a means to follow the tumor over time. PET is most helpful in the determination of transformation of a lower-grade tumor (primarily glial) to a higher-grade neoplasm and the separation of post-therapy, especially postradiation, treatment effects from tumor progression.

Classification

Because of the histologic variability of childhood brain and spinal cord tumors, classification is often difficult and, at times, subjective [11]. In most cases, diagnosis continues to be made predominantly upon light

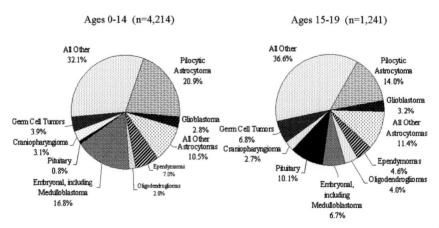

Fig. 1. Distribution of childhood primary brain and other central nervous system tumors by histology from the Central Brain Tumor Registry of the United States (CBTRUS) 1998–2002.

microscopy findings. In selective situations, such as in embryonal tumors, especially atypically teratoid/rhabdoid lesions, immunohistochemistry has aided diagnosis greatly. Although the molecular underpinnings of childhood brain tumors increasingly have been unraveled, molecular techniques have not been incorporated extensively into most classification systems. Evaluation of the mitotic activity of the tumor, assessed by mitotic indices, usually does not change classification, but may be helpful, in selected situations, in determining prognosis and approach to therapy.

Specific tumor types

Discussions of the biology of the tumor, its growth pattern, management, and prognosis are discussed best within individual tumor types. For most tumors, the same modalities of treatment are used (ie, surgery, radiation, and in an increasing number of patients chemotherapy), but the use of each of these types of treatment is not only dependent on the type of tumor present, but also on its location in the CNS tumor and the age of the child. Biologic therapies are just being introduced into management, and to date, have been reserved primarily for those patients who fail initial treatment.

Medulloblastoma

Medulloblastoma, which by definition arises in the posterior fossa, is the most common malignant brain tumor of childhood (Fig. 2a). Medulloblastomas usually are diagnosed in children less than 15 years of age, and they have a bimodal distribution, peaking at 3 to 4 years of age and then again between 8 and 9 years of age [12]. For unknown reasons, there is a male predominance [12]. Ten percent to 15% of patients are diagnosed in infancy. The classical, or undifferentiated, type of medulloblastoma, comprising 70% or more of medulloblastomas, is composed of densely packed cells with hyperchromatic, round, oval, or carrot-shaped nuclei and minimal cytoplasm [11]. The large-cell, or anaplastic variant, which has pleomorphic nuclei, prominent nucleoli and more abundant cytoplasm, as well as possibly higher mitotic and apoptotic indices, increasingly has been recognized and may carry a poorer prognosis [13]. By contrast, the desmoplastic, at times nodular, medulloblastoma variant seems more responsive to therapy and may have a better prognosis [14].

Biology

Medulloblastoma is thought to originate from a primitive cell type in the cerebellum, arising from one of the two cerebellar germinal zones, the ventricular zone that forms the innermost boundary of the cerebellum or the external germinal layer that lines the outside of the cerebellum [15]. The

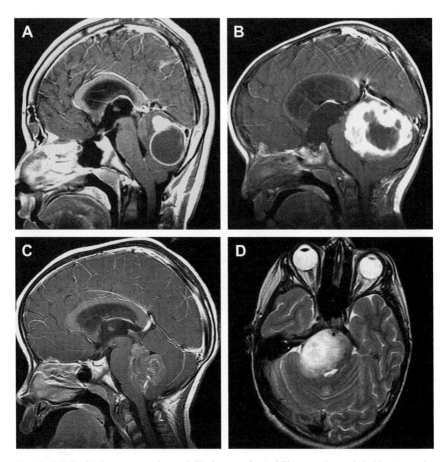

Fig. 2. (*A*) Sagittal contrast-enhanced T1 image of a midline, cystic medulloblastoma. An enhancing solid nodule is seen superiorly within the vermis; the cystic component (with a thin enhancing wall) is inferior. (*B*) Sagittal contrast-enhanced T1 image of a midline, mixed solid–cystic pilocytic astrocytoma. A large enhancing mass occupies the upper half of the vermis. Central, nonenhancing cystic/microcystic elements are evident. Severe hydrocephalus is caused by compression of the fourth ventricle. (*C*) Sagittal contrast-enhanced T1 image of a fourth ventricular ependymoma. A lobulated mass expands the fourth ventricle and shows irregular moderate enhancement. (*D*) Axial T2 weighted image of an infiltrative brainstem (pontine) glioma. An intrinsic T2 bright mass replaces most of the pons and infiltrates the right middle cerebellar peduncle.

multipotent progenitor cells of the ventricular zone have been postulated to be the primary site of development of classical medulloblastomas, and the classical tumor is more likely to express more primitive, possibly stem cell markers. Medulloblastomas arising from the external granular layer on the other hand are believed to originate from a more neuronally restricted granular cell precursor, and are more likely to be desmoplastic and express markers of granular cell lineage.

Various genes and signaling pathways have been identified as active in medulloblastoma and support progenitor cell theories. The nevoid basal cell carcinoma syndrome, which is caused by an inherited germ line mutation of the PTCH gene on chromosome 22, encodes the sonic hedgehog (SHH) receptor PATCHED1 (PTC1), which normally represses SHH signaling [15]. Somatic mutation of PTC1 has been associated predominantly with the desmoplastic variant, possibly from external granular layer precursors, and this pathway is likely a potential therapeutic target for 10% to 20% of medulloblastomas [13,16]. Classical medulloblastomas are less likely to have abnormalities in the SHH pathway and may be more likely to arise from the internal granular layer. Another signaling pathway that has been identified in a subset of patients with medulloblastoma has been the WNT pathway, which is aberrant in Turcot's syndrome [17]. Patients who have this molecular abnormality, which has been noted in as many as 15% of patients and may affect growth and survival of multipotential cerebellar progenitor cells, have been demonstrated to have better prognosis.

Specific molecular genetic abnormalities have been associated with medulloblastoma and variably correlated with survival [13,18]. Amplification of the MYCC oncogene has been associated with the large-cell variant and poorer outcome. Similarly, expression of the tyrosine kinase receptor ERBB2 has been demonstrated in 40% of medulloblastomas and is also predictive of poor outcome [19]. Increased expression of the neurotrophin-3 receptor (TRKC), which regulates proliferation, differentiation, and granular layer cell death, has been associated with better survival [20,21]. Amplification of the OXT2 homeobox gene, a retinoid target, has been identified in the anaplastic medulloblastoma variant [22]. Gene expression profiling has demonstrated differences in metastatic and nonmetastatic tumors, as platelet-derived growth factor receptor beta and members of the RAS-MAP kinase pathway are up-regulated significantly in metastatic tumors [23].

These and other biologic alterations have allowed a significant better understanding of medulloblastoma. In time, it is likely that they will be incorporated into staging schema for medulloblastoma and also will act as therapeutic targets [24,25]. To date, however, medulloblastomas predominantly are staged and treated based on clinical parameters.

Management

In most patients who have medulloblastomas, the initial step in treatment is surgical resection. Total or near-total resection of the primary tumor site has been correlated with better survival, predominantly in nondisseminated patients [26]. Such resections will result in avoidance of permanent ventriculoperitoneal cerebrospinal drainage in over 60% of patients. Significant postoperative complications may occur, including both septic and aseptic meningitis, postoperative cerebrospinal fluid leaks, and increased neurologic morbidity caused by direct cerebellar or brain stem damage. The cerebellar mutism syndrome has been identified in up to 25% of patients following resection of midline cerebellar tumors [27]. This syndrome presents as the late (delayed) onset of mutism associated with a variable constellation of nystagmus, truncal hypotonia, dysmetria, dysphagia, other supranuclear cranial nerve palsies, and marked emotional lability. The neurophysiologic mechanism underlying this syndrome is unclear, but it is believed to be related to vermian damage and possibly impaired dentatorubrothalamic connections to the supplementary motor cortex. Symptoms may persist from weeks to months and approximately 50% of those affected will have significant sequelae 1 year after surgery. Neurosurgery-related complications have not been related clearly to more aggressive surgery.

Following surgery, patients usually are stratified into one of two risk groups, based on extent of surgical resection and disease extent at the time of diagnosis (Table 2). Neuroradiographic staging, although critical, remains problematic, as central review of international studies has demonstrated inadequate spinal neuroimaging or misinterpreted studies in nearly 25% of patients [12,25]. Adequate staging requires meticulous, multiplanar neuro-axis imaging and lumbar cerebrospinal fluid analysis. In time, as these risk groups are modified by the inclusion of other factors, including histological features and molecular genetic parameters, an intermediate risk group of patients may become more apparent (see Table 2).

Patients greater than 3 years of age with average-risk disease are treated conventionally with craniospinal (2400 cGy) and local boost radiotherapy (5580 cGy), supplemented with adjuvant chemotherapy [28]. The dose of craniospinal radiation therapy for children who have nondisseminated disease has been decreased by one-third (from 3600 cGy) with maintained efficacy, as long as chemotherapy is given during and after radiotherapy. Studies are underway attempting to determine if a further reduction of the dose of craniospinal radiotherapy from 2340 cGy to 1800 cGy will result in equivalent survival figures and better neurocognitive outcome.

Different chemotherapeutic regimens have shown benefit in medulloblastoma. Probably the best tested is the use of vincristine during radiotherapy and the combination of CCNU, cisplatin and vincristine, or cyclophosphamide, cisplatin, and vincristine following radiotherapy [28,29]. Another approach, demonstrating similar survival, has used essentially the same agents

Table 2
Staging of medulloblastoma in children older than 3 years of age

	Average-risk	High-risk
Tumor extent	Localized	Disseminated
Tumor resection	Total; near total	Subtotal; biopsy
Histology	Classical; desmoplastic/nodular	Anaplastic/large cell
Biologic parameters	Neurotrophin-3 receptor expression; sonic hedgehog lineage markers	↑ MYCC amplification; ↑ ERBB2 expression; OXT2 amplification

in a truncated, higher-dose fashion supported by peripheral stem cell rescue [30]. With such combination approaches used during and after radiotherapy, over 80% of children with average-risk medulloblastoma are alive and free of disease five years following diagnosis, most of whom are apparently cured from their disease. The use of preradiotherapy chemotherapy has resulted in inferior survival [28–32].

Children older than 3 years who have high-risk medulloblastoma have approximately a 50% to 60% 5-year disease-free survival after treatment with higher doses of craniospinal radiation therapy (3600 cGy) and similar doses of local radiotherapy, as used for children with average-risk disease, and chemotherapy during and after radiation therapy [30]. Recent trials have included the use of carboplatin as a radiosensitizer during radiation therapy and the delivery of higher-dose chemotherapy, essentially an intensified cisplatin, cyclophosphamide, vincristine, and etoposide regimen, supported by peripheral stem cell rescue, following radiotherapy, with possibly better results [30]. The added efficacy of biologic therapy, such as retinoic acid and tyrosine kinase inhibitors, is being explored in this subset of patients.

Treatment of children younger than 3 years of who have medulloblastoma is problematic. Because of the immaturity of the brain and the resultant deleterious effects of whole brain irradiation on the very young child, there is significant reluctance to use craniospinal radiation therapy. Management of infants is complicated further by the increased likelihood of dissemination at the time of diagnosis in younger patients, because as many as 40% of children younger than 3 years who have medulloblastoma will have disseminated disease at diagnosis [12]. Although various chemotherapeutic approaches have been used, and others are under active study, the most important predictor of outcome is likely not the type of regimen employed, but rather the biology of the tumor [33–35]. Infants who have desmoplastic/nodular tumors are quite responsive to chemotherapy, and 75% or greater of patients harboring this histologic variant may be cured by chemotherapy alone. Outcome is less favorable in infants who have classical, undifferentiated medulloblastoma, especially in those who have disseminated disease at the time of diagnosis. More intensive chemotherapeutic regimens using peripheral stem cell support or regimens that have been supplemented with high-dose, intravenous, and intrathecal methotrexate have shown possible increased efficacy [34,35]. The safety and efficacy of focal radiation therapy to the primary tumor site also is being explored in this age group.

Children of all ages with medulloblastoma who survive are at risk for significant long-term sequelae. The whole brain portion of craniospinal radiation therapy has been implicated as the primary cause of long-term neurocognitive deficits. Other factors, however, may play a significant role in sequelae encountered. These include: the tumor's location extent and the presence of hydrocephalus at diagnosis, postsurgical complications, the age of the patient, the potential deleterious effects of concomitant chemotherapy, and the additive toxicity of local radiotherapy [36,37]. Neu-rocognitive difficulties are the most common sequelae seen, and even after reduction of whole-brain radiotherapy from 3600 cGy to 2340 cGy, most children, especially those younger than 7 years of age, will have significant intellectual difficulties [36,37]. Deficits include demonstrable post-treatment drop in overall intelligence, as well as deficits in perceptual motor ability, memory tasks, verbal learning, and executive function. Moderate-to-severe learning difficulties are common.

Neuroendocrine sequelae are also relatively common, but these seem to be somewhat less frequent in those children who have been treated with re-duced doses of craniospinal radiation therapy [12]. Of the endocrinologic sequelae, growth hormone insufficiency is the most common, occurring in almost all prepubertal children who have received 3600 cGy of cranio-spinal radiation and probably 50% or more of those children receiving 2340 cGy of whole-brain irradiation therapy [12,38]. Thyroid dysfunction also occurs frequently and is caused not only by the dose of radiotherapy delivered to the hypothalamic region, but also by scatter radiation to the thyroid gland.

Permanent neurologic sequelae, including motor difficulties, sensory dysfunction, hearing impairments caused by the tumor, chemotherapy (especially cisplatinum), or radiation therapy, and visual abnormalities in-creasingly have been recognized in long-term survivors [39]. Late-onset cere-brovascular damage resulting in stroke-like episodes is not uncommon, and can cause devastating long-term complications [39]. Survivors are at risk for small vessel microangiopathy and more subtle vascular-related sequelae, such as seizures. Secondary tumors are another long-term complication of medulloblastoma and may be related to the underlying genetic predisposi-tion of these patients to tumors and/or to the radiotherapy employed. Both meningiomas and gliomas can occur at any time following successful treatment, and, in general, high-grade gliomas tend to predominate in the first 5 to 10 years following therapy, while the risk of meningiomas con-tinues to increase over time [40].

Supratentorial primitive neuroectodermal tumors

Supratentorial primitive neuroectodermal tumors are characterized by undifferentiated or poorly differentiated neuroepithelial cells that may show some degree of differentiation. Although similar histologically, they are biologically different from medulloblastomas [21]. Various different names, including cerebral neuroblastomas, have been used for these tumors, which, by definition, must occur above the tentorium, primarily in the cere-bral cortex and less frequently in the diencephalic region. They are infre-quent, comprising 2.5% of all childhood brain tumors. The tumors are staged based predominantly on tumor extent at diagnosis, although approx-imately 20% or less of lesions have evidence of dissemination.

The degree of surgical resection has been related variably to outcome [41–44]. Postsurgical management has been similar to that employed for high-risk medulloblastoma patients, with most children being treated with craniospinal and local boost radiotherapy and aggressive adjuvant chemotherapy. The need for craniospinal radiation therapy has never been demonstrated clearly, although it is used frequently. Reported 5-year progression-free survival rates have ranged from 30% to 60%, with most series finding that approximately 50% of affected patients survive [41–44].

Pineoblastomas

Although pineoblastomas are classified as pineal parenchymal tumors, they are conceptualized most commonly as a subvariant of embryonal tumors and are managed similarly to high-risk medulloblastomas. They represent approximately 25% of tumors that occur in the pineal region. Dissemination at the time of diagnosis is present in 20% to 30% of patients [41–44].

Total resections before the initiation of adjuvant treatment are uncommon because of tumor location. Survival figures after treatment with craniospinal plus local boost radiation therapy and adjuvant chemotherapy, similar to that being used for high-risk medulloblastoma patients, have been quite variable, with some studies reporting relatively optimistic 5-year progression-free survival rates of as high as 60% [41–44]. Other series have reported much less favorable outcomes, especially in very young children who are not treated with craniospinal radiotherapy.

Atypical teratoid/rhabdoid tumors

Atypical teratoid/rhabdoid tumors (AT/RTs) first were recognized as a discreet entity in the late 1980s [45]. These lesions, which predominantly occur in children younger than 3 years, but may be first diagnosed in older children and adolescents, histologically are characterized by rhabdoid cells intermixed with a variable component of primitive neuroectodermal, mesenchymal, and epithelial cells. The rhabdoid cell is a medium-sized round-to-oval cell with distinct borders, an eccentric nucleus, and a prominent nucleolus. The primitive neuroectodermal component of AT/RTs is indistinguishable from that found in other forms of primitive neuroectodermal tumors. Immunohistochemical studies demonstrated that AT/RTs were different from medulloblastomas, because the rhabdoid component of the tumor characteristically stained positive for epithelial membrane antigen, vimentin, cytokeratin, glial fibrillary acidic protein, and, at times, smooth muscle actin and neurofilament protein. Molecular genetic studies have demonstrated that AT/RTs are distinct from other embryonal tumors and are characterized by deletions or mutations of the tumor suppressor gene hSNF5/INI1 located in the chromosomal region 22q11.2 [46].

Management of AT/RTs has been extremely problematic. The tumor arises equally in the posterior fossa or supratentorium [47]. Dissemination has been reported in approximately 25% of patients at diagnosis. Outcome after treatment of infants on protocols used for children younger than 3 years with medulloblastoma, including high-dose chemotherapy protocols, has been disappointing, with prolonged survival occurring in less than 20% of patients who had nondisseminated tumors, primarily in those who had undergone a total or near-total resection. Various different chemotherapeutic approaches are under study, including adding methotrexate to the drug regimen or using protocols that are hybrids of the infant medulloblastoma and sarcoma treatment regimens. Survival seems more favorable in patients older than 3 years at diagnosis treated with extensive resections, craniospinal and local boost radiotherapy, and chemotherapy.

Gliomas

High-grade gliomas

These tumors present most frequently between 5 and 10 years of age [48]. Patients may present with headaches, motor weakness, personality changes and seizures; however, seizures are more typical of low-grade cortical lesions [49]. On CT and MRI, high-grade gliomas (HGG) typically appear as irregularly shaped lesions with partial contrast enhancement and peritumoral edema with or without mass effect [49].

Radical (greater than 90%) surgical resection is the most powerful predictor of favorable outcome in HGG when followed by irradiation [50,51]. Only 49% of tumors in the superficial hemisphere and 8% of tumors in the midline or deep cerebrum are amenable to radical resection, however. Local or wide-field irradiation to 5000 cGy to 6000 cGy is the mainstay of therapy. The addition of radiation therapy has improved 5-year survival rates (10% to 30%) compared with surgery alone (0%) [50]. Although initial reports demonstrated a benefit of adjuvant chemotherapy with prednisone, CCNU, and vincristine (pCV) compared with radiotherapy alone (46% versus 18%), a subsequent trial comparing pCV with the eight-in-one regimen failed to show the same benefit (26%) [52,53]. A review of the histology from the original trial with pCV suggested that a significant portion of patients (69/250) actually did not meet the central consensus definition of HGG. Most recently, temozolamide and concurrent radiation followed by maintenance temozolomide therapy has been used; however this regimen has shown no improvement in survival. To date, no large randomized clinical trial has demonstrated a benefit of chemotherapy clearly. High-dose chemotherapy for HGG has shown effective responses, and despite significant associated toxicity, may warrant further investigation [54,55].

Biologic therapy, such as drugs that target angiogenesis, is being investigated as an alternative approach. Specific biologic therapeutic targets have not been defined well for childhood HGG. For example, although 80% of pediatric HGG overexpress the EGFR protein, amplification of the EGFR gene is rare compared with EGFR amplification in one-third of adult glioblastomas [56–58]. A more recent expression profiling study of childhood HGG revealed increased expression of the EGFR/HIF/IGFBP2 pathway [57]. The TP53 gene is mutated in 34% of HGG in children younger than 3 years and only 12% of HGG in children older than 3 years, while the 5-year progression-free survival in those with low expression of p53 protein is 44% compared with 17% in those with high expression [59,60]. Deletions for p16INK4a and p14ARF of the Rb pathway are observed in only 10% of pediatric HGG [61]. These data indicate that the development of pediatric HGG may follow different pathways from the primary or secondary paradigm of adult glioblastomas and as such may require differently tailored biologic therapy than is being employed for adults with HGG.

Low-grade gliomas

Most low-grade cortical gliomas in children are juvenile pilocytic astrocytoma (JPA) or diffuse fibrillary astrocytoma. Other forms, such as oligodendroglioma, oligoastrocytoma and mixed glioma are much less common [62]. Low-grade cortical gliomas (LGG) most commonly present with headache and seizure. On CT, diffuse astrocytomas appear as ill-defined, homogeneous masses of low density without contrast enhancement. MRI usually shows a mass that is hypodense on T1 weighted and hyperintense on T2 weighted images with little enhancement. Imaging of JPA lesions is similar to the cerebellar counterpart [63].

Complete surgical resection is curative for most, and even with incomplete excision, long-term progression-free survival is common [64]. If subsequent progression occurs, then re-resection generally is undertaken. For patients who have progressive disease not amenable to resection, irradiation with 5000 cGy to 5500 cGy is warranted. Chemotherapy is reserved for very young children and infants and most commonly includes carboplatin and vincristine.

Overall 5-year survival is 95%, while progression-free survival is 88%. Less favorable results have been seen in patients who have nonpilocytic astrocytoma [65].

Chiasmatic gliomas

Gliomas of the visual pathway, which also may extend to the hypothalamus and thalamus, comprise a relatively common form of childhood glioma. Tumors of the optic chiasm are usually low-grade. Twenty percent of children who have (NF-1) will develop visual pathway tumors, predominantly JPA, during childhood [66]. Visual pathway tumors may cause visual loss, strabismus, proptosis and/or nystagmus. Extension to the hypothalamus may present with endocrinologic disturbances, including precocious puberty. Imaging demonstrates similar characteristics of low-grade gliomas that present elsewhere (Fig. 3). Optic pathway lesions have limited capacity to spread, as they are confined to migrate between the optic nerve and chiasm [66].

Radiation therapy with 5000 cGy to 5500 cGy generally is reserved for older children who have progressive or symptomatic tumors. Therapy with carboplatin and vincristine has demonstrated tumor shrinkage and/or stabilization in over 90% of children younger than 5 years of age [67,68]. In children who have NF-1, tumor biopsy for histologic confirmation is not necessary because of the highly characteristic appearance on MRI. In these children, lesions may be detected by routine screening before the onset of symptoms, and treatment is often withheld until there is clear radiographic or clinical progression.

Brain stem gliomas

Brain stem gliomas (BSGs) comprise 10% to 15% of all pediatric CNS tumors and are generally uncommon in the adult population. Peak incidence is between 5 and 9 years of age, but may occur anytime during childhood [62]. BSGs most commonly arise in the pons (diffuse intrinsic), in which location they typically resemble adult glioblastomas multiforme (GBM) and have an almost uniformly dismal prognosis (see Fig. 2). In contrast, those arising from midbrain or medulla are likely to be low-grade lesions that have a more indolent course and better outcome. BSGs commonly present with multiple cranial nerve deficits, especially sixth and

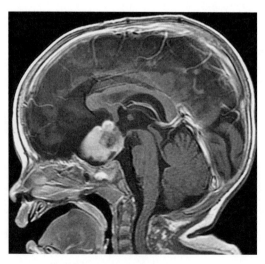

Fig. 3. Sagittal contrast-enhanced T1 image a of a chiasmatic glioma. A large, enhancing suprasellar mass is evident, which replaces the chiasm. Nonenhancing cystic/microcystic components are evident posteriorly.

seventh nerve palsies, long track signs, and cerebellar deficits [69]. Diffuse pontine gliomas show CT and MRI characteristics similar to HGG within an enlarged pons. Low-grade BSGs are relatively discrete, often exophytic, and contrast, enhancing with cyst formation [11].

Treatment is local irradiation with 5500 cGy to 6000 cGy. Over 90% of patients who have diffuse intrinsic lesions transiently respond, but ultimately succumb to disease progression within 18 months of diagnosis. Neither hyperfractionated radiotherapy nor chemotherapy has been shown to add benefit [70]. Low-grade lesions are treated with similar irradiation doses but overall respond less favorably than their counterparts in other locations [69,71].

Cerebellar gliomas

Cerebellar glioma is found almost exclusively in children, occurring most frequently between ages 4 and 9. JPA is the most common subtype, accounting for 85% of cerebellar gliomas [72]. Diffuse astrocytoma is the next most common, while malignant astrocytoma is rare in this location. Children typically present with headache, vomiting, papilledema, and gait disturbance. CT and MRI reveal either a large solid (20%) or mixed solid and cystic (80%) circumscribed mass that enhances with contrast (see Fig. 2b) [73,74]. Pilocytic tumors are circumscribed well and characterized by a biphasic pattern with varying proportion of bipolar cells with Rosenthal fibers and loose multipolar cells with microcysts [11].

Total surgical resection is curative in 95% to 100% of cases [73,74]. JPAs may stabilize for long periods of time or even spontaneously regress. however, the behavior of cerebellar gliomas in children who have NF-1 may be more aggressive. Those children whose lesions are inoperable because of brain stem involvement may require additional therapy, although residual tumor may remain quiescent for years. Thus irradiation and/or chemotherapy should be reserved for tumors that demonstrate clear growth or symptomatic change [73,74]. Rare malignant cerebellar astrocytomas have a poor outcome and require aggressive treatment similar to supratentorial HGG.

Ependymomas

Ependymomas comprise 5% to 10% of all childhood brain tumors [75,76]. Most (70% to 80%) arise in the posterior fossa and, because of a relative predilection for the cerebellopontine angle and lateral portion of the lower brainstem, often cause multiple cranial nerve deficits including sixth and seventh nerve palsies, hearing loss, and swallowing difficulties. Ependymomas tend to present more insidiously than medulloblastomas and at the time of diagnosis, despite their lateral posterior fossa location, frequently cause obstructive hydrocephalous (see Fig. 2c). Various histological subtypes of ependymoma are recognized; however, clinically, the most important distinction is between anaplastic lesions and somewhat lower grade, usually cellular tumors [77]. The myxopapillary ependymoma, which occurs predominantly in the conus and cauda equina region of the spinal cord, is likely a biologically different subtype of tumor with an even more indolent natural history.

Although probably no greater than 5% of ependymomas are disseminated at the time of diagnosis, staging for extent of disease usually is undertaken either before or after surgery [78]. The degree of surgical resection is a critical determinant of outcome for children who have ependymomas, as those who have total or near-total resections have the highest likelihood of long-term disease control [79]. Infratentorial tumors notoriously extend along the upper cervical cord, making total resection and radiotherapy planning difficult. Such contiguous extension has been related to poorer disease control, especially if radiation planning does not take into consideration the tendency of these tumors to contiguously spread.

The need for radiotherapy in totally resected nonanaplastic ependymomas is somewhat controversial. Small series have suggested that totally resected supratentorial lesions can be treated with surgery alone. most patients with completely resected infratentorial tumors have received radiotherapy, with resultant 5-year progression-free survival rates of 75% to 80% [79]. Local radiotherapy, using conformal treatment planning and doses ranging between 5500 cGy and 5960 cGy, is as effective as craniospinal and local boost radiotherapy. Patients who have anaplastic tumors may fare less well. Patients who have subtotally resected ependymomas, after local radiotherapy, have 5-year progression-free survival rates of probably no higher than 50%. Combination therapy with radiation and chemotherapy has been reserved predominantly for children older than 3 years and those patients who have subtotally resected and/or anaplastic tumors [80,81]. Randomized studies, using chemotherapy as an adjuvant after radiotherapy, have not demonstrated significant improvements in survival, although more recent preirradiation phase 2 investigations suggest there may be a role for adjuvant, predominantly cisplatin-based combination drug regimens.

Because of the apparent crucial role of extensive surgery in patients with ependymomas, studies are underway evaluating the feasibility, safety, and utility of second-look surgery after chemotherapy before radiation. Postsurgical neurologic complications due to the location of the tumor and its involvement of multiple lower cranial nerves are a major risk, however, and the need for total resection has to be counterbalanced by the risk of surgically induced long-term neurologic impairment.

Ependymomas are relatively common in younger patients, as they comprise 20% or more of infantile infratentorial tumors. Chemotherapy usually is used in attempts to delay the need for radiotherapy, although there has been renewed interest in using local radiotherapy in children as young as

1 year who have infratentorial tumors, especially for patients who have tumors not amenable to total surgical resection [82].

Craniopharyngiomas

Craniopharyngiomas account for 5% to 10% of all childhood brain tumors and are believed to arise from embryonic remnants of Rathke's pouch in the sellar region [83]. Clinical presentation is variable, and symptoms may be secondary to blockage of cerebrospinal fluid and resultant increased intracranial pressure or direct chiasmatic or hypothalamic damage from the solid tumor and associated cyst. Visual symptoms are variable and may include decreased visual acuity in one or both eyes and visual field deficits. Endocrinologic abnormalities at the time of diagnosis are common and may include failure of growth, delayed sexual maturation, weight gain, and, in a significant minority of patients, diabetes insipidus. Craniopharyngiomas peak at 6 to 10 years and then later at 11 to 15 years. They are notoriously large at the time of diagnosis and are often multilobulated heterogeneous masses with cystic and solid components and significant amounts of calcification (Fig. 4).

The tumor's size and its proximity to the hypothalamus, visual pathway, and carotid vessels, as well as craniopharyngioma's tendency to be quite gritty and adherent to these critical brain structures and the undersurface of the frontal lobes, make surgical removal difficult [83,84]. Despite decades of clinical experience, controversy exists over optimal management. Complete tumor removal results in an 80% to 95% 10-year progression-free survival rate and cure, but this also may be associated with significant

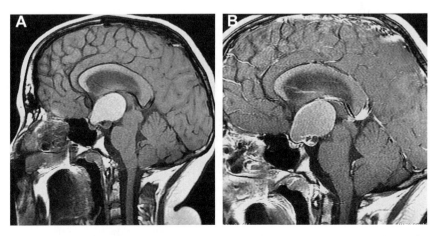

Fig. 4. Sagittal precontrast (A) and postcontrast (B) T1 images of a cystic suprasellar craniopharyngioma. The proteinaceous contents of the dominant, superior cyst are very bright on the precontrast image (A); following contrast (B), the capsule surrounding the large cyst and a more solid nodule (inferior) enhance and become hyperintense to the cyst contents.

behavioral and neurocognitive difficulties and, in most patients, permanent hormonal deficits [83]. After total removal, most patients will require growth, thyroid, and cortisol supplementation; chronic DDAVP replacement to correct diabetes insipidus will be needed in up to 75% of patients. The degree of neurocognitive/psychological damage, manifested by severe memory loss, behavioral difficulties, and associated obesity secondary subfrontal and hypothalamic damage can be severe and, in the cases of severe obesity, can be life-threatening [85]. Alternative approaches, which include partial tumor resection and/or cyst aspiration followed by radiotherapy, may be nearly as effective in controlling disease and result in less morbidity [86]. Intercavitary brachytherapy using p^{32} or y^{90}, repeated cyst aspiration, or the use of intracyst bleomycin may be useful in selected situations [87,88]. Even after less aggressive surgery and other means of treatment, sequelae may occur. Hormonal deficits are less likely if the pituitary stalk is preserved [89].

Germ cell tumors

Germ cell tumors, which comprise approximately 2% to 5% of all childhood brain tumors, arise predominantly in the pineal and suprasellar region, but may occur throughout the brain [90]. Despite their relatively rapid growth rate, they may present insidiously and delays of 6 months to 1 year between initial onset of symptoms, which may include school difficulties, polyuria, and behavioral problems, occurs in up to one-third of patients. Germinomas and mixed germ cell tumors account for approximately 60% of all pineal region masses. Germinomas may present in both the pineal region and the suprasellar region in 10% to 20% of patients. Those patients with pineal region symptomatology, which is classically manifested by symptoms of hydrocephalus and/or direct tectal damage (Parinaud's syndrome), with associated diabetes insipidus or other hormonal deficits, are considered to have both pineal and suprasellar involvement, even in the case of equivocal neuroradiographic findings. Tumors in the thalamic region and those disseminated throughout the brain and spinal cord may be more difficult to diagnose neuroradiographically and may not show characteristic enhancement.

Histological confirmation is usually, but not always, required for the diagnosis of germinomas and distinction from other pineal region tumors such as pineoblastomas, pineocytomas, and teratomas [90,91]. Elevated cerebrospinal fluid and, in selected cases, blood levels of alpha-feta protein and β-HCG can be used to confirm a mixed germ cell tumor. Highly elevated levels of beta-human chorionic gonadotrophin (β-HCG) alone are diagnostic of a choriocarcinoma. A subvariety of germinoma, the syncytiotrophoblastic variant, secretes moderate levels of β-HCG into the cerebrospinal fluid. Surgery for patients who have presumed germ cell tumors usually is preserved for those patients for whom a diagnosis cannot be made by cerebrospinal fluid markers or when the tumor is very large and requires debulking.

Radiation therapy has been the primary modality of therapy for patients who have pure germinomas, and craniospinal plus local boost radiotherapy can result in cure in 95% or more of patients, including those with disseminated disease at the time of diagnosis [92,93]. Germinomas, however, are also chemosensitive, and treatment with preradiation chemotherapy followed by more localized radiotherapy, usually whole ventricular therapy, may be as effective and result in somewhat less sequelae because of the avoidance of whole-brain radiation [94–96]. In contradistinction, patients with mixed germ cell tumors have only a 40% to 60% likelihood of long-term disease control after treatment with radiotherapy alone. In these patients, multidrug chemotherapeutic regimens, either given before or after radiotherapy, have seemed to result in improved survival rates [97].

Choroid plexus tumors

Tumors of the choroid plexus are relatively uncommon, contributing 1% to 5% of all pediatric tumors [98–100]. Choroid plexus papillomas, because of their intraventricular location and associated cerebrospinal fluid overproduction, and blockage of cerebrospinal fluid reabsorbtion pathways, predominantly result in hydrocephalus. Papillomas notoriously occur in very young infants and result in massive hydrocephalus. They increasingly are being diagnosed during prenatal ultrasound evaluations. Unlike the situation in older patients and adults, where the tumor more commonly arises in the fourth ventricle, infantile tumors classically arise in the lateral ventricles and may be bilateral. The treatment of choice for choroid plexus papillomas is surgical removal. Because of the marked vascularity of these tumors, the massive hydrocephalus often present, and the age of the patient, however, there may be considerable surgical mortality.

Choroid plexus carcinomas are much more likely to invade the contiguous brain parenchyma than papillomas. Despite their histological aggressivity, gross total resections alone can result in long-term disease control. Optimal treatment for subtotally resected choroid plexus carcinomas is unclear. Although adjuvant chemotherapy and radiotherapy have been used and may result in tumor response, the long-term efficacy of such approaches has been difficult to demonstrate [98–100].

Spinal cord tumors

Spinal cord tumors may be extremely difficult to diagnose in young children who may present with delays in walking and, in older patients, who develop difficult-to-characterize gait disturbances [101,102]. Back pain is frequent but often nonspecific and initially nonlocalizing, and sensory abnormalities are often hard to characterize in children. Tumors in the conus region result in early bowel and bladder difficulties. In total, spinal cord tumors account for less than 10% of all CNS neoplasms. The most common primary central nervous system lesions are gliomas and ependymomas. Patients who have NF-1 are prone to develop intramedullary astrocytomas, and are at high risk for extrinsic cord compression by neurofibromas. Children who have neurofibromatosis type 2 are more likely to harbor intramedulllary ependymomas, which are often indolent lesions requiring little therapy for many years.

In patients who have low-grade gliomas, MRI usually reveals an enlarged hypointense cord, at times associated with a thin syrinx. There may be focal enhancement, especially in pilocytic tumors. In general, ependymomas are somewhat more circumscribed than astrocytomas.

Low-grade spinal astrocytomas can be treated effectively by extensive surgical resections or by partial resections followed by radiotherapy, or possibly, in very young children, chemotherapy [103,104]. The outcome for patients who have ependymomas is somewhat more variable, although long-term control after resection and usually adjuvant radiotherapy is possible. High-grade lesions may be very difficult to resect, and even after treatment with radiation therapy, most patients will suffer tumor relapse within 3 to 5 years of diagnosis, often associated with neuro-axis dissemination [103].

References

[1] CBTRUS 2005. Statistical report: primary brain tumors in the United States, 1995–1999. Published by the Central Brain Tumor Registry of the United States.
[2] Lindor NM, Greene MH. Mayo Familial Cancer Program. The concise handbook of family cancer syndromes. J Natl Cancer Inst 1998;90:1039–71.
[3] McGaughran JM, Harris DL, Donnai E, et al. A clinical study of type 1 neurofibromatosis in northwest England. J Med Genet 1999;36:197–203.
[4] Webb DW, Fryer AE, Osborne JP. Morbidity associated with tuberous sclerosis: a population study. Dev Med Child Neurol 1996;38:146–55.
[5] Varley JM, Evans DGR, Birch JM. Li-Fraumeni syndrome—a molecular and clinical review. Br J Cancer 1997;76:1–14.
[6] Cowan R, Hoban P, Kelsey A, et al. The gene for the nevoid basal cell carcinoma syndrome acts as a tumour suppressor gene in medulloblastoma. Br J Cancer 1997;76:141–5.
[7] Paraf F, Jothy S, van Meir EG. Brain tumor polyposis syndrome: two genetic diseases? J Clin Oncol 1997;15:2744–58.
[8] Ron E, Modan B, Boice JD, et al. Tumors of the brain and nervous system after radiotherapy in childhood. N Engl J Med 1988;319:1033–9.
[9] Pollack IF. Brain tumors in children. N Engl J Med 1994;331:1500–7.
[10] Vézina L-G. Neuroradiology of childhood brain tumors: new challenges. J Neuro-Oncol 2005;75:243–52.
[11] Kleihues P, Cavenee WK. Survival and prognostic factors following radiation therapy and chemotherapy for ependymoma in children: a report of the Children's Cancer Group. Lyon, France: IARC Press; 2000.
[12] Packer RJ, Cogen P, Vézina G, et al. Medulloblastoma: clinical and biologic aspects. Neuro Oncol 1999;1:232–50.
[13] Eberhart CG, Kratz J, Wang Y, et al. Histopathological and molecular prognostic markers in medulloblastoma: c-myc, N-myc, TrkC, and anaplasia. J Neuropathol Exp Neurol 2004; 63(5):4441–9.

[14] Giangaspero F, Rigobello L, Badiali M, et al. Large-cell medulloblastomas. a distinct variant with highly aggressive behavior. Am J Surg Pathol 1992;16(7):687–93.

[15] Read T-A, Hegedus B, Wechsler-Reya R, et al. The neurobiology of neuro-oncology. Ann Neurol 2006;6:3–11.

[16] Raffel C, Jenkins RB, Frederick L, et al. Sporadic medulloblastomas contain PTCH mutation. Cancer Res 1997;57:842–5.

[17] Ellison DW, Onilude OE, Lindsey JC, et al. Beta-catenin status predicts a favorable outcome in childhood medulloblastoma: the United Kingdom Children's Cancer Study Group brain tumour committee. J Clin Oncol 2005;23:7951–7.

[18] Grotzer MA, Hogarty MD, Janss AJ, et al. MYC messenger RNA expression predicts survival outcome in childhood primitive neuroectodermal tumor/medulloblastoma. Clin Cancer Res 2001;7:2425–33.

[19] Gilbertson S, Wickramasinghe C, Hernan R, et al. Clinical and molecular stratification of disease risk in medulloblastoma. Br J Cancer 2001;85:705–12.

[20] Grotzer MA, Janss AJ, Fung K, et al. TrkC expression predicts good clinical outcome in primitive neuroectodermal brain tumors. J Clin Oncol 18:1027–1035.

[21] Pomeroy S, Tamayo P, Gaasenbeek M, et al. Prediction of central nervous system embryonal tumour outcome based on gene expression. Nature 2002;415(6870):436–42.

[22] MacDonald TJ, Rood B, Santi MR, et al. Advances in the diagnosis, molecular genetics, and treatment of pediatric embryonal CNS tumors. Oncologist 2003;8:174–86.

[23] MacDonald TJ, Brown KM, LaFleur B, et al. Expression profiling of medulloblastoma: PDGFRA and the RAS/MAPK pathway as therapeutic targets for metastatic disease. Nat Genet 2001;29:143–52.

[24] Gajjar A, Hernan R, Kocak M, et al. Clinical, histopathologic, and molecular markers of prognosis: toward a new disease risk stratification system for medulloblastoma. J Clin Oncol 2004;22(6):984–93.

[25] Ray A, Ho M, Ma J, et al. A clinicobiological model predicting survival in medulloblastoma. Clin Cancer Res 2004;10:7613–20.

[26] Albright AL, Sposto R, Holmes E, et al. Correlation of neurosurgical subspecialization with outcomes in children with malignant brain tumors. Neurosurgery 2000;47:879–87.

[27] Robertson PL, Muraszko KM, Holmes EJ, et al. Incidence and severity of postoperative cerebellar mutism syndrome in children with medulloblastoma: a prospective study by the Children's Oncology Group. J Neurosurg 2006;105(S6 Pediatrics):444–51.

[28] Packer RJ, Gajjar A, Vézina G, et al. Phase III study of craniospinal radiation therapy followed by adjuvant chemotherapy for newly diagnosed average-risk medulloblastoma. J Clin Oncol 2006;24(25):4202–8.

[29] Packer RJ, Sutton LN, Elterman R, et al. Outcome for children with medulloblastoma treated with radiation and cisplatin, CCNU, and vincristine chemotherapy. J Neurosurg 81(5): 690–8.

[30] Gajjar A, Chintagumpala M, Ashley D, et al. Risk-adapted craniospinal radiotherapy followed by high-dose chemotherapy and stem cell rescue in children with newly diagnosed medulloblastoma (St Jude Medulloblastoma-96): long-term results from a prospective, multicentre trial. Lancet 2006;7:813–20.

[31] Taylor RE, Bailey CC, Robinson K, et al. Results of a randomized study of preradiation chemotherapy versus radiotherapy alone for nonmetastatic medulloblastoma: The International Society of Paediatric Oncology/United Kingdom Children's Cancer Study Group PNET-3 Study. J Clin Oncol 2003;21(8):1582–91.

[32] Kuhl J, Muller HL, Berthold F, et al. Preradiation chemotherapy of children and young adults with malignant brain tumors: results of the German pilot trial HIT '88/'89. Klin Padiatr 1998;210(4):227–33.

[33] Duffner PK, Horowitz ME, Krischer JP, et al. Postoperative chemotherapy and delayed radiation in children less than three years of age with malignant brain tumors. N Engl J Med 1993;328(24):1725–31.

[34] Rutkowski S, Bode U, Deinlein F, et al. Treatment of early childhood medulloblastoma by postoperative chemotherapy alone. N Engl J Med 2005;352(10):978–86.

[35] Geyer JR, Jennings M, Sposto, et al. Multiagent chemotherapy and deferred radiotherapy in infants with malignant brain tumors: a report from the Children's Cancer Group. J Clin Oncol 2005;23:7621–31.

[36] Ris MD, Packer R, Goldwein J, et al. Intellectual outcome after reduced-dose radiation therapy plus adjuvant chemotherapy for medulloblastoma: a Children's Cancer Group study. J Clin Oncol 2001;19:3470–6.

[37] Mulhern RK, Kepner JL, Thomas PR, et al. Neuropsychologic functioning of survivors of childhood medulloblastoma randomized to receive conventional or reduced-dose cranio-spinal irradiation: a Pediatric Oncology Group study. J Clin Oncol 1889;16:1723–8.

[38] Gurney JG, Kadan-Lottick NS, Packer RJ, et al. Endocrine and cardiovascular late effects among adult survivors of childhood brain tumors: Childhood Cancer Survivor Study. Cancer 2003;47:663–73.

[39] Packer RJ, Gurney JG, Punyko JA, et al. Longterm neurologic and neurosensory sequelae in adult survivors of a childhood brain tumor: Childhood Cancer Survivor Study. J Clin Oncol 2003;21:3255–61.

[40] Neglia JP, Robison LL, Stovall M, et al. New primary neoplasms of the central nervous system in survivors of childhood cancer: a report from the Childhood Cancer Survivor Study. J Natl Cancer Inst 2006;98:1528–37.

[41] Reddy AT, Janss AJ, Phillips PC, et al. Outcome for children with supratentorial primitive neuroectodermal tumors treated with surgery, radiation, and chemotherapy. Cancer 2000; 88(9):2189–93.

[42] Massimino M, Gandola L, Spreafico F, et al. Supratentorial primitive neuroectoder-mal tumors (S-PNEET) in children: a prospective experience with adjuvant intensive chemotherapy and hyperfractionated accelerated radiotherapy. Int J Radiat Oncol Biol Phys 2006;64:1031–7.

[43] Jakacki R, Zeltzer PM, Boyett JM, et al. Survival and prognostic factors following radia-tion and/or chemotherapy for primitive neuroectodermal tumors of the pineal region in in-fants and children: a report of the Children's Cancer Group. J Clin Oncol 1995;13(6): 1377–83.

[44] Timmermann B, Kortmann RD, Kuhl J, et al. Role of radiotherapy in the treatment of supratentorial primitive neuroectodermal tumors in childhood: results of the prospective German brain tumor trials HIT 88/89 and 91. J Clin Oncol 2002;20:842–9.

[45] Rorke LB, Packer RJ, Biegel JA. Central nervous system atypical teratoid/rhabdoid tumors of infancy and childhood: definition of an entity. J Neurosurg 1996;85:56–65.

[46] Biegel JA, Zhou J-Y, Rorke LB, et al. Germ-line and acquired mutations of INI1 in atypical teratoid and rhabdoid tumours. Cancer Res 1999;59:74–9.

[47] Packer RJ, Biegel JA, Blaney S, et al. Atypical teratoid/rhabdoid tumor of the central ner-vous system: report on workshop. J Ped Hem/Onc 2002;24(5):337–42.

[48] Ciurea AV, Vasilescu G, Nuteanu L, et al. Neurosurgical management of cerebral astrocy-tomas in children. Ann N Y Acad Sci 1997;824:237–40.

[49] Marchese MJ, Chang CH. Malignant astrocytic gliomas in children. Cancer 1990;65: 2771–8.

[50] Wolff JE, Gnekow AK, Kortmann RD, et al. Preradiation chemotherapy for pediatric pa-tients with high-grade glioma. Cancer 2002;94:264–71.

[51] Wisoff JH, Boyett JM, Berger MS, et al. Current neurosurgical management and the impact of the extent of resection in the treatment of malignant gliomas of childhood: a report of the Children's Cancer Group trial no. CCG-945. J Neurosurg 1998;89: 52–9.

[52] Sposto R, Ertel IJ, Jenkin RD, et al. The effectiveness of chemotherapy for treatment of high-grade astrocytoma in children: results of a randomized trial. A report from the Children's Cancer Study Group. J Neurooncol 1989;7:165–77.

[53] Finlay JL, Boyett JM, Yates AJ, et al. Randomized phase III trial in childhood high-grade astrocytoma comparing vincristine, lomustine, and prednisone with the eight drugs- in 1 day regimen. Children's Cancer Group. J Clin Oncol 1995;13:112–23.

[54] MacDonald TJ, Arenson E, Sposto R, et al. Phase II study of high-dose chemotherapy before radiation in children with newly diagnosed high-grade astrocytoma: final analysis of Children's Cancer Group study 9933. Cancer 2005;104:2862–71.

[55] Coppes MJ, Lau R, Ingram LC, et al. Open-label comparison of the antiemetic efficacy of single intravenous doses of dolasetron mesylate in pediatric cancer patients receiving moderately to highly emetogenic chemotherapy. Med Pediatr Oncol 1999;33:99–105.

[56] Sung T, Miller DC, Hayes RL, et al. Preferential inactivation of the p53 tumor suppressor pathway and lack of EGFR amplification distinguish de novo high-grade pediatric astrocytomas from de novo adult astrocytomas. Brain Pathol 2000;10:249–59.

[57] Khatua S, Peterson KM, Brown KM, et al. Overexpression of the EGFR/FKBP12/HIF-2alpha pathway identified in childhood astrocytomas by angiogenesis gene profiling. Cancer Res 2003;63:1865–70.

[58] Bredel M, Pollack IF, Hamilton RL, et al. Epidermal growth factor receptor expression and gene amplification in high-grade nonbrainstem gliomas of childhood. Clin Cancer Res 1999;5:1786–92.

[59] Pollack IF, Finkelstein SD, Burnham J, et al. Age and TP53 mutation frequency in childhood malignant gliomas: results in a multi-institutional cohort. Cancer Res 2001;61:7404–7.

[60] Pollack IF, Finkelstein SD, Woods J, et al. Expression of p53 and prognosis in children with malignant gliomas. N Engl J Med 2002;346:420–7.

[61] Newcomb EW, Alonso M, Sung T, et al. Incidence of p14ARF gene deletion in high-grade adult and pediatric astrocytomas. Hum Pathol 2000;31:115–9.

[62] Gurney JG, Bunin GR. CNS and miscellaneous intracranial and intraspinal neoplasms. In: Ries LAG, S M, Gurney JG, et al, editors. Cancer incidence and survival among children and adolescents: United States SEER Program 1975–1995. NIH Pub No 99–4649. Bethesda (MD): National Cancer Institute SEER program; 1999. p. 51–63.

[63] Finizio FS. CT and MRI aspects of supratentorial hemispheric tumors of childhood and adolescence. Childs Nerv Syst 1995;11:559–67.

[64] Pollack IF. The role of surgery in pediatric gliomas. J Neurooncol 1999;42:271–88.

[65] Pollack IF, Claassen D, al-Shboul Q, et al. Low-grade gliomas of the cerebral hemispheres in children: an analysis of 71 cases. J Neurosurg 1995;82:536–47.

[66] Burger PC, Cohen KJ, Rosenblum MK, et al. Pathology of diencephalic astrocytomas. Pediatr Neurosurg 2000;32:214–9.

[67] Gropman AL, Packer RJ, Nicholson HS, et al. Treatment of diencephalic syndrome with chemotherapy: growth, tumor response, and long-term control. Cancer 1998;83:166–72.

[68] Packer RJ. Chemotherapy: low-grade gliomas of the hypothalamus and thalamus. Pediatr Neurosurg 2000;32:259–63.

[69] Farmer JP, Montes JL, Freeman CR, et al. Brainstem gliomas. a 10-year institutional review. Pediatr Neurosurg 2001;34:206–14.

[70] Mandell LR, Kadota R, Freeman C, et al. There is no role for hyperfractionated radiotherapy in the management of children with newly diagnosed diffuse intrinsic brainstem tumors: results of a pediatric oncology group phase III trial comparing conventional vs. hyperfractionated radiotherapy. Int J Radiat Oncol Biol Phys 1999;43:959–64.

[71] Rubin G, Michowitz S, Horev G, et al. Pediatric brain stem gliomas: an update. Childs Nerv Syst 1998;14:167–73.

[72] Rickert CH, Paulus W. Epidemiology of central nervous system tumors in childhood and adolescence based on the new WHO classification. Childs Nerv Syst 2001;17:503–11.

[73] Undjian S, Marinov M, Georgiev K. Long-term follow-up after surgical treatment of cerebellar astrocytomas in 100 children. Childs Nerv Syst 1989;5:99–101.

[74] Kayama T, Tominaga T, Yoshimoto T. Management of pilocytic astrocytoma. Neurosurg Rev 1996;19:217–20.

[75] Robertson PL, Zeltzer PM, Boyett JM, et al. Survival and prognostic factors following radiation therapy and chemotherapy for ependymoma in children: a report of the Children's Cancer Group. J of Neurosurg 1998;88:695–703.

[76] Horn B, Heideman R, Geyer R, et al. A multi-institutional retrospective study of intracranial ependymoma in children: identification of risk factors. J Pediatr Hematol Oncol 1999; 21:203–11.

[77] Merchant TE, Jenkins JJ, Burger PC, et al. Influence of tumor grade on time to progression after irradiation for localized ependymoma in children. Int J Radiat Oncol Biol Phys 2002; 53:52–7.

[78] Bouffet E, Perilongo G, Canete A, et al. Intracranial ependymomas in children: a critical review of prognostic factors and a plea for cooperation. Med Pediatr Oncol 1998;30: 319–29.

[79] Pollack IF, Gerszten PC, Martinez AJ, et al. Intracranial ependymomas of childhood: long-term outcome and prognostic factors. Neurosurgery 1995;37:655–66.

[80] Merchant TE, Mulhern RK, Krasin MJ, et al. Preliminary results from a phase II trial of conformal radiation therapy and evaluation of radiation-related CNS effects for pediatric patients with localized ependymoma. J Clin Oncol 2004;22:3156–62.

[81] Needle MN, Goldwein JW, Grass J, et al. Adjuvant chemotherapy for the treatment of intracranial ependymoma of childhood. Cancer 1997;80:341–7.

[82] Massimino M, Giangaspero F, Garre ML, et al. Salvage treatment for childhood ependymoma after surgery only: pitfalls of omitting at once adjuvant treatment. Int J Radiat Oncol Biol Phys 2006;65(4):1440–5.

[83] Grill J, Le Lelay Mc, Gambarell D, et al. Postoperative chemotherapy without irradiation for ependymoma in children under 5 years of age: a multicenter trial of the French Society of Pediatric Oncology. J Clin Oncol 2001;19:1288–96.

[84] Müller HL, Albanese A, Calaminus G, et al. Consensus and perspectives on treatment strategies in childhood craniopharyngioma: results of a meeting of the craniopharyngioma study group (SIOP), Genova, 2004. J Pediatr Endocrinol Metab 2006;19:453–4.

[85] Puget S, Garnett M, Wray A, et al. Pediatric craniopharyngiomas: classification and treatment according to the degree of hypothalamic involvement. J Neurosurg 2007; 106(Peds 1):3–12.

[86] Sands SA, Milner JS, Goldberg J, et al. Quality of life and behavioral follow-up study of pediatric survivors of craniopharyngioma. J Neurosurg 2005;103(Peds 4):302–11.

[87] Merchant TE, Kiehna EN, Kun LE, et al. Phase II trial of conformal radiation therapy for pediatric patients with craniopharyngioma and correlation of surgical factors and radiation dosimetry with change in cognitive function. J Neurosurg 2006;104(Peds 2):94–102.

[88] Kobayashi T, Kida Y, Mori Y, et al. Long-term results of gamma knife surgery for the treatment of craniopharyngioma in 98 consecutive cases. J Neurosurg 2005;102(Peds 6): 428–88.

[89] Cáceres A. Intracavitary therapeutic options in the management of cystic craniopharyngioma. Childs Nerv Syst 2005;21:705–18.

[90] Müller HL, Bruhnken G, Emser A, et al. Longitudinal study on quality of life in 102 survivors of childhood craniopharyngioma. Childs Nerv Syst 2005;21:975–80.

[91] Balmaceda C, Modak S, Finlay J. Central nervous system germ cell tumors. Semin Oncol 1998;25(2):243–50.

[92] Packer RJ, Cohen BH, Cooney K. Intracranial germ cell tumors. Oncologist 2000;5: 312–20.

[93] Legido A, Packer RJ, Sutton LN, et al. Suprasellar germinomas in childhood. A reappraisal. Cancer 1989;63:340–4.

[94] Bamberg M, Kortmann RD, Calaminus G, et al. Radiation therapy for intracranial germinoma: results of the German cooperative prospective trials MAKEI 83/86/89. J Clin Oncol 1999;17:2585–92.

[95] Bouffet E, Baranzelli MC, Patte C, et al. Combined treatment modality for intracranial germinomas: results of a multicentre SFOP experience. Sociééet Francaise d'Oncologie Pédiatrique. Br J Cancer 1999;79:1199–204.

[96] Balmaceda C, heller G, Rosenblum M, et al. Chemotherapy without irradiation—a novel approach for newly diagnosed CNS germ cell tumors: results of an international cooperative trial. The First International Central Nervous System Germ Cell Tumor Study. J Clin Oncol 1996;14:2908–15.

[97] Yoshida J, Sugita K, Kobayashi T. Treatment of intracranial germ cell tumors: effectiveness of chemotherapy with cisplatin and etoposide (CDDP and VP16). Acta Neurochir (Wien) 1993;120:111–7.

[98] Berger C, Thiesse P, Lellouch-Tubiana A, et al. Choroid plexus carcinoma in childhood: clinical features and prognostic factors. Neurosurgery 1998;42:470 5.

[99] Pencalet P, Sainte-Rose C, Lellouch-tubiana A, et al. Papillomas and carcinomas of the choroid plexus in children. J Neurosurg 1998;88:521–8.

[100] McEvoy AW, Harding BN, Phipps KP, et al. Management of choroid plexus tumours in children: 20 years experience at a single neurosurgical center. Pediatr Neurosurg 2000;32:192–9.

[101] Merchant TE, Kiehna EN, Thompson SJ, et al. Pediatric low-grade and ependymal spinal cord tumors. Pediatr Neurosurg 2000;32:30–6.

[102] Epstein F, Constantini S. Spinal cord tumors of childhood. In: Pang D, editor. Disorders of the pediatric spine. New York: Raven Press; 1995. p. 55–76.

[103] Constantini S, Miller DC, Allen JC, et al. Radical excision of intramedullary spinal cord tumors: surgical morbidity and long-term follow-up evaluation in 164 children and young adults. J Neurosurg 2000;93:183–93.

[104] Bouffet E, Pierre-Kahn A, Marchal JC, et al. Prognostic factors in pediatric spinal cord astrocytoma. Cancer 1998;83:2391–9.

ELSEVIER
SAUNDERS

PEDIATRIC CLINICS
OF NORTH AMERICA

Pediatr Clin N Am 55 (2008) 147–167

Cancer Immunotherapy: Will Expanding Knowledge Lead to Success in Pediatric Oncology?

Terry J. Fry, MD[a],*, Arjan C. Lankester, MD, PhD[b]

[a]Division, Blood/Marrow Transplantation and Immunology, Center for Cancer and Blood
Disorders, Children's National Medical Center, 111 Michigan Ave., NW,
Washington, DC 10010, USA
[b]Department of Pediatrics, BMT-Unit, Leiden University Medical Center,
Leiden, the Netherlands

The initial use of immunotherapy for cancer occurred in the early 1900s when Coley [1] used bacterial products to treat patients who had Ewing sarcoma based on the observation that postoperative infections seemed to diminish the likelihood of tumor recurrence. A number of patients were treated with these bacterial products, resulting in regression in a few [2]. James Ewing was simultaneously testing radiation as a means to treat these sarcomas, and controversy as to which approach was superior ensued. The consistency in response seen with radiation led to this treatment being more widely accepted, and the field of immunotherapy would need to wait approximately 50 years until it was explored further. The past 25 years have seen an increase in our understanding of immunology and further expansion in the clinical use of immunotherapeutic modalities. How immunotherapy will be integrated with chemotherapy, radiation, and surgery remains to be established. Although there have been successes in the field of immunotherapy, they have been inconsistent, and it is hoped that increased understanding of the basic principles of immunology will improve the consistency of beneficial effects. In this article, we briefly provide a general overview of our current understanding of the immune system, with a focus on concepts in tumor immunology, followed by a discussion of how these concepts are being used in the clinic. Although this overview illustrates the highly integrated nature of the immune system, we divide the clinical section into specific arms of the immune response. It is likely that, as with the

* Corresponding author.
E-mail address: tfry@cnmc.org (T.J. Fry).

doi:10.1016/j.pcl.2007.10.015   pediatric.theclinics.com natural immune response, immunotherapy is most effective when the components of the immune armamentarium are used in combination.

Principles of the immune response

The immune system evolved to protect the host from invading pathogens. These processes can effectively clear aberrant self-antigens, including malignant cells [3]. A complete description of the immune response is beyond the scope of this article, but we highlight areas relevant to cancer immunotherapy. In general, the immune system can be divided into the innate response, which allows rapid, nonspecific protection, and the adaptive response, which develops more slowly but provides specific recognition of antigens via expression of carefully rearranged receptors. Fig. 1 illustrates the various components of the immune response. Although the innate system is an essential part of successful immune clearance, this article focuses on adaptive immunity.

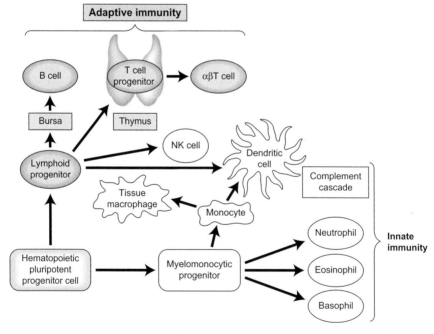

Fig. 1. The immune response can be divided into innate and adaptive components. The innate system provides rapid and relatively nonspecific protection, whereas the adaptive response is delayed but more specific. Innate and adaptive responses are critical for effective immunity, although each plays more or less prominent roles depending on the nature of the immune response (viral, bacterial, etc.). Monocytes/macrophages, neutrophils, basophils, and eosinophils serve as the primary players in innate immunity. B cells and αβ T cells represent the central components of adaptive immunity. NK cells are generally considered a member of the innate response, although there is some specificity to NK cell recognition.

The adaptive immune system contains millions of potential specificities requiring amplification upon initial antigen encounter, which results in delayed onset but allows for a memory effect such that subsequent exposures to antigen result in a more rapid clearance. One potential danger of this type of system is the recognition of self-antigens resulting in autoimmunity. To prevent this, a number of strategies have evolved, including central deletion of specificities directed against self-antigens (in the thymus for T cells); the development of a complex network of regulatory cell types that maintain tolerance to self-antigens in the periphery (outside the thymus); and the requirement for professional antigen-presenting cells, such as dendritic cells (DCs), to effectively initiate the adaptive immune response. DCs are capable of sensing, filtering, and interpreting signals for the adaptive immune cells, providing an important link between the innate and adaptive immune response [4].

T cells and B cells

Developing T cells and B cells rearrange germline DNA to generate receptors that are maintained throughout subsequent progeny and are capable of recognizing specific antigens. For B cells, gene rearrangement initially occurs in the bone marrow, with further rearrangements possible in the germinal center of the lymph node during maturation of the immune response after antigen encounter. For T cells, this process occurs in the thymus, where specificities are selected on the basis of recognition of self–human leukocyte antigens (HLAs) followed by deletion of T cells with high affinity for self-antigens. Although this process is complex and results in loss of greater than 95% of all rearranged T cells in the thymus, it allows for sufficient repertoire to protect throughout the lifespan of the host without causing autoimmunity in most individuals. Naive T cells and B cells circulate in a resting state until they encounter an antigen that binds to the specific receptor expressed on the surface of a responding cell. For T cells, this antigen is presented in the context of self HLA molecules on specialized antigen-presenting cells (APCs), such as DCs. CD4+ T cells recognize antigen in the context of HLA class II molecules, and for CD8+ T cells this recognition occurs on HLA class I molecules. Effective stimulation of the immune response also requires a second costimulatory signal provided by the APCs. The nature of a costimulatory signal (positive, negative, and how strong) is modulated by factors sensed by the APCs, such as bacterial products or inflammatory substances produced during the innate immune response (also referred to as "danger signals" [4]). An important group of receptors known as toll-like receptors (TLRs) recognizes these products and modulates the capacity for the APCs to stimulate a T-cell response, thus demonstrating one important link between innate and adaptive immunity [5]. Once activated, T and B lymphocytes undergo rapid clonal expansion, providing large numbers of effectors. T cells mediate an immune response via direct cytotoxicity of the target cell (perforin, granzyme, fas/fasL) or by secretion of effector cytokines, such as interferons, whereas B cells differentiate into antibody-secreting plasma cells. T and B lymphocytes also "talk" to other immune cells (innate and adaptive) by secretion of cytokines or through expression of surface molecules, resulting in further refinement in the immune response. Cytokines such as interleukin (IL)-2, IL-7, or IL-15 have been administered in clinical and preclinical studies to enhance antitumor immune responses [6–8]. In addition, agents that interfere with regulatory signals generated by surface receptors on responding immune cells, such as CTLA-4 (a negative regulator of T-cell immunity), have been used in patients who have cancer and who have demonstrated clinical activity [9]. Fig. 2 demonstrates a schematic of the immune response.

An important subset of T cells generated in the thymus acquires a regulatory phenotype before export into the periphery, providing further protection against autoimmunity [10]. These naturally occurring regulatory T cells (Tregs) can be identified by expression of CD4 and CD25 (a component of the IL-2 receptor), low or absent expression of the IL-7 receptor, and the FoxP3 transcription factor. There is a subset of Tregs that can be induced during an immune response that may express the CD4 or CD8 co-receptor [10]. Our growing understanding of Tregs has led to the recognition that these cells may be detrimental to an effective antitumor immune response, particularly when the antigens targeted are self-antigens for which these regulatory networks are well developed [11]. Current immunotherapeutic protocols are exploring depletion or the modulation of Tregs as a means to enhance adaptive immune responses [12].

Natural killer cells

Natural killer (NK) cells are bone-marrow–derived lymphocytes that do not bear clonally rearranged antigen-specific receptors. In humans, NK cells are phenotypically defined as $CD3^-/CD56^+$ lymphocytes, which can be divided into $CD56^{dim}$ ($CD16^+$) cytotoxic and $CD56^{bright}$ immunoregulatory NK-cell subsets [13]. NK cells have the potential to recognize and eliminate a wide range of tumors and virally infected cells. Besides acting as cytotoxic effector cells in immune responses, evidence is accumulating that NK cells play a crucial role in the translation of signals from innate toward adaptive immunity via bidirectional interaction with DCs [14]. Recent evidence indicates that type I interferon (IFN)-experienced DCs prime NK cells in an IL-15–dependent manner [15]. Primed NK cells can promote maturation of DCs in an IFN-γ–dependent manner, thereby facilitating further induction of T_{H1} (cellular) T-cell responses [16,17]. Therefore, NK cells may exert a dual function in antitumor responses by acting as direct effector cells and as initiators of T-cell–mediated antitumor responses [18].

The functional status of NK cells is regulated by the balance of inhibitory and activating NK-cell ligands on the target cells. Inhibitory signals are

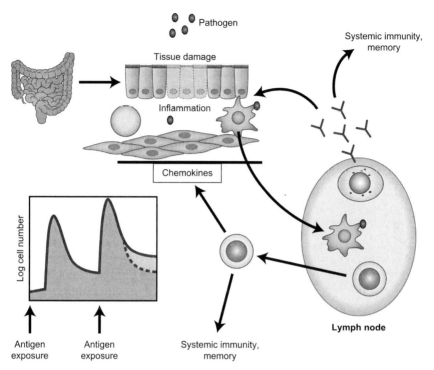

Fig. 2. Representation of the immune response to a gut pathogen. Initial pathogen-induced tissue damage results in invasion of submucosa by the pathogen and the generation of inflammation mediated, in part by the initial innate response. DCs resident in the gut acquire pathogen-derived antigens and signals from the inflammatory environment, resulting in further activation. The loaded and activated DCs migrate to the lymph node and initiate antigen-specific B-cell activation. B cells secrete antibodies directed against pathogen-derived antigens and activated T cells with pathogen specificity traffic to the gut directed, in part, by chemokines. Inset: Graphical representation of sequential adaptive immune responses to the same antigen. The response to the initial encounter is delayed, followed by a rapid amplification and subsequent contraction. The response does not return to initial baseline, instead remaining at a higher-level reflective of memory, which allows for a more rapid response upon subsequent encounter. One principal of vaccination against infections or tumors is that repeated boosting results in greater and greater amplification and a larger memory pool. Responses to tumors likely follow a similar pattern, although there is the added complexity of immune evasion as described in the section on immune escape.

provided by classical and nonclassical HLA class I molecules, which bind to killer immunoglobulin- like receptors (KIRs) or NKG2A/CD94 on NK cells [19]. Within the human population, there is a wide variation in the repertoire of KIR genes. Together with the clonal distribution within the NK repertoire, this results in a wide diversity of expression profiles between and within individuals.

The inhibitory signals can be decreased in patients who have solid tumors caused by a down-regulation of HLA class I on the tumor cells (see

"Immune escape"). Lack of HLA-dependent inhibitory signals may permit recognition and elimination of tumor cells by NK cells according to mechanism of "missing self" recognition [20]. In addition, interaction between NK-cell–activating receptors and their specific ligands on target cells seems necessary for adequate NK cell stimulation [21]. NK cells can be triggered by stress-induced ligands that are expressed by the tumor itself, such as the MIC (MICA/B) and ULBP (ULBP1-4) family of proteins. The expression of these molecules on tumors can be induced by DNA damage. The activating receptor NKG2D on the NK cell can bind to these ligands and lead to an activating signal [22]. Other activating NK cell receptors include the DNAX accessory molecule-1, which is activated by the CD112 (Nectin-2) and CD155 (PVR) molecules [23]. A third group of activating receptors is represented by the natural cytotoxicity receptors NKp30, NKp44, and NKp46. Their physiologic ligands remain to be identified [14].

Many preclinical studies have provided evidence that a broad spectrum of human and murine tumor cell lines are susceptible to NK-cell cytotoxicity, albeit with different efficacy. The variation in NK-cell susceptibility seems related to differences in expression levels of the aforementioned activating and inhibitory ligands on tumor cells [24,25]. In addition to tumor cell lines, NK cells have been shown to have the potential to eliminate or prevent outgrowth of murine tumors in in vivo models [26]. In humans, the clinical significance of NK cells in the control of solid tumors is unresolved and is the subject of many studies.

NK-cell activation and cytolytic potential can be increased upon stimulation with various cytokines (eg, IL-2, IL-12, and IL-15) and type I IFN [27]. In various clinical trials, in vivo administration of some of these agents has been used to induce NK-cell–mediated antitumor responses with limited clinical efficacy [28]. Further insight in the role of these agents in NK cell regulation will provide tools to manipulate NK-cell function and will be of benefit in future adoptive transfer studies.

Another dimension of NK tumor target recognition may be seen in an allogeneic setting where a KIR–HLA mismatch between donor and patient may result in the absence of tumor cells of ligands for inhibitory KIR on donor NK cells. In this setting of "missing self-recognition," the available alloreactive donor NK-cell repertoire may be exploited to eliminate recipient tumor cells. Combined with the preferential expression of activating NK-cell ligands on malignant cells, this might result in a selective elimination of these targets without the risk of inducing concurrent graft-versus-host disease (GvHD). The first evidence for the clinical implication of this model has been reported by Ruggeri and colleagues in patients who have acute myeloid leukemia undergoing haploidentical stem cell transplantation [29]. In their experience, KIR-HLA mismatch was associated with a better clinical outcome, lower relapse rate, and reduced frequency of GvHD [30]. In subsequent studies, conflicting results have been reported on the advantage of KIR-HLA that may be related to the level of T-cell depletion and the repertoire of alloreactive donor NK cells [31]. Further insight into reconstitution, regulation, and functional properties of the (alloreactive) NK-cell repertoire after allogeneic stem cell transplantation (SCT) is needed to optimize exploitation of its potential. Altogether, the mode of action of NK cells indicates that they have the potential to exert potent antitumor immunity and may act complementary to and in synergy with T cells.

Immune escape

As first proposed by Burnett [32], tumors are not passive targets for cellular immune responses and are capable of escaping from and disabling the host immune system [3,15]. Changes in tumor phenotype not only permit tumor escape from normal immunologic surveillance but may also negatively influence the susceptibility and response to antitumor immunotherapy. In the setting of clinically established tumors, initial immune surveillance has failed to eliminate tumor cells. Immune pressure may have resulted in the generation of immune escape variants via the mechanism of immuno-editing [33,34]. General mechanisms of immune escape include interference with specific recognition of tumors by the immune system, reduced susceptibility of tumors to the apoptosis-inducing capacity of cytotoxic effector cells, and immunosuppressive potential of the tumor. These mechanisms have been described in detail elsewhere [35,36] and are therefore only be briefly discussed here.

Immune cell recognition of tumors

Appropriate expression of HLA/peptide complexes on tumor cells plays a crucial role in the effector phase of cellular immunotherapy because they present antigenic epitopes to CTLs. A commonly known mechanism of immune escape involves impaired antigen processing or presentation. Total or selective loss of HLA I expression has been reported in a large variety of human tumors, including sarcomas, carcinomas, and lymphomas. The clinical relevance has been demonstrated by the observation that a lack of HLA expression often relates to metastatic disease and an unfavorable outcome [37]. The basis of aberrant HLA expression has been reported to be genetic, regulatory, or epigenetic in origin. Lack of HLA expression in tumors may be caused by loss of heterozygosity, mutations, or deletions in individual HLA genes and in genes encoding $\beta 2$ microglobulin and components of the antigen-processing machinery, including peptide transporters TAP1 and TAP2, tapasin, and the proteosomal subunits LMP-2 and LMP-7 [38]. The aberrant HLA expression pattern in tumors at diagnosis, which may be heterogeneous within individual tumors, indicates that a process of selection pressure has occurred. Evidence that immune surveillance and immune pressure may result in selective outgrowth of tumor variants has come from observations in clinical trials in which progressive disease after cellular immunotherapy revealed total or allelic loss of HLA expression [39–41].

Recently, a unique category of CTLs has been identified in mice bearing TAP-deficient tumors. These tumors were found to express peptides derived from self-antigens in the context of classical and nonclassical MHC class I molecules, named T-cell epitopes, associated with impaired peptide processing, which may serve as alternative tumor-specific CTL targets [42]. Together with conventional tumor-specific T cells, T cell epitopes associated with impaired peptide processing (TEIPP)-specific CTLs might be considered in future studies to prevent outgrowth of or treat TAP-deficient tumors.

In addition to genetic causes, aberrant HLA expression may be the result of transcriptional regulation. During normal immune responses, HLA class I and II expression is strictly orchestrated and mediated by several immune regulators, including IFN-γ and TNF-α [43], that have the potential to increase HLA expression in a variety of HLA-deficient tumor cell lines. Another possible mechanism responsible for transcriptional regulation of HLA expression is represented by epigenetic modifications, including histone acetylation and DNA methylation. Treatment with histone deacetylase inhibitors and methyltransferase inhibitors has been demonstrated to restore HLA expression in a variety of tumors and hematologic malignancies [44]. Whether this category of agents, which has been used as anticancer therapy in clinical trials, may be beneficial in future clinical immunotherapy studies remains to be resolved.

Tumors may specifically down-regulate expression of CTL tumor target antigens, which result in antigenic loss variants [45]. The clinical significance of this mechanism has been clearly observed in immunotherapy trials with patients who have melanoma in whom metastases occurring after treatment were found to selectively lack expression of CTL target antigens [46]. This illustrates the biological mechanism that selective pressure has the potential to generate immune escape variants. In addition, it shows that antigen-specific therapies, although elegant, may be vulnerable to the process of immune editing, especially in cases where tumor target antigens are used that are not essential for tumor biology and survival. Another potential hurdle for antigen-specific therapy is the often heterogeneous expression of target antigens, such as cancer-testis antigens, within individual tumors. Epigenetic regulation has been found to play a significant role in the expression of these genes, and treatment with the aforementioned hypomethylating agents has the potential to restore or increase expression, which may be beneficial in future immunotherapy studies [47].

Although partial or complete loss of HLA/peptide complex expression impairs T-cell–mediated recognition, it may increase susceptibility to NK cells, which may be inhibited by self-HLA (see section on NK cells). Aberrant expression on the tumor of the ligands for NK-cell–activating receptors or expression of HLA-surrogate molecules can protect tumor cells from NK-cell–mediated recognition and killing. Several mechanisms leading to this so-called "NK-cell tolerance" have been described. First, sustained expression of its ligand induced down-regulation of NKG2D in a murine tumor model [48], resulting in increased tumorigenesis. This process seemed to be reversible by stimulating innate immunity through TLRs. Similarly, expression of natural cytotoxicity receptors was found to be reduced in patients who have acute myelogenous leukemia (AML) compared with healthy control subjects, which was in part reversible by cytokine stimulation [49]. Second, NKG2D expression and consequent NK-cell (but also T-cell) function may be blocked and thus impaired by tumor-derived soluble ligands, as reported for soluble MICA in various human tumors [50]. Third, expression of the non-classical HLA-E and G molecules on tumors has the potential to inhibit NK-cell function via interaction with their respective receptors [51,52]. A fourth potential mechanism is the aberrant expression of NK co-receptors and (soluble) adhesion molecules, which may prevent a functional interaction [38].

Tumor susceptibility to immune cell-mediated killing

Interference with the induction of apoptosis is a frequently observed phenomenon in tumors and may be caused by a variety of mechanisms. This article focuses on the mechanisms directly related to the mode of action used by cytotoxic effector lymphocytes and particularly those reported in human tumors. Tumor cells may interfere with the cytolytic pathways used by NK and T cells by overexpression of antiapoptotic genes or by down-regulation of proapoptotic molecules.

Overexpression of serine protease-inhibitor 9 has been shown to irreversibly inactivate GrB, resulting in defective apoptosis in tumor cell lines via the granule exocytosis pathway. The clinical significance has been suggested by the correlation between protease inhibitor–9 overexpression and clinical outcome in lymphomas and the outcome after tumor vaccination in patients who have melanoma [53,54]. Escape from death receptor (DR)-mediated apoptosis by overexpression of cellular FLICE inhibitory protein, which is a catalytic inactive homolog of procaspase 8, has been demonstrated in various types of tumors in vitro and in vivo [27,28]. Negatively affecting the same pathway, lack of caspase 8 expression has been reported to interfere with DR-mediated apoptosis in several human tumors and to favor formation of metastases [55,56].

Other possible mechanisms to escape from DR pathway–mediated apoptosis include the expression of soluble (eg, soluble CD95; [57]) and decoy receptors (eg, DcR 3; [58]) and the presence of mutations in proteins involved in the DR cascade that may interfere with DR-mediated apoptosis [59]. Although the presence of these mechanisms was found to be correlated with clinical outcome of various tumors, their direct involvement in escape from immune pressure in vivo is remains to be resolved.

Tumor-induced immune suppression

It has been extensively reported that cancer patients are often characterized by a general state of decreased immune competence by mechanisms that are only partially understood. These mechanisms have been described in detail in several recent reviews [15,60]. Therefore, only a selection of mechanisms actively induced by the tumor is mentioned here. First, tumors may actively secrete immune suppressive cytokines (eg, IL-10, TGF-β and Indolamine 2,3-Dioxygenase [IDO]) that are able to interfere in various ways with innate and adaptive immune responses. Second, an increased frequency of circulating Tregs and their migration to the tumor environment has been reported in cancer patients [11]. The influx of Tregs in tissue or the surrounding stroma varied among different tumor types and between individuals. An association between Tregs numbers and clinical behavior (progressive disease) was first described in ovarian cancer patients [61]. The immunosuppressive effect induced by Tregs involves several potential mechanisms mediated via soluble factors and direct cell–cell contact as described in the previous sections on T-cell–mediated responses. Third, tumors have the potential to attract myeloid suppressor cells that may exert multiple inhibitory functions, including suppression of tumor infiltrated lymphocytes [62]. Fourth, down-regulation of T-cell receptor signaling molecules that may be reversible upon removal of the tumor has been reported in cancer patients [63].

Lymphocyte migration

For cellular immunotherapy to be effective, migration of effector T or NK cells to the tumor site, extravasation, and invasion into the tumor are pivotal. The presence of and variability in the amount of tumor-infiltrating lymphocytes (TILs) have been reported in many human tumors. In some studies, the presence of these TILs was reported to be correlated with the pattern of HLA expression. Recent studies in colorectal, ovarian, and cervical tumors have shown that the phenotypical profile of the TIL at diagnosis was a strong predictor of clinical outcome [64–66]. Particularly, the CD8/Treg ratio was found to be positively correlated with a favorable prognosis. These findings illustrate that insight into the molecular mechanisms involved in tumor site–directed migration are important to the understanding of the quantitative and qualitative differences in the naturally occurring TIL responses. This provides knowledge required to develop strategies to manipulate the natural immune response and to support (adoptive) immunotherapy interventions.

Site-directed migration of T/NK cells is a nonrandom process induced by inflammatory and other pathogenic stimuli. In lymphoid and in inflamed nonlymphoid tissues, lymphocyte adherence and tissue influx are facilitated by specialized high-endothelial venules (HEVs). HEVs express various adhesion molecules (eg, VCAM-1 and ICAM-1) and chemokines (eg, CCL21, CXCL9, and CXCL25), which create a highly regulated interface between lymphocytes and endothelial cells [67]. In contrast, intratumoral vessels are characterized by squamous endothelial cells with low expression of these molecules [68]. Generally, lymphocyte extravasation at the tumor site is limited. Significant differences have been reported between intratumoral-(low) and peritumoral- (dense) vessel lymphocyte extravasation. The molecular basis for these differences remains to be resolved, but a regulatory role has been suggested for pro- and antiangiogenic factors (eg, vascular endothelial growth factor), anti-inflammatory cytokines (eg, TGF-β), and the tumor cells themselves [69]. Transformation of squamous "nonattractive" tumor vessel endothelium into endothelial cells with a HEV-like appearance could have a beneficial effect on lymphocyte migration at the tumor site. Potential approaches include stimulation with inflammatory mediators (eg, TLR ligands), ionizing irradiation, and transgenic expression of recruiting cytokines [70].

Chemokines are a superfamily of small molecules that regulate this selective process of migration. Directional migration of T/NK cells expressing the appropriate chemokine receptor(s) occurs along a chemical gradient of ligand(s) [71]. In cancer, chemokines produced by the tumor may play a role in the pattern of leukocyte infiltration [72]. Several recent studies on human tumors have provided evidence for the significance of tumor-secreted chemokines on TIL responses and clinical outcome. Immune stimulatory and inhibitory effects have been proposed depending on the extent and by which cells the chemokines are produced in the tumor environment [71,72]. Identification of the relevant chemokines involved in the attraction of cytotoxic effector T or NK cells and Tregs combined with insight in the patterns of expression and regulation of these chemokines in human tumors may provide tools to manipulate the attractive capacity of the tumor and thereby improve the process of tumor-site–directed migration during T/NK-cell–mediated immunotherapy studies.

Clinical experience with immune-based therapies for cancer

T-cell therapy

A number of strategies have been developed to use T cells as immunotherapeutic tools against tumors. Adoptive therapies involve the infusion of large numbers of T cells into patients (autologous or allogeneic). Vaccine therapy attempts to expand T cells, recognizing tumor associated antigens in vivo. Finally, cytokines have been used alone or combined with other strategies to expand or enhance the function of antitumor T cells.

Autologous

The use of autologous T cells to target malignancy can involve the infusion of manipulated or unmanipulated T cells or the administration of vaccines to expand tumor-reactive T cells in vivo. The existence of tumor-specific or tumor-associated antigens that can be targeted using these approaches has been clearly demonstrated [73]. The majority of these antigens are self-antigens expressed during a restricted period of development or in restricted tissues. Therefore, the process of inducing effective antitumor T-cell immunity requires that the self-tolerance mechanisms previously described be overcome [10,74]. This has presented one of the major obstacles to effective T-cell–based therapies.

For adoptive T-cell therapies, the source can be peripheral blood T cells or tumor-infiltrating T cells, which can then be harvested and reinfused into patients. T cells reactive against tumor antigens are present but infrequent in the blood of cancer patients. Although these T cells may be present at higher frequency in tumor infiltrates, the total number of cells that can be harvested is insufficient. Thus, effective adoptive immunotherapy requires manipulation and expansion in vitro to increase the frequency of T-cell–recognizing tumor antigens in the infused product. This approach has been used in the clinic and has resulted in regression in patients who have melanoma. A number of other clinical trials using adoptive immunotherapy have been undertaken, some demonstrating clinical benefit [75]. The experience of Dudley and colleagues [76] suggested that regression required that extremely high doses of T cells be infused such that a high percentage of circulating T cells recognized the tumor (~ 20–30%). These important findings indicate proof of the principle that, at least for melanoma, adoptive T-cell therapies represent a promising immunotherapeutic modality [77,78]. An alternative method to overcome the low frequency of tumor reactive T cells in autologous products that is being explored is gene transfer of T-cell receptors known to recognize tumor antigens into cells with cytotoxic potential, such as T cells or NK cells [79–81]. Although there has been much progress in the area of autologous adoptive immunotherapy for cancer in adults, there are limited data in pediatric patients [82].

Another approach that can be used alone or in combination with adoptive T-cell therapy is the use of vaccines to expand tumor-reactive T cells. The types of vaccines used include whole tumor cells, peptides derived from known tumor antigens, replication-deficient viruses expressing tumor antigens, and DCs loaded with tumor antigens [83]. A large and growing number of clinical trials have been undertaken using each of these vaccine strategies resulting in vaccine responses and some evidence of clinical response, but the potency and consistency of these responses has been poor [84,85]. Most of these trials have been undertaken in the setting of bulky tumors where immune-based therapies may be less effective due to the tumor suppressive mechanisms discussed previously. Furthermore, the magnitude of the immune response generated by vaccines alone suggests that combining vaccines with adoptive therapies or T-cell–active cytokines may be necessary. Another strategy is the use of adjuvants to amplify weak vaccine-induced T-cell responses. There is the most clinical experience with Freund's adjuvant, but newer agents are being explored that specifically target innate immune cells via TLRs [86,87]. It is likely that effective vaccination protocols will need to incorporate multiple strategies to generate sufficient immune responses to induce clinically meaningful responses [88].

As with adoptive immunotherapy, experience in pediatrics is limited, but there has been one promising clinical response in pediatric sarcoma [89–92].

Allogeneic

Perhaps the most potent form of immune-based therapy is the graft-versus-tumor reaction that occurs after allogeneic transplantation [93]. T cells and NK cells contribute to this response. The T-cell contribution is evident from the increased risk of relapse that occurs after transplantation of stem cell products that are depleted of T lymphocytes and when patients are treated with T-cell immunosuppressants. For chronic myeloid leukemia (CML) that recurs after transplant, remissions can be induced in up 50% or more of patients by stopping immunosupression or infusing donor lymphocytes (DLI) [94]. For AML, responses to donor lymphocyte infusions occur, but the frequency of responses is substantially lower than for CML (~20–30%). For pediatric acute lymphocytic leukemia, 5-year disease-free survival after allogeneic transplantation ranges from approximately 40% to 80%, depending on risk status and type of donor used [95]. If relapse occurs, the poor response to immune manipulation suggests that the graft-versus-leukemia effect is far less potent than for AML or CML, although the reasons for this are not clear. Acute lymphocytic leukemia blasts are inferior at initiating immune responses but are susceptible to autologous T-cell–mediated immune responses [96]. Thus, for the most common form of pediatric leukemia, strategies to enhance the graft-versus-leukemia response are needed if outcomes are to be improved.

The effectiveness of the graft-versus-malignancy response is, to a large extent, due to the ability to target minor histocompatibility antigens that are disparate between the donor and recipient because these antigens do not require the immune response to overcome tolerance to self-antigens [97]. Another advantage of allogeneic transplant is the availability of donor-immune cells that have not been depleted or exposed to cytotoxic therapy and are not contaminated by tumor cells. Finally, it is possible that tumor restricted immune responses induced in the allogeneic transplant environment may be more potent than similar responses induced using the autologous environment. Thus, there are a number of potential benefits in considering allogeneic transplantation as a platform for immune-based therapies.

The main hurdle to overcome when using allogeneic transplantation as immunotherapy is the induction of GvHD. Most of the available approaches to enhance graft-versus-tumor reactions are nonspecific, such that the antitumor reaction is closely linked to GvHD. The use of strategies such as vaccines [98,99] or adoptive therapy with antitumor T-cell–enriched donor lymphocytes may be potential mechanisms to overcome this hurdle. An alternative would be to develop strategies to selectively modulate alloresponses against GvHD target organs. For example, selective depletion of alloreactive T cells in vitro before infusion of stem cells has been explored in preclincial and clinical settings [100–102]. The ability to manipulate the post-transplant environment to enhance the graft-versus-malignancy reaction would result in less reliance on pretransplant conditioning for cure, potentially allowing the use of reduced-intensity conditioning regimens, which have been used successfully for pediatric nonmalignant diseases and adult malignancies. Given the long-term morbidity associated with myeloablative transplantation for pediatric patients, this would be a desirable scenario.

Natural killer cell therapy

Autologous

The first studies in this field were performed in the 1980s by the Rosenberg team [103]. Autologous IL-2/lymphokine-activated killer cells, combined with high-dose IL-2 in vivo, were used to treat cancer patients who had refractory disease, including melanoma and renal cell carcinoma.

In subsequent years, many more patients were included in similar studies receiving lymphokine activated killer cells combined with IL-2 or IL-2 alone, resulting in a response rate of 10% to 20% [104]. The limited efficacy and substantial toxicity of this approach together with the identification of tumor antigens as targets has shifted attention to T-cell–mediated strategies. Progress in our understanding of NK-cell biology and the aforementioned implications of KIR-HLA (mis)matching in allogeneic SCT have resulted in renewed attention for the clinical application of allogeneic NK-cell–mediated immunotherapy strategies.

Allogeneic

The use of haploidentical NK cells in a nontransplant setting was first explored by Miller and colleagues [105] in patients who had refractory hematologic malignancies and solid tumors. For this purpose, NK-cell preparations were obtained from leukapheresis products using immunomagnetic CD3 depletion followed by overnight IL-2 stimulation. From this and subsequent studies, they concluded that a high-dose cyclophosphamide/fludarabine regimen was required to obtain long-term survival and expansion of the infused cells. In addition, NK-cell expansion was found to be correlated with endogenous IL-15 levels, which is in agreement with its role in survival and homeostatic proliferation. Infusion of the NK-cell products did not result in GvHD or other toxicity events. Clinical efficacy was demonstrated by achievement of a CR in a subgroup of patients who had AML. This was only observed in the patients receiving high-dose NK-cell treatment and was correlated with KIR–ligand mismatch in the GvHD direction. This and other pilot studies have provided evidence for the safety and feasibility of allogeneic NK-cell infusions [106]. Further studies are required to investigate the antitumor efficacy in vivo and to unravel the relevant mechanisms involved. In addition to primary NK cells, adoptive transfer studies have been performed using the NK cell line NK-92, expressing activating receptors and lacking inhibitory receptors. The use of these cells was found to be safe, and antitumor responses have been observed [107].

Several important issues remain unresolved and require further study to optimize the clinical use of allogeneic NK-cell preparations [108]. One of these issues includes the technical approach used to obtain a defined number of NK cells from leukapheresis products and to reduce the amount of contaminating alloreactive T cells. Several procedures, including negative (ie, T and B cells) and positive (ie, CD56) selection steps, which are available under clinical grade conditions, are being investigated by several groups. Second, the absolute number and functional status of NK cells required for efficacy needs to be established. Little is known about dose-response ratios and the in vivo behavior of infused NK cells, but it is likely that this is influenced by multiple factors. Miller and colleagues [105] have demonstrated that a leuko/lymphopenia-inducing preparative regimen seems required to permit engraftment and expansion of adoptively transferred NK cells. Substantial evidence obtained from in vitro and in vivo studies indicates that the functional properties and survival of NK-cell populations, including responses toward tumor cells, can be increased after cytokine stimulation. This seems to justify the preferential use of ex vivo–stimulated NK-cell populations. Endogenous production of cytokines that influence NK-cell activation and survival (eg, IL-15) could play a significant role and is probably dependent on the preparative regimen, timing of NK-cell infusion, and postinfusion therapeutic regimens. By definition, the NK-cell repertoire is phenotypically and functionally heterogeneous, implying that significant interindividual differences will probably be encountered when these cells are used in adoptive transfer studies. In the allogeneic KIR-ligand mismatched setting, the interindividual variability in the amount of alloreactive NK cells is an additional factor that may influence outcome [30]. The challenge is to obtain further insight in the impact of all these parameters on clinical immune and antitumor responses in the scheduled and ongoing clinical trials. Given the reported favorable outcome of KIR-ligand mismatched haploidentical SCT in patients who have refractory AML and the apparent safety profile of allogeneic NK-cell infusions, it seems interesting to investigate exploitation of the NK-cell effect in patients who have NK-cell–permissive solid tumors in a similar haploidentical setting.

B cells

Antibody therapy

Although this review has emphasized cellular therapies, the use of monoclonal antibodies targeting malignancy is rapidly expanding. Although the majority of these antibodies has been developed for adult cancers, some have demonstrated utility in pediatric malignancy [109]. For example, anti-CD20 has been used in pediatric lymphomas. Although this agent may theoretically target CD20-expressing pediatric B-cell leukemias,

responses in this setting have been less promising. One difficulty with monoclonal antibodies alone is that, unless they interfere with receptor signaling
on which the tumor is dependant, they require a mechanism such as antibody-dependant cytotoxicity to clear tumor cells. To overcome this, a newer
generation of antibodies has been conjugated to radioisotopes or toxins to
deliver these directly to the tumor [110,111]. A number of these antibodies
are in clinical trials in pediatric malignancies.

Summary

Although the immune system has long been recognized as providing
a strategy to treat cancer, the full potential of immune-based therapies for
malignancy has not been realized. Rapid increases in our understanding
of basic immunologic principles and mechanisms by which tumors evade
the immune response have served as a basis for improving on these
approaches. Current strategies have used numerous arms of the adaptive
and innate immune response. It will likely require a multipronged approach
incorporating combination therapy to maximize the potential of the immune
response against cancer. In addition, it will be important to establish how
immunotherapy is to be best integrated into the standard armamentarium
of chemotherapy therapy, radiation therapy, and surgery. This will be particularly true for pediatric cancers, where remissions can be induced using
standard treatments in the majority of patients and preventing relapse presents the major obstacle to cure. Immunotherapy may ultimately prove most
effective in this setting.

References

[1] Coley WB. Sarcoma of the long bones: the diagnosis, treatment and prognosis, with a report
    of sixty-nine cases. Ann Surg 1907;45(3):321–68.
[2] Brunschwig A. The efficacy of "Coley's Toxin" in the treatment of sarcoma: an experimen-
    tal study. Ann Surg 1939;109(1):109–13.
[3] Dunn GP, Old LJ, Schreiber RD. The immunobiology of cancer immunosurveillance and
    immunoediting. Immunity 2004;21(2):137–48.
[4] Matzinger P. An innate sense of danger. Ann N Y Acad Sci 2002;961:341–2.
[5] Iwasaki A, Medzhitov R. Toll-like receptor control of the adaptive immune responses. Nat
    Immunol 2004;5(10):987–95.
[6] Waldmann TA. The biology of interleukin-2 and interleukin-15: implications for cancer
    therapy and vaccine design. Nat Rev Immunol 2006;6(8):595–601.
[7] Fry TJ, Mackall CL. The many faces of IL-7: from lymphopoiesis to peripheral T cell main-
    tenance. J Immunol 2005;174(11):6571–6.
[8] Rosenberg SA, Sportes C, Ahmadzadeh M, et al. IL-7 administration to humans leads to
    expansion of CD8+ and CD4+ cells but a relative decrease of CD4+ T-regulatory cells.
    J Immunother (1997) 2006;29(3):313–9.
[9] Langer LF, Clay TM, Morse MA. Update on anti-CTLA-4 antibodies in clinical trials.
    Expert Opin Biol Ther 2007;7(8):1245–56.

[10] Zou W. Regulatory T cells, tumour immunity and immunotherapy. Nat Rev Immunol 2006;6(4):295–307.

[11] Beyer M, Schultze JL. Regulatory T cells in cancer. Blood 2006;108(3):804–11.

[12] Banham AH, Powrie FM, Suri-Payer E. FOXP3+ regulatory T cells: current controversies and future perspectives. Eur J Immunol 2006;36(11):2832–6.

[13] Cooper MA, Fehniger TA, Caligiuri MA. The biology of human natural killer-cell subsets. Trends Immunol 2001;22(11):633–40.

[14] Moretta L, Ferlazzo G, Bottino C, et al. Effector and regulatory events during natural killer-dendritic cell interactions. Immunol Rev 2006;214:219–28.

[15] Whiteside TL. Immune suppression in cancer: effects on immune cells, mechanisms and future therapeutic intervention. Semin Cancer Biol 2006;16(1):3–15.

[16] Lucas M, Schachterle W, Oberle K, et al. Dendritic cells prime natural killer cells by trans-presenting interleukin 15. Immunity 2007;26(4):503–17.

[17] Degli-Esposti MA, Smyth MJ. Close encounters of different kinds: dendritic cells and NK cells take centre stage. Nat Rev Immunol 2005;5(2):112–24.

[18] Raulet DH. Interplay of natural killer cells and their receptors with the adaptive immune response. Nat Immunol 2004;5(10):996–1002.

[19] Parham P. MHC class I molecules and KIRs in human history, health and survival. Nat Rev Immunol 2005;5(3):201–14.

[20] Ljunggren HG, Karre K. In search of the 'missing self': MHC molecules and NK cell recognition. Immunol Today 1990;11(7):237–44.

[21] Bryceson YT, March ME, Ljunggren HG, et al. Activation, coactivation, and costimulation of resting human natural killer cells. Immunol Rev 2006;214:73–91.

[22] Hayakawa Y, Smyth MJ. NKG2D and cytotoxic effector function in tumor immune surveillance. Semin Immunol 2006;18(3):176–85.

[23] Pende D, Bottino C, Castriconi R, et al. PVR (CD155) and Nectin-2 (CD112) as ligands of the human DNAM-1 (CD226) activating receptor: involvement in tumor cell lysis. Mol Immunol 2005;42(4):463–9.

[24] Castriconi R, Dondero A, Corrias MV, et al. Natural killer cell-mediated killing of freshly isolated neuroblastoma cells: critical role of DNAX accessory molecule-1-poliovirus receptor interaction. Cancer Res 2004;64(24):9180–4.

[25] Pende D, Spaggiari GM, Marcenaro S, et al. Analysis of the receptor-ligand interactions in the natural killer-mediated lysis of freshly isolated myeloid or lymphoblastic leukemias: evidence for the involvement of the Poliovirus receptor (CD155) and Nectin-2 (CD112). Blood 2005;105(5):2066–73.

[26] Wu J, Lanier LL. Natural killer cells and cancer. Adv Cancer Res 2003;90:127–56.

[27] Becknell B, Caligiuri MA. Interleukin-2, interleukin-15, and their roles in human natural killer cells. Adv Immunol 2005;86:209–39.

[28] Smyth MJ, Cretney E, Kershaw MH, et al. Cytokines in cancer immunity and immunotherapy. Immunol Rev 2004;202:275–93.

[29] Ruggeri L, Capanni M, Urbani E, et al. Effectiveness of donor natural killer cell alloreactivity in mismatched hematopoietic transplants. Science 2002;295(5562):2097–100.

[30] Ruggeri L, Mancusi A, Capanni M, et al. Donor natural killer cell allorecognition of missing self in haploidentical hematopoietic transplantation for acute myeloid leukemia: challenging its predictive value. Blood 2007;110(1):433–40.

[31] Farag SS, Bacigalupo A, Eapen M, et al. The effect of KIR ligand incompatibility on the outcome of unrelated donor transplantation: a report from the center for international blood and marrow transplant research, the European blood and marrow transplant registry, and the Dutch registry. Biol Blood Marrow Transplant 2006;12(8):876–84.

[32] Burnett FM. The concept of immunological surveillance. Prog Exp Tumor Res 1970;13:1–27.

[33] Khong HT, Restifo NP. Natural selection of tumor variants in the generation of "tumor escape" phenotypes. Nat Immunol 2002;3(11):999–1005.

[34] Zitvogel L, Tesniere A, Kroemer G. Cancer despite immunosurveillance: immunoselection and immunosubversion. Nat Rev Immunol 2006;6(10):715–27.

[35] Malmberg KJ, Ljunggren HG. Escape from immune- and nonimmune-mediated tumor surveillance. Semin Cancer Biol 2006;16(1):16–31.

[36] Kim R, Emi M, Tanabe K. Cancer immunoediting from immune surveillance to immune escape. Immunology 2007;121(1):1–14.

[37] Algarra I, Garcia-Lora A, Cabrera T, et al. The selection of tumor variants with altered expression of classical and nonclassical MHC class I molecules: implications for tumor immune escape. Cancer Immunol Immunother 2004;53(10):904–10.

[38] Chang CC, Ferrone S. Immune selective pressure and HLA class I antigen defects in malignant lesions. Cancer Immunol Immunother 2007;56(2):227–36.

[39] Lehmann F, Marchand M, Hainaut P, et al. Differences in the antigens recognized by cytolytic T cells on two successive metastases of a melanoma patient are consistent with immune selection. Eur J Immunol 1995;25(2):340–7.

[40] Restifo NP, Marincola FM, Kawakami Y, et al. Loss of functional beta 2-microglobulin in metastatic melanomas from five patients receiving immunotherapy. J Natl Cancer Inst 1996;88(2):100–8.

[41] Seliger B, Cabrera T, Garrido F, et al. HLA class I antigen abnormalities and immune escape by malignant cells. Semin Cancer Biol 2002;12(1):3–13.

[42] van Hall T, Wolpert EZ, van Veelen P, et al. Selective cytotoxic T-lymphocyte targeting of tumor immune escape variants. Nat Med 2006;12(4):417–24.

[43] van den Elsen PJ, Gobin SJ, van Eggermond MC, et al. Regulation of MHC class I and II gene transcription: differences and similarities. Immunogenetics 1998;48(3):208–21.

[44] van den Elsen PJ, Holling TM, van der Stoep N, et al. DNA methylation and expression of major histocompatibility complex class I and class II transactivator genes in human developmental tumor cells and in T cell malignancies. Clin Immunol 2003;109(1):46–52.

[45] Ohnmacht GA, Marincola FM. Heterogeneity in expression of human leukocyte antigens and melanoma-associated antigens in advanced melanoma. J Cell Physiol 2000;182(3): 332–8.

[46] Yee C, Thompson JA, Byrd D, et al. Adoptive T cell therapy using antigen-specific CD8+ T cell clones for the treatment of patients with metastatic melanoma: in vivo persistence, migration, and antitumor effect of transferred T cells. Proc Natl Acad Sci U S A 2002; 99(25):16168–73.

[47] Meklat F, Li Z, Wang Z, et al. Cancer-testis antigens in haematological malignancies. Br J Haematol 2007;136(6):769–76.

[48] Oppenheim DE, Roberts SJ, Clarke SL, et al. Sustained localized expression of ligand for the activating NKG2D receptor impairs natural cytotoxicity in vivo and reduces tumor immunosurveillance. Nat Immunol 2005;6(9):928–37.

[49] Fauriat C, Just-Landi S, Mallet F, et al. Deficient expression of NCR in NK cells from acute myeloid leukemia: evolution during leukemia treatment and impact of leukemia cells in NCRdull phenotype induction. Blood 2007;109(1):323–30.

[50] Gonzalez S, Groh V, Spies T. Immunobiology of human NKG2D and its ligands. Curr Top Microbiol Immunol 2006;298:121–38.

[51] Menier C, Riteau B, Carosella ED, et al. MICA triggering signal for NK cell tumor lysis is counteracted by HLA-G1-mediated inhibitory signal. Int J Cancer 2002;100(1): 63–70.

[52] Malmberg KJ, Levitsky V, Norell H, et al. IFN-gamma protects short-term ovarian carcinoma cell lines from CTL lysis via a CD94/NKG2A-dependent mechanism. J Clin Invest 2002;110(10):1515–23.

[53] Bladergroen BA, Meijer CJ, ten Berge RL, et al. Expression of the granzyme B inhibitor, protease inhibitor 9, by tumor cells in patients with non-Hodgkin and Hodgkin lymphoma: a novel protective mechanism for tumor cells to circumvent the immune system? Blood 2002;99(1):232–7.

[54] van Houdt IS, Oudejans JJ, van den Eertwegh AJ, et al. Expression of the apoptosis inhibitor protease inhibitor 9 predicts clinical outcome in vaccinated patients with stage III and IV melanoma. Clin Cancer Res 2005;11(17):6400–7.

[55] Harada K, Toyooka S, Shivapurkar N, et al. Deregulation of caspase 8 and 10 expression in pediatric tumors and cell lines. Cancer Res 2002;62(20):5897–901.

[56] Stupack DG, Teitz T, Potter MD, et al. Potentiation of neuroblastoma metastasis by loss of caspase-8. Nature 2006;439(7072):95–9.

[57] Ugurel S, Rappl G, Tilgen W, et al. Increased soluble CD95 (sFas/CD95) serum level correlates with poor prognosis in melanoma patients. Clin Cancer Res 2001;7(5):1282–6.

[58] Roth W, Isenmann S, Nakamura M, et al. Soluble decoy receptor 3 is expressed by malignant gliomas and suppresses CD95 ligand-induced apoptosis and chemotaxis. Cancer Res 2001;61(6):2759–65.

[59] Gronbaek K, Straten PT, Ralfkiaer E, et al. Somatic Fas mutations in non-Hodgkin's lymphoma: association with extranodal disease and autoimmunity. Blood 1998;92(9):3018–24.

[60] Ben-Baruch A. Inflammation-associated immune suppression in cancer: the roles played by cytokines, chemokines and additional mediators. Semin Cancer Biol 2006;16(1):38–52.

[61] Curiel TJ, Coukos G, Zou L, et al. Specific recruitment of regulatory T cells in ovarian carcinoma fosters immune privilege and predicts reduced survival. Nat Med 2004;10(9):942–9.

[62] Serafini P, Borrello I, Bronte V. Myeloid suppressor cells in cancer: recruitment, phenotype, properties, and mechanisms of immune suppression. Semin Cancer Biol 2006;16(1):53–65.

[63] Baniyash M. TCR zeta-chain downregulation: curtailing an excessive inflammatory immune response. Nat Rev Immunol 2004;4(9):675–87.

[64] Galon J, Costes A, Sanchez-Cabo F, et al. Type, density, and location of immune cells within human colorectal tumors predict clinical outcome. Science 2006;313(5795):1960–4.

[65] Sato E, Olson SH, Ahn J, et al. Intraepithelial CD8+ tumor-infiltrating lymphocytes and a high CD8+/regulatory T cell ratio are associated with favorable prognosis in ovarian cancer. Proc Natl Acad Sci U S A 2005;102(51):18538–43.

[66] Piersma SJ, Jordanova ES, van Poelgeest MI, et al. High number of intraepithelial CD8+ tumor-infiltrating lymphocytes is associated with the absence of lymph node metastases in patients with large early-stage cervical cancer. Cancer Res 2007;67(1):354–61.

[67] von Andrian UH, Mempel TR. Homing and cellular traffic in lymph nodes. Nat Rev Immunol 2003;3(11):867–78.

[68] Chen Q, Wang WC, Evans SS. Tumor microvasculature as a barrier to antitumor immunity. Cancer Immunol Immunother 2003;52(11):670–9.

[69] Carriere V, Colisson R, Jiguet-Jiglaire C, et al. Cancer cells regulate lymphocyte recruitment and leukocyte-endothelium interactions in the tumor-draining lymph node. Cancer Res 2005;65(24):11639–48.

[70] Fisher DT, Chen Q, Appenheimer MM, et al. Hurdles to lymphocyte trafficking in the tumor microenvironment: implications for effective immunotherapy. Immunol Invest 2006;35(3–4):251–77.

[71] Zlotnik A, Yoshie O. Chemokines: a new classification system and their role in immunity. Immunity 2000;12(2):121–7.

[72] Balkwill F. Cancer and the chemokine network. Nat Rev Cancer 2004;4(7):540–50.

[73] Dunn GP, Old LJ, Schreiber RD. The three Es of cancer immunoediting. Annu Rev Immunol 2004;22:329–60.

[74] Mapara MY, Sykes M. Tolerance and cancer: mechanisms of tumor evasion and strategies for breaking tolerance. J Clin Oncol 2004;22(6):1136–51.

[75] June CH. Adoptive T cell therapy for cancer in the clinic. J Clin Invest 2007;117(6):1466–76.

[76] Dudley ME, Wunderlich JR, Robbins PF, et al. Cancer regression and autoimmunity in patients after clonal repopulation with antitumor lymphocytes. Science 2002;298(5594):850–4.

[77] Gattinoni L, Powell DJ Jr, Rosenberg SA, et al. Adoptive immunotherapy for cancer: building on success. Nat Rev Immunol 2006;6(5):383–93.

[78] June CH. Principles of adoptive T cell cancer therapy. J Clin Invest 2007;117(5):1204–12.

[79] Berger C, Berger M, Feng J, et al. Genetic modification of T cells for immunotherapy. Expert Opin Biol Ther 2007;7(8):1167–82.

[80] Morgan RA, Dudley ME, Wunderlich JR, et al. Cancer regression in patients after transfer of genetically engineered lymphocytes. Science 2006;314(5796):126–9.

[81] Dotti G, Heslop HE. Current status of genetic modification of T cells for cancer treatment. Cytotherapy 2005;7(3):262–72.

[82] Savoldo B, Goss JA, Hammer MM, et al. Treatment of solid organ transplant recipients with autologous Epstein Barr virus-specific cytotoxic T lymphocytes (CTLs). Blood 2006;108(9):2942–9.

[83] Banchereau J, Palucka AK. Dendritic cells as therapeutic vaccines against cancer. Nat Rev Immunol 2005;5(4):296–306.

[84] Figdor CG, de Vries IJ, Lesterhuis WJ, et al. Dendritic cell immunotherapy: mapping the way. Nat Med 2004;10(5):475–80.

[85] Rosenberg SA, Yang JC, Restifo NP. Cancer immunotherapy: moving beyond current vaccines. Nat Med 2004;10(9):909–15.

[86] Paulos CM, Kaiser A, Wrzesinski C, et al. Toll-like receptors in tumor immunotherapy. Clin Cancer Res 2007;13(18):5280–9.

[87] Krieg AM. Development of TLR9 agonists for cancer therapy. J Clin Invest 2007;117(5): 1184–94.

[88] Schlom J, Arlen PM, Gulley JL. Cancer vaccines: moving beyond current paradigms. Clin Cancer Res 2007;13(13):3776–82.

[89] Dagher R, Long LM, Read EJ, et al. Pilot trial of tumor-specific peptide vaccination and continuous infusion interleukin-2 in patients with recurrent Ewing sarcoma and alveolar rhabdomyosarcoma: an inter-institute NIH study. Med Pediatr Oncol 2002;38(3):158–64.

[90] Geiger JD, Hutchinson RJ, Hohenkirk LF, et al. Vaccination of pediatric solid tumor patients with tumor lysate-pulsed dendritic cells can expand specific T cells and mediate tumor regression. Cancer Res 2001;61(23):8513–9.

[91] Rousseau RF, Brenner MK. Vaccine therapies for pediatric malignancies. Cancer J 2005; 11(4):331–9.

[92] Rousseau RF, Haight AE, Hirschmann-Jax C, et al. Local and systemic effects of an allogeneic tumor cell vaccine combining transgenic human lymphotactin with interleu-kin-2 in patients with advanced or refractory neuroblastoma. Blood 2003;101(5):1718–26.

[93] Nash RA, Storb R. Graft-versus-host effect after allogeneic hematopoietic stem cell trans-plantation: GVHD and GVL. Curr Opin Immunol 1996;8(5):674–80.

[94] Gilleece MH, Dazzi F. Donor lymphocyte infusions for patients who relapse after alloge-neic stem cell transplantation for chronic myeloid leukaemia. Leuk Lymphoma 2003;44(1): 23–8.

[95] Hahn T, Wall D, Camitta B, et al. The role of cytotoxic therapy with hematopoietic stem cell transplantation in the therapy of acute lymphoblastic leukemia in children: an evidence-based review. Biol Blood Marrow Transplant 2005;11(11):823–61.

[96] Cardoso AA, Schultze JL, Boussiotis VA, et al. Pre-B acute lymphoblastic leukemia cells may induce T-cell anergy to alloantigen. Blood 1996;88(1):41–8.

[97] Bleakley M, Riddell SR. Molecules and mechanisms of the graft-versus-leukaemia effect. Nat Rev Cancer 2004;4(5):371–80.

[98] Molldrem JJ. Vaccinating transplant recipients. Nat Med 2005;11(11):1162–3.

[99] Rousseau RF, Biagi E, Dutour A, et al. Immunotherapy of high-risk acute leukemia with a recipient (autologous) vaccine expressing transgenic human CD40L and IL-2 after chemotherapy and allogeneic stem cell transplantation. Blood 2006;107(4):1332–41.

[100] Amrolia PJ, Muccioli-Casadei G, Yvon E, et al. Selective depletion of donor alloreactive T cells without loss of antiviral or antileukemic responses. Blood 2003;102(6):2292–9.

[101] Solomon SR, Mielke S, Savani BN, et al. Selective depletion of alloreactive donor lymphocytes: a novel method to reduce the severity of graft-versus-host disease in older

patients undergoing matched sibling donor stem cell transplantation. Blood 2005;106(3): 1123–9.

[102] Mielke S, Nunes R, Rezvani K, et al. A clinical scale selective allodepletion approach for the treatment of HLA-mismatched and matched donor-recipient pairs using expanded T lymphocytes as antigen-presenting cells and a TH9402-based photodepletion technique. Blood 2007; [epub ahead of print].

[103] Rosenberg SA, Lotze MT, Muul LM, et al. Observations on the systemic administration of autologous lymphokine-activated killer cells and recombinant interleukin-2 to patients with metastatic cancer. N Engl J Med 1985;313(23):1485–92.

[104] Atkins MB, Lotze MT, Dutcher JP, et al. High-dose recombinant interleukin 2 therapy for patients with metastatic melanoma: analysis of 270 patients treated between 1985 and 1993. J Clin Oncol 1999;17(7):2105–16.

[105] Miller JS, Soignier Y, Panoskaltsis-Mortari A, et al. Successful adoptive transfer and in vivo expansion of human haploidentical NK cells in patients with cancer. Blood 2005; 105(8):3051–7.

[106] Passweg JR, Koehl U, Uharek L, et al. Natural-killer-cell-based treatment in haematopoietic stem-cell transplantation. Best Pract Res Clin Haematol 2006;19(4):811–24.

[107] Klingemann HG. Natural killer cell-based immunotherapeutic strategies. Cytotherapy 2005;7(1):16–22.

[108] Ljunggren HG, Malmberg KJ. Prospects for the use of NK cells in immunotherapy of human cancer. Nat Rev Immunol 2007;7(5):329–39.

[109] Wayne AS, Kreitman RJ, Pastan I. Monoclonal antibodies and immunotoxins as new therapeutic agents for childhood acute lymphoblastic leukemia. American Society of Clinical Oncology 2007 Educational Book. Alexandria (VA): ASCO; 2007. p. 596–601.

[110] Pastan I, Hassan R, Fitzgerald DJ, et al. Immunotoxin therapy of cancer. Nat Rev Cancer 2006;6(7):559–65.

[111] Boerman OC, Koppe MJ, Postema EJ, et al. Radionuclide therapy of cancer with radiolabeled antibodies. Anticancer Agents Med Chem 2007;7(3):335–43.

PEDIATRIC CLINICS

OF NORTH AMERICA

Pediatr Clin N Am 55 (2008) 169–186

Vaccinations in Children Treated with Standard-Dose Cancer Therapy or Hematopoietic Stem Cell Transplantation

Soonie R. Patel, MBChB, MRCP, MD[a],*,
Julia C. Chisholm, MBChB, PhD, FRCPCH[b],
Paul T. Heath, MBBS, FRACP, FRCPCH[c]

[a]*Paediatric Department, Mayday University Hospital, Croydon, CR7 7YE, UK*
[b]*Department of Haematology/Oncology, Great Ormond Street Hospital,
London, WC1N 3JH, UK*
[c]*Vaccine Institute and Child Health, St George's, University of London,
London, SW17 0QT, UK*

Most children with cancer are immuncompromised. The cancer itself may cause a variable degree of immunosuppression, but it is the cytotoxic antineoplastic therapy that is the main contributor. Many pediatric cancers are highly chemosensitive and radiosensitive, and their treatment usually involves chemotherapy or radiotherapy or both. The majority of children with cancer are treated with standard-dose chemotherapy, but children with high-risk hematologic malignancy, children with certain solid tumors, and children with disease relapse require high dose chemotherapy or radiotherapy followed by hematopoietic stem cell transplant (HSCT). These different forms of treatment have different influences on the immune system and the degree of immunodeficiency. Immune alteration is reflected by decrease in neutrophils, lymphocytes, immunoglobulin levels, and specific antibody against previous vaccinations. This results in increased susceptibility to and severity of infections.

Most of the vaccine-preventable diseases are now fortunately rare; however, the risk for some remains significant, in part because of increases in migration and travel. Furthermore, they can be associated with high

---

* Corresponding author.
E-mail address: soonie.patel@mayday.nhs.uk (S.R. Patel).

0031-3955/08/$ - see front matter © 2008 Elsevier Inc. All rights reserved.
doi:10.1016/j.pcl.2007.10.012   *pediatric.theclinics.com*

morbidity and mortality, particularly in immunocompromised patients (eg, varicella zoster, measles). In view of the secondary immunodeficiency of children treated for cancer, particularly HSCT recipients, and their improved long-term survival after completion of treatment, it is important to ensure that they are protected against vaccine-preventable diseases. This can be achieved by optimizing the immunization strategy in children during immunosuppressive therapy and by reimmunization of children after completion of treatment. In view of the diversity of malignant diseases and their treatment protocols, it would be difficult to propose different immunization schedules for each disease. Rather, it is sensible to divide them into children treated with standard-dose chemotherapy and children treated with intensive chemotherapy followed by allogeneic or autologous HSCT.

Vaccinations in children treated with standard-dose chemotherapy

Children treated with standard-dose chemotherapy are at increased risk of infection. However, there are few data on the precise incidence of specific infections in this population. With regard to vaccine-preventable disease, there are data demonstrating an increase in incidence and severity of *Haemophilus influenzae* type b (Hib), pneumococcal, measles, and varicella infections [1–4].

Influence of cancer on immune function

Cancer itself, particularly leukemia and lymphoma, can have an adverse influence on immune function. Patients with acute leukemia may have myelosuppression at diagnosis; of particular significance is granulocytopenia. Some cancers may also affect adaptive immune functions; for example, leukemia and Hodgkin lymphoma, by the nature of their pathology, may have an adverse influence on lymphocyte function. However, there are few data to substantiate this assumption. Several studies show that total immunoglobulin concentrations, as well as specific antibody concentrations, to vaccine-preventable infections are normal at the time of diagnosis, suggesting that the effect of the cancer itself on the adaptive immune system is likely to be relatively small [5,6].

Influence of standard chemotherapy on immune function

Different cancers require treatment with different combinations of chemotherapy agents. Therapy for a single disease is risk-stratified based on patient factors, extent of disease, and tumor biology, so there may be variation in intensity of therapy for a single disease type. Therapy regimens that include agents such as cyclophosphamide, purine nucleoside analogs, or corticosteroids are immunosuppressive; they particularly have an effect on lymphocyte function. For example, treatment regimens for acute lymphoblastic leukemia (ALL) are targeted against lymphoid cells and can have an adverse influence on lymphocyte function, while the chemotherapy agents used for the treatment of low stage Wilms tumor (actinomycin and vincristine) are not particularly immunosuppressive. The extent and duration of immune dysfunction following the completion of standard-dose chemotherapy will depend on the antineoplastic agent used and its dose intensity, and can therefore vary widely. This may influence immunity to vaccine antigens and responses to vaccination.

B-lymphocyte levels decrease during treatment for ALL [7,8], with an increase in number occurring 1 month after completion of chemotherapy [7]. There is a decrease of T-helper (CD4$^+$) lymphocytes and T-suppressor (CD8$^+$) lymphocytes, with CD4$^+$ lymphocytes recovering more slowly than CD8$^+$ lymphocytes [9]. Total B- and T-lymphocytes usually recover fully, quantitatively and functionally, 6 months after completion of chemotherapy, although in some cases recovery may take up to 1 year [7,9]. There is a reduction of immunoglobulin levels after completion of chemotherapy, particularly of IgG2 levels [5,10,11]. Normalization of immunoglobulin levels can take up to 1 year after completion of treatment [11]. Younger patients are more likely to have immune suppression after completion of chemotherapy, and this includes the loss of protective serum antibody concentrations against vaccines [12,13].

Immunity to vaccine antigens after completion of chemotherapy

Depending on their age at diagnosis, some children may not have completed their primary vaccination series before starting chemotherapy. This will influence the concentrations of vaccine-antigen specific antibodies at completion of therapy. The chemotherapy regimen will also have an influence on immunity to vaccine antigens. For example, children treated for acute leukemia may have greater loss of antibody than children treated for solid tumors, and the more intensive ALL chemotherapy regimens can result in a greater reduction of antibody concentrations than the less intensive ALL regimens [14–16]. The treatment regimens of some solid tumors are not particularly immunosuppressive, so that there may be no loss of immunity to vaccine antigens after completion of treatment. However, until further studies are done to evaluate immunity to vaccine antigens in specific disease types and treatment regimens, it is wise to follow the same reimmunization recommendations for all patients.

There is a reduction in vaccine-antigen specific antibody concentrations after completion of chemotherapy [12–19], although the degree of reduction varies from one study to another, and with it the proportions of children who have protective concentrations. A recent study looking at immunity to vaccines at a median time of 7 months after completion of treatment for acute leukemia in British children, demonstrated protective antibody concentrations for all patients to tetanus, 87% to Hib, 71% to measles, 12% to *Neisseria meningitidis* group C (meningococcus C), and 11% to all three poliovirus-serotypes [18]. Therefore, this and other studies demonstrate a need for reimmunization of patients after completion of chemotherapy.

Immunization during chemotherapy

During treatment for cancer children are immunosuppressed, therefore live vaccines, such as measles-mumps-rubella (MMR), oral polio (OPV), Bacillus Calmette-Guerin (BCG), oral typhoid, and yellow fever vaccines, are not recommended. A possible exception to this is the live attenuated varicella zoster virus (VZV) vaccine. Many of the early VZV vaccine immunogenicity studies evaluated responses in children with ALL in disease remission and during the maintenance phase of chemotherapy [20,21]. The vaccine proved to be immunogenic and safe. Currently however, VZV vaccine is not routinely recommended during chemotherapy. If considered appropriate to give the VZV vaccine, then chemotherapy should be suspended for 1 week before and 1 week after vaccination and the patient should not be receiving steroids. Two doses are required [20,21]. Cases of vaccine-associated varicella have been reported and oral or intravenous acyclovir, as appropriate, should be used if the child develops a skin rash consistent with varicella [22].

Children are immunosuppressed during chemotherapy and are particularly susceptible to infections. However, this is also the time that they are less likely to achieve a good immune response to vaccines. Regardless, nonlive vaccines can be administered during chemotherapy. Studies have evaluated antibody response to vaccines during chemotherapy; most of these studies have evaluated antibody response during the maintenance phase of ALL chemotherapy. Antibody responses during chemotherapy are usually impaired. A significantly lower response rate and antibody concentration has been demonstrated to Hib, for example [1]. Nevertheless, the current recommendations are that nonlive vaccines should be given according to routine childhood immunization schedules, provided that the child's general health is stable and is expected to remain stable for 3 weeks after immunization [23]. This is particularly important for infant immunizations to ensure immunity in an otherwise nonimmune child. The trivalent influenza vaccine should be given annually before the influenza season to patients receiving chemotherapy [23,24].

Immunization after completion of chemotherapy

In view of the reduction in vaccine-antigen specific antibody levels after completion of chemotherapy, and increases in migration and travel, it is sensible to reimmunize children after completion of chemotherapy. In terms of timing, the aim is to balance safety and efficacy of immunization. Generally, 3 to 6 months after completion of treatment should be safe and elicit good antibody responses. Reimmunization of children after completion of chemotherapy results in a good immune response, with most recipients achieving protective levels of antibody [13,14,18,25]. The immune response to a single dose of vaccine after completion of treatment, as per the British acute leukemia protocols, has recently been shown to be very satisfactory. There was a significant rise in antibody to each vaccine antigen studied, with 100% achieving protection to tetanus, 93% to Hib, 94% to measles, 96% to meningococcus C, and 85% to the three poliovirus-serotypes. Interestingly, this study demonstrated that children treated for ALL achieved better antibody responses than children treated for acute myeloid leukemia (although the number of children treated for acute myeloid leukemia was relatively small) [18]. This difference is worthy of further study.

The immunization program in the child's country of residence should guide the vaccines to be administered. For example, the British guidelines recommend a booster dose of each routine childhood vaccine (Hib-conjugate, diphtheria/tetanus/acellular pertussis [DTaP], MMR, inactivated poliovirus [IPV] and meningococcal C-conjugate [MCC]) 6 months after completion of chemotherapy [23]. The American guidelines recommend reimmunization no sooner than 3 months after completion of chemotherapy [26]. The heptavalent pneumococcus-conjugate vaccine (PCV7) is now included in childhood immunization schedules in several countries and should also be included in the schedule after completion of chemotherapy. However, there are no published studies looking at immune responses to PCV7 in children treated for cancer. Additionally, the BCG vaccine should only be considered for children to be at high risk of tuberculosis, and Hepatitis B (HepB) vaccine should be considered if it is part of the routine childhood immunization schedule in the child's country of residence.

It is not generally recommended to routinely screen for immunity to vaccine antigens or immune responses to vaccination after completion of chemotherapy. From a pragmatic point of view, most children will require one or more vaccines anyway, few laboratories are able to perform these assays, and the use of specific concentrations to guide reimmunization may not be helpful: for example, when protective levels are not clearly established (such as pertussis). Additionally, so-called "protective" levels are derived from studies in healthy children and may not be applicable in this population.

Most studies have examined reimmunization at or more than 6 months after completion of treatment. However, immune function recovery appears to be occurring as early as 3 months following therapy, depending on the treatment regimen used. Therefore earlier reimmunization may be possible, for example 3 months after finishing chemotherapy. The optimal timing of reimmunization should be the subject of new studies.

Influence of radiation therapy on immune function

Some treatment regimens include radiation therapy. There are relatively few data on the effects of radiotherapy on immune function; its effect is likely to be less significant than that of chemotherapy. However irradiation of the spleen, for example, may cause functional hyposplenia and asplenia that increases susceptibility to infections with polysaccharide encapsulated bacteria, such as *Streptococcus pneumoniae* [27].

Vaccinations in hematopoietic stem cell transplant recipients

In recent years HSCT has become increasingly used to allow the administration of potentially curative high-dose chemotherapy and radiotherapy to patients with hematologic and nonhematologic malignancies. HSCT is classified as either allogeneic or autologous. Allogeneic HSCT is the infusion of hematopoeitic stem cells (HSC) from a donor to a patient. Autologous HSCT is the reinfusion of the patient's own HSC. HSCT procedures vary; the source of HSC cells can be bone marrow, umbilical cord blood, or peripheral blood. For allogeneic HSCT, the HSC donor can be related or unrelated to the recipient and may be human leukocyte antigen (HLA)-identical, HLA-mismatched, or haplo (half)-identical. Grafts may be T-cell depleted (TCD) to reduce the severity of graft-versus-host disease (GvHD). The most commonly used pretransplant conditioning regimen for children over the age of 2 years, with a hematologic malignancy, is cyclophosphamide and total body irradiation (TBI) [28]. This combination causes profound immunosuppression. Functional hypospenia or asplenia and thymic atrophy are recognized complications after allogeneic HSCT, particularly with TBI containing regimens [29,30]. GvHD, particularly chronic-GvHD, is immunosuppressive, as are its prophylaxis and treatment [31]. Chronic-GvHD targets the lymphoid system; it diminishes thymic-dependent T-cell development and causes functional hypospenia and asplenia [32]. All of these HSCT-related factors can have an influence on immune reconstitution after HSCT and on immune responses to vaccination.

Immune reconstitution after hematopoietic stem cell transplant

HSCT recipients are profoundly immunosuppressed for several months, even years after transplantation. Immune reconstitution after HSCT occurs in a well-defined manner [33]. The various components of the new immune system develop and mature at different rates, and this dictates the timing and type of specific infections, as well as the response to different antigens.

Immune reconstitution after autologous HSCT occurs faster than after allogeneic HSCT [34]. For allogeneic HSCT, immunosuppression is secondary to a combination of pretransplant conditioning regimen, GvHD, and immunosuppressive therapy given following transplant. For autologous HSCT, the immunosuppression is primarily related to the pretransplant treatment. Innate immune function recovers earlier than adaptive immune function; innate immune function recovers in weeks to months after transplant. A prolonged immune deficiency arises from a deficiency of the more specialized functions of the adaptive immune system, in particular, the reconstitution of CD4$^+$ lymphocytes [32,35,36].

B-lymphocytes reach age-matched levels 3 to 6 months after transplant [35,37]. Recovery is slower in TCD-graft recipients and recipients with chronic-GvHD [36,38,39]. Immunoglobulin isotypes start normalizing 6 months after transplant and are produced in accordance with that seen in normal immune development: that is, IgM → IgG1+IgG3 → IgG2+IgG4 → IgA [35]. Total IgG levels can be normal, but there is an IgG subclass imbalance, with low IgG2 levels for 18 months or more after transplant [40]. Antibody responses to recall antigens can begin to be elicited 3 to 6 months after transplantation [41].

T-lymphocyte reconstitution occurs in two stages: first the thymus-independent pathway, followed by the thymus-dependent pathway [32,42]. During the first 6 months after transplant, T-lymphocytes are predominantly repopulated through peripheral expansion of mature T-lymphocytes, with recovery starting 1 to 2 months after transplant and peaking at 3 to 6 months [42]. This pathway is responsible for the rapid reconstitution of memory T-lymphocytes of limited repertoire diversity. At 6 to 12 months after transplant T-lymphocyte neogenesis is evident. Lymphocytes from this pathway have a diverse receptor repertoire and should be capable of responding to a range of antigens; this pathway is important in the reconstitution of CD4$^+$ lymphocytes [32,42]. Reconstitution to normal levels can occur 1 to 2 years after transplant and occurs more rapidly in younger HSCT recipients [32,36,39,43,44].

Immunization schedules for hematopoietic stem cell transplant recipients

As transplant-related mortality has improved, long-term complications of HSCT have become more evident. There are many published studies demonstrating the loss of pretransplant-acquired natural and vaccine-acquired immunity. Reimmunization is therefore an important strategy for maintaining long-term health in such children. Although the loss of immunity is likely to be lower for autologous than allogeneic HSCT recipients, it is difficult to predict this for an individual child, and therefore it is wise to reimmunize both groups with similar schedules.

A survey of reimmunization schedules in Europe and North America revealed wide variations in practice. Most programs began administering vaccines 1 year after transplant, and only a small number administered multiple doses [45,46]. There are few controlled studies in this area on which recommendations can be based, and guidelines are therefore often the result of a combination of expert opinion and the limited published data. This was the basis of the British guidelines, published in 2002 [23]. These guidelines recommend that reimmunization should commence 12 months after an autologous and HLA-identical related donor allogeneic HSCT, and 18 months after any other allogeneic HSCT, provided there is no evidence of active chronic-GvHD, the child is off all immunosuppressive therapy for at least 6 months (12 months for live vaccines), and has not received intravenous immunoglobulin for at least 3 months. The guidelines recommend that autologous and allogeneic HSCT recipients should receive the full complement of primary routine childhood vaccines, as well as the influenza vaccine, every autumn while the patient is considered immunocompromised. Details of the schedule are summarized in Table 1.

Hepatitis A and B, and BCG vaccines, may be considered for individual cases. Hepatitis B vaccine is recommended for HSCT recipients residing in countries where it is included in the routine childhood immunization schedule [47]. There are limited supportive data to incorporate VZV vaccine into the reimmunization schedule for HSCT recipients; VZV vaccine should be considered for their VZV-seronegative family members [47]. There are few data about the safety and effectiveness of BCG immunization after HSCT. Its

Table 1
A suggested reimmunization schedule for hematopoietic stem cell transplant recipients

Time after HSCT	HLA-identical sibling, syngeneic, autologous HSCT	Any other allogeneic HSCT
From 6 months	Influenza vaccine every autumn (for as long as patient considered immunocompromised)	
At 12 months	3 doses at 1–2 monthly intervals: - DTaP - IPV - Hib-conjugate - MCC (or MQC) 3 doses at 0-, 1-, 6-month schedule: - HepB[a]	
At 12–15 months	2 doses of PCV7 at 1–2 monthly intervals	
At 18 months	MMR-1	3 doses at 1–2 monthly intervals: - DTaP - IPV - Hib-conjugate - MCC (or MQC) 3 doses at 0-, 1-, 6-month schedule: - HepB
At 18–21 months		2 doses of PCV7 at 1–2 monthly intervals
At 24 months	MMR-2 + Pn-PS23	MMR-1
At 30 months		MMR-2 + Pn-PS23

Based on Royal College of Pediatrics and Child Health guidelines [23]. Specific vaccines to be used will be dictated by current recommendations in different countries.

Abbreviations: DTaP, Diphtheria/tetanus/acellular pertussis; HepB, Hepatitis B; Hib-conjugate, *Haemophilus influenzae* type b-conjugate; IPV, Inactivated poliovirus; MCC, Meningococcal C-conjugate; MMR, Measles-mumps-rubella; MQC, Meningococcal quadravalent (A, C, Y, W135) conjugate; PCV7, Heptavalent pneumococcal conjugate; Pn-PS23, 23-valent pneumococcal conjugate.

[a] HepB is not part of the Royal College of Paediatrics and Child Health schedule, but for use in countries where HepB is part of the routine schedule or in specific circumstances.

use is not recommended unless there is a clear case of need, such as travel to or residence in an area with a high incidence of tuberculosis (greater than 40 per 100,000 per year), no active chronic-GvHD, and where there is evidence of recovery of immune function (such as normal serum immunoglobulin concentrations, normal lymphocyte function, and normal CD4-lymphocyte numbers) [23]. Prior to administering BCG, particularly in patients that have previously had BCG, a tuberculin skin test should be performed [23].

European Blood and Marrow Transplantation guidelines were updated in 2005; they do not differentiate between transplant type and suggest earlier immunization than the British guidelines (from 6 months after HSCT for most vaccines and 24 months for MMR) [48].

Factors that influence immunity to vaccines in hematopoietic stem cell transplant recipients

A number of factors have an influence on antibody level to previous vaccinations and immunogenicity of vaccines in HSCT recipients: whether the HSC graft is autologous or allogeneic, time after HSCT, chronic-GvHD, recipient age, the number of vaccine doses, and donor immunization status. Studies looking at immune response to vaccines after HSCT show that the time elapsed after transplantation [49–52] and the number of vaccine doses are important determinants [53–56]. There is some evidence that chronic-GvHD adversely effects the decline of specific antibody levels and the immunogenicity of vaccines [57], although other studies demonstrate little influence [52,58,59]. Two studies have demonstrated that younger recipient age is associated with a higher chance of being seronegative to vaccine antigens [57,60]. Additionally, younger recipients may not have had the opportunity to receive a particular vaccine or the full schedule of childhood vaccines, and this may be reflected in their pre- and posttransplant antibody levels. Whether immunity has been acquired naturally or through active immunization can also influence maintenance of immunity after HSCT; for example, those with naturally acquired measles immunity are more likely to retain immunity after transplant than those who have been vaccinated [56,60].

A possible strategy to enhance vaccine efficacy is donor preharvest immunization. Some studies indicate that donor immune status does not influence recipient antibody levels [51,53,61], while others demonstrate that donor immunization before HSC harvest has a positive influence on the recipient's antibody response to immunization [62–64]. This has been particularly demonstrated for polysaccharide-protein conjugate Hib and pneumococcal vaccines and tetanus and diphtheria vaccines [62–64]. For allogeneic HSCT, the practical and ethical implications limit the use of this strategy, and for autologous HSCT there is currently insufficient evidence. Further studies in this area are required before any recommendations can be made.

In summary, the aim in HSCT recipients is to commence revaccination as soon as it is safe and as soon as a protective immune response can be achieved. Potentially, this would be once the patient is off immunosuppressive therapy and may be as early as 6 months after HSCT. In most published studies, however, immunization schedules have been started at 12 months or longer after HSCT.

Vaccines currently recommended in reimmunization schedules following hematopoietic stem cell transplant

Tetanus toxoid vaccine

There is variable evidence regarding the persistence of immunity to tetanus after HSCT. Some studies have observed well-maintained immunity against tetanus [51,59], and some have shown a significant decline after HSCT [53]. Early studies have recommended the need for three doses of tetanus-toxoid vaccine [53,65]. A recent study of British pediatric HSCT recipients demonstrated that all achieved optimal (greater or equal to 0.1 IU/mL) antitetanus antibody concentrations after three doses, suggesting that fewer doses might be sufficient [59].

Diphtheria toxoid

There are limited published studies on immunity against diphtheria after HSCT [66]. As diphtheria toxoid is invariably part of a combined vaccine preparation; its timing and number of doses will be dictated by that of the other vaccine components.

Pertussis vaccine

As pertussis vaccine has not been routinely administered to individuals older than 7 to 10 years (until recently in some countries), and the correlation between antibody concentration and clinical efficacy of the vaccine is not established, data are not available on pertussis immunity and the immune response to pertussis vaccine in HSCT recipients. A recent case report suggests that consideration should be given to its routine inclusion for revaccination in HSCT recipients older than 7 years [67]. In practice, as the acellular pertussis vaccine is often part of a combined vaccine preparation, its timing and number of doses will again be dictated by that of the other vaccine components.

Poliovirus vaccine

OPV is a live attenuated vaccine that has, in rare cases, been associated with vaccine-associated paralytic polio. Persons with immunodeficiency are at an increased risk of vaccine-associated paralytic polio, and therefore OPV is not recommended for HSCT recipients or their household contacts. IPV is recommended instead.

Immunity to poliovirus declines after HSCT [54,59,66,68]. A recent study of British pediatric HSCT recipients demonstrated that only 11% of patients were immune to the three poliovirus serotypes after HSCT [59]. Reimmunization with IPV after HSCT is effective [52,54,59]. Three doses of IPV are recommended [59].

Measles-mumps-rubella vaccine

MMR vaccine is a live attenuated vaccine and poses a risk of viral replication and dissemination of infection in children with immunodeficiency. Of the three diseases preventable with MMR, measles is associated with serious morbidity and mortality in immunosuppressed patients [3]. MMR is only recommended for HSCT recipients, 18 months following transplant, and who are no longer receiving immunosuppressive treatment [23,45,69]. The time interval between HSCT and immunization is not only of importance for the potential risk of clinical measles, but also for the quality of immune response to the measles component.

A loss of immunity has been demonstrated to all three vaccine antigens after HSCT [56,59,69,70]. There is considerable variation between studies with regard to retention of immunity to measles and protective antibody concentrations being retained in 13% to over 70% of patients [56,59,71]. It is generally recommended to administer MMR, provided HSCT recipients do not have chronic-GvHD and are not on immunosuppressive therapy. However, studies by Machado and colleagues [70,71], have demonstrated that measles vaccine can be safely administered to HSCT recipients on immunosuppressive therapy within 2 years of transplant. There is a range in immune response to measles vaccination; some studies demonstrate over 75% of subjects responding to one dose [58,59,69], while one study demonstrated only 50% responding [56]. Seroconversion to rubella is generally higher [69,72].

In addition to primary vaccine failure [56,72], secondary vaccine failure has been demonstrated to measles vaccination [56,70]. This, together with the fact that two doses of MMR are recommended for healthy children, suggests that two doses should also be offered to HSCT recipients. Only one published study has looked at the response to two doses of MMR; the first dose resulted in 91% and the second dose resulted in 100% achieving protective measles-neutralizing antibody concentrations [59].

Influenza vaccine

Annual influenza vaccine is recommended starting 6 months after transplant. There are sparse data on the epidemiology of influenza infections after HSCT, or on influenza vaccination after HSCT. Influenza causes annual world-wide epidemics, and HSCT recipients will have a higher risk of severe influenza-related complications. One study demonstrated that seasonal exposure and more aggressive HSCT conditioning regimens increase the risk of influenza morbidity [73]. The time interval between HSCT and vaccination is correlated with antibody response; response within the first 6 months of HSCT is poor [49]. Therefore, vaccination after 6 months would be advisable [73]. In view of the poor responses of HSCT recipients in the early period after HSCT, the time of greatest risk, it would be wise to protect HSCT recipients by immunizing family members and hospital staff.

Polysaccharide-encapsulated bacteria

HSCT recipients are at increased risk of infection with polysaccharide-encapsulated bacteria such as *Streptococcus pneumoniae, Haemophilus influenzae* type b, and *Neisseria meningitidis,* particularly *S. pneumoniae.* There are no data regarding the incidence of Hib and meningococcal C infection, but an increased incidence of pneumococcal infection is well documented [27]. The increased susceptibility of HSCT recipients is related to a number of host factors: functional hyposplenia and asplenia, low serum IgG2 levels, and impaired opsonization by specific antibodies.

The traditional approach to preventing infection with *S. pneumoniae* is the lifelong administration of prophylactic penicillin and use of pneumococcal-polysaccharide vaccines. Despite the use of such measures, HSCT recipients continue to have a higher incidence of pneumococcal disease than healthy individuals [74,75]. There are concerns about the strategy of penicillin prophylaxis, which include compliance, and the increasing number of penicillin resistant *S. pneumoniae* isolates being recorded [76]. Polysaccharide vaccines induce a T-cell independent immune response and are poorly immunogenic in HSCT recipients, particularly during the first 2 years after transplant, and even longer in recipients with chronic-GvHD [50,66,77,78]. The development of polysaccharide-protein conjugate vaccines offers a new strategy for protection against polysaccharide-encapsulated bacteria. By stimulating an IgG1 response, the conjugate vaccine can induce higher antibody levels (IgG1 recovers earlier than IgG2 in HSCT recipients) [35,77,78]. HSCT recipients should therefore be offered immunization with polysaccharide-protein conjugate vaccines against *S. pneumoniae, H. influenzae* type b, and *N. meningitidis* group C, rather than with the polysaccharide vaccines alone.

Haemophilus influenzae type b vaccine

There are limited data available regarding the incidence of Hib disease in HSCT recipients, and on immunity to Hib after HSCT. A recent study found that 63% of subjects had protective anti-Hib antibody concentrations before revaccination, and that three doses of Hib-conjugate vaccine resulted in all subjects achieving protective antibody concentrations [59]. At least two doses of Hib-conjugate are required to elicit protective antibody concentrations in HSCT recipients [55,65]. The timing of vaccination after HSCT may be an important determinant of immune response. In two studies, vaccination 18 months after transplant elicited a better response than earlier vaccination [78,79], but in two other studies immune responses were similar when Hib-conjugate was administered at 6 and 18 months after HSCT [65,66].

Neisseria meningitidis group C vaccine

There are very limited data on meningococcus C immunity in HSCT recipients. A recent study demonstrated that only 11% of HSCT recipients were immune to group C meningococcus [59]. There is one published study looking at response to MCC vaccines: three doses of MCC vaccine resulted in significant increase of antibody, with all recipients achieving optimal protective antibody titers [59]. It is possible that two doses may suffice and further studies looking at response to two doses of MCC would be useful. There are no published data on the meningococcal quadravalent conjugate vaccine in this population, and responses to the four serogroups in this vaccine are worthy of study.

Streptococcus pneumoniae vaccines

S. pneumoniae is an important cause of infection, occurring relatively late (at or more than 100 days), often over 6 to 12 months after HSCT [74,80–82]. It is more frequent in allogeneic than autologous HSCT recipients, and in allogeneic HSCT recipients with chronic-GvHD [75,81,82], and those that develop pneumococcal disease usually have low IgG2 levels [82]. Antipneumococcal antibody levels decline from pre-transplant levels and are lower than in healthy controls [83]. The serotypes and antimicrobial susceptibilities of pneumococcal isolates in transplant recipients appear to be similar to those from healthy children [80]. Increasing antimicrobial resistance, variation in the administration of penicillin, and patient compliance may explain the occurrence of pneumococcal disease in HSCT recipients despite prophylaxis with penicillin [75]. This demonstrates the need for additional protection by the most effective available pneumococcal vaccines.

Data from studies looking at pneumococcal polysaccharide vaccines in HSCT recipients demonstrate that the time of vaccination after transplant is an important factor in determining the immune response [50,66,77,83]. Recipients vaccinated 18 months after transplant have a better immune response than those vaccinated earlier [50,77]. In general, the studies show variable and often poor immunogenicity to the 23-valent-pneumococcal polysaccharide vaccine (Pn-PS23) [50,55,66,83]. Nonetheless, until recently recommendations have been that this group should receive two doses of Pn-PS23 [47]. A combination of PCV7 and Pn-PS23 has recently been shown to result in protective antibody responses, with a suggestion that two doses of conjugate vaccine are more immunogenic than one dose of polysaccharide vaccine [59]. Another study has demonstrated good responses to two doses of PCV7 when administered 6 to 9 months after HSCT [84]. Donor immunization with PCV7 also has a positive influence on the recipients' antibody response to PCV7 [62]. Further studies are needed to evaluate immune responses to PCV7 at earlier time points after HSCT, as well as the influence of preharvest immunization.

Summary

Children are immunosuppressed after completion of standard dose chemotherapy and after HSCT. They are at increased risk of infections, including vaccine-preventable infections. Revaccination is therefore important. After completion of standard dose chemotherapy, children should receive one dose of each childhood vaccine as per the immunization schedule of their country of residence.

HSCT recipients have extensive immune alterations and are particularly susceptible to infection with polysaccharide-encapsulated organisms. It is important that they receive the full schedule (usually two to three doses) of childhood vaccines as per the immunization schedule of their country of residence, and this should include PCV7 and Pn-PS23.

Further studies are required to evaluate immune responses to fewer doses of certain vaccines, and the efficacy of administering them at earlier time points after completion of standard chemotherapy and after HSCT. Further work also needs to be done to evaluate preharvest immunization for allogeneic and autologous HSCT.

References

[1] Feldman S, Gigliotti F, Shenep JL, et al. Risk of *Haemophilus influenzae* type b disease in children with cancer and response of immunocompromised leukemic children to a conjugate vaccine. J Infect Dis 1990;161:926–31.
[2] Meisel R, Toschke M, Heiligensetzer C, et al. Increased risk for invasive pneumococcal disease in children with acute lymphoblastic leukaemia. Br J Haematol 2007;137:457–60.
[3] Kaplan LJ, Daum RS, Smaron M, et al. Severe measles in immunocompromised patients. JAMA 1992;267:1237–41.
[4] Feldman S, Lott L. Varicella in children: impact of antiviral therapy and prophylaxis. Pediatrics 1987;80(4):465–72.
[5] Martin Ibáñez I, Arce Casas A, Cruz Martinez O, et al. Humoral immunity in pediatric patients with acute lymphoblastic leukaemia. Allergol Immunopathol (Madr) 2003;31:303–10.
[6] Ercan TE, Soycan LY, Apak H, et al. Antibody titers and immune response to diphtheria-tetanus-pertussis and measles-mumps-rubella vaccination in children treated for acute lymphoblastic leukaemia. J Pediatr Hematol Oncol 2005;27:273–7.
[7] Alanko S, Pelliniemi TT, Salmi TT. Recovery of blood B-lymphocytes and serum immunoglobulins after chemotherapy for childhood acute lymphoblastic leukaemia. Cancer 1992;69:1481–6.
[8] Caver TE, Slobod KS, Flynn PM, et al. Profound abnormality of the B/T lymphocyte ratio during chemotherapy for pediatric acute lymphoblastic leukaemia. Leukemia 1998;12:619–22.
[9] Alanko S, Salmi TT, Pelliniemi TT. Recovery of blood T-cell subsets after chemotherapy for childhood acute lymphoblastic leukaemia. Pediatr Hematol Oncol 1994;11:281–92.
[10] Abrahamsson J, Marky I, Mellander L. Immunoglobulin levels and lymphocyte response to mitogenic stimulation in children with malignant disease during treatment and follow-up. Acta Paediatr 1995;84:177–82.
[11] Kristinsson VH, Kristinsson JR, Jonmundsson GK, et al. Immunoglobulin class and subclass concentrations after treatment of childhood leukaemia. Pediatr Hematol Oncol 2001;18:167–72.
[12] Nilsson A, De Milito A, Engström P, et al. Current chemotherapy protocols for childhood acute lymphoblastic leukaemia induce loss of humoral immunity to viral vaccination antigens. Pediatrics 2002;109:1–6.

[13] Zignol M, Peracchi M, Tridello G, et al. Assessment of humoral immunity to poliomyelitis, tetanus, hepatitis B, measles, rubella, and mumps in children after chemotherapy. Cancer 2004;101:635–41.

[14] Ek T, Mellander L, Hahn-Zoric M, et al. Intensive treatment for childhood acute lymphoblastic leukaemia reduces immune responses to diphtheria, tetanus and *Haemophilus influenzae* type b. J Pediatr Hematol Oncol 2004;26:727–34.

[15] Fioredda F, Plebani A, Hanau G, et al. Re-immunisation schedule in leukaemic children after intensive chemotherapy: a possible stratergy. Eur J Haematol 2005;74:20–3.

[16] Ridgway D, Wolff LJ, Deforest A. Immunisation response varies with intensity of acute lymphoblastic leukaemia therapy. Am J Dis Child 1991;145:887–91.

[17] Feldman S, Andrew M, Norris B, et al. Decline in rates of seropositivity for measles, mumps, and rubella antibodies among previously immunised children treated for acute leukaemia. Clin Infect Dis 1998;27:388–90.

[18] Patel SR, Ortin M, Cohen B, et al. Re-immunization of children after completion of standard chemotherapy for acute leukemia. Clin Infect Dis 2007;44(5):635–42.

[19] von der Hardt K, Jungert J, Beck JD, et al. Humoral immunity against diphtheria, tetanus and poliomyelitis after antineoplastic therapy in children and adolescents—a retrospective analysis. Vaccine 2000;18:2999–3004.

[20] Leung TF, Li CK, Hung EC, et al. Immunogenicity of a two-dose regime of varicella vaccine in children with cancers. Eur J Haematol 2004;72(5):353–7.

[21] Gershon AA, Steinberg SP. Persistence of immunity to varicella in children with leukemia immunized with live attenuated varicella vaccine. N Engl J Med 1989;320(14):892–7.

[22] American Academy of Pediatrics Committee on Infectious Diseases. Prevention of varicella: recommendations for use of varicella vaccines in children, including a recommendation for a routine 2-dose varicella immunization schedule. Pediatrics 2007;120(1):221–31.

[23] Royal College of Paediatrics and Child Health. Immunisation of the immunocompromised child, best practice statement. United Kingdom: Royal College of Paediatrics and Child Health; 2002.

[24] Chisholm JC, Devine T, Charlett A, et al. Response to influenza immunisation during treatment for cancer. Arch Dis Child 2001;84:496–500.

[25] Smith S, Schiffman G, Karayalcin G, et al. Immunodeficiency in long-term survivors of acute lymphoblastic leukaemia treated with Berlin-Frankfurt-Munster therapy. J Pediatr 1995; 127:68–75.

[26] American Academy of Pediatrics Committee on Infectious Diseases. Red book, Section 1, Immunization of immunocompromised children. Elk Grove Village (IL): American Academy of Pediatrics; 2006.

[27] Krivit W. Overwhelming postsplenectomy infection. Am J Hematol 1977;2:193–201.

[28] Woolfrey AE, Anasetti C, Storer B, et al. Factors associated with outcome after unrelated marrow transplantation for treatment of acute lymphoblastic leukaemia in children. Blood 2002;99:2002–8.

[29] Knecht H, Jost R, Gmur J, et al. Functional hyposplenia after allogeneic bone marrow transplantation is detected by epinephrine stimulation test and splenic ultrasonography. Eur J Haematol 1988;41:382–7.

[30] Adkins B, Gandour D, Strober S, et al. Total irradiation leads to transient depletion of the mouse thymic medulla and persistent abnormalities among medullary stromal cells. J Immunol 1988;140:3373–9.

[31] Lum LG, Seigneuret MC, Storb RF, et al. In vitro regulation of immunoglobulin synthesis after marrow transplantation. I. T-cell and B-cell deficiencies in patients with and without chronic graft-versus-host disease. Blood 1981;58:431–9.

[32] Fallen PR, McGreavey L, Madrigal JA, et al. Factors affecting reconstitution of the T cell compartment in allogeneic haematopoietic cell transplant recipients. Bone Marrow Transplant 2003;32:1001–14.

[33] Lum LG. The kinetics of immune reconstitution after human marrow transplantation. Blood 1987;69:369–80.

[34] Ueda M, Harada M, Shiobara S, et al. T lymphocyte reconstitution in long-term survivors after allogeneic and autologous marrow transplantation. Transplantation 1984;37:552–6.

[35] Foot AB, Potter MN, Donaldson C, et al. Immune reconstitution after BMT in children. Bone Marrow Transplant 1993;11(1):7–13.

[36] de Vries E, Van Tol MJD, Langlois van den Bergh R, et al. Reconstitution of lymphocyte subpopulations after paediatric bone marrow transplantation. Bone Marrow Transplant 2000;25:267–75.

[37] Steingrimsdottir H, Gruber A, Bjorkholm M, et al. Immune reconstitution after autologous hematopoietic stem cell transplantation in relation to underlying disease, type of high dose therapy and infectious complications. Haematologica 2000;85:832–8.

[38] Chakraverty R, Robinson S, Peggs K, et al. Excessive T-cell depletion of peripheral blood stem cells has an adverse effect upon outcome following allogeneic stem cell transplantation. Bone Marrow Transplant 2001;2899:827–34.

[39] Kalwak K, Gorcynska E, Toporski J, et al. Immune reconstitution after haematopoietic stem cell transplantation in children: immunophenotype analysis with regard to factors affecting the speed of recovery. Br J Haematol 2002;118:74–89.

[40] Hammarström V, Pauksen K, Svensson H, et al. Serum immunoglobulin levels in relation to levels of specific antibodies in allogeneic and autologous bone marrow transplant recipients. Transplantation 2000;69:1582–6.

[41] Lum LG, Munn NA, Schanfield MS, et al. The detection of specific antibody formation to recall antigens after human marrow transplantation. Blood 1986;67:582–7.

[42] Hochberg EP, Chillemi AC, Wu CJ, et al. Quantitation of T-cell neogenesis in vivo after allogeneic bone marrow transplantation in adults. Blood 2001;98:1116–21.

[43] Mackall CL, Fleisher TA, Brown MR, et al. Age, thymopoiesis, and CD4$^+$ T-lymphocyte regeneration after intensive chemotherapy. N Engl J Med 1995;332:143–9.

[44] Storek J, Joseph A, Dawson MA, et al. Factors influencing T-lymphopoiesis after allogeneic hematopoietic cell transplantation. Blood 2002;73:1154–8.

[45] Ljungman P, Cordonnier C, de Bock R, et al. Immunisations after bone marrow transplantation: results of a European survey and recommendations from the Infectious Diseases Working Party of the European Group for Blood and Marrow Transplantation. Bone Marrow Transplant 1995;15:455–60.

[46] Henning KJ, White MH, Sepkowitz KA, et al. A national survey of immunisation practices following allogeneic bone marrow transplantation. JAMA 1997;277:1148–51.

[47] Centers for Disease Control and Prevention. Guidelines for preventing opportunistic infections among hematopoietic stem cell transplant recipients: Recommendations of CDC, Infectious society of America and the American society of Blood and Marrow Transplantation. MMWR Morb Mortal Wkly Rep 2000;49(RR-10):1–125.

[48] Ljungman P, Engelhard D, Cámara R de la, et al. Vaccination of stem cell transplant recipients: recommendations of the Infectious Diseases Working Party of the EBMT. Bone Marrow Transplant 2005;35:737–46.

[49] Engelhard D, Nagler A, Hardan I, et al. Antibody response to a two-dose regimen of influenza vaccine in allogeneic T-cell-depleted and autologous BMT recipients. Bone Marrow Transplant 1993;11(1):1–5.

[50] Avanzini MA, Carra AM, Maccario R, et al. Antibody response to pneumococcal vaccine in children receiving bone marrow transplantation. J Clin Immunol 1995;15:137–44.

[51] Parkkali T, Olander R-M, Ruutu T, et al. A randomised comparison between early and late vaccination with tetanus toxoid vaccine in allogeneic BMT. Bone Marrow Transplant 1997;19:933–8.

[52] Parkkali T, Stenvik M, Ruutu T, et al. Randomised comparison of early and late vaccination with inactivated poliovirus vaccine after allogeneic BMT. Bone Marrow Transplant 1997;20:663–8.

[53] Ljungman P, Wiklund-Hammarsten M, Duraj V, et al. Response to tetanus toxoid immunisation after allogeneic bone marrow transplantation. J Infect Dis 1990;162:496–500.

[54] Ljungman P, Duraj V, Magnius L. Response to immunisation against polio after allogeneic marrow transplantation. Bone Marrow Transplant 1991;7(2):89–93.

[55] Guinan EC, Molrine DC, Antin JH, et al. Polysaccharide conjugate vaccine responses in bone marrow transplant patients. Transplantation 1994;57:677–84.

[56] Spoulou V, Giannaki M, Vounatsou M, et al. Long-term immunity to measles, mumps and rubella after MMR vaccination among children with bone marrow transplants. Bone Marrow Transplant 2004;33:1187–90.

[57] Ljungman P, Aschan J, Gustafsson B, et al. Long-term immunity to poliovirus after vaccination of allogeneic stem cell recipients. Bone Marrow Transplant 2004;34:1067–9.

[58] Ljungman P, Fridell E, Lonnqvist B, et al. Efficacy and safety of vaccination of marrow transplant recipients with a live attenuated measles, mumps and rubella vaccine. J Infect Dis 1989;159:610–5.

[59] Patel SR, Ortín M, Cohen BJ, et al. Re-immunization with Measles, Tetanus, Poliovirus, *Haemophilus influenzae* type b, Meningococcus C and Pneumococcal vaccines in children after hematopoietic stem cell transplantation. Clin Infect Dis 2007;44(5):625–34.

[60] Ljungman P, Aschan J, Barkholt L, et al. Measles immunity after allogeneic stem cell transplantation; influence of donor-type, graft type, intensity of conditioning and GvHD. Bone Marrow Transplant 2004;34:589–93.

[61] Ljungman P, Lewensohn-Fuchs I, Hammarstrom V, et al. Long-term immunity to measles, mumps and rubella after allogeneic bone marrow transplantation. Blood 1994;84:657–63.

[62] Molrine DC, Antin JH, Guinan EC, et al. Donor immunisation with pneumococcal conjugate vaccine allows early protective antibody responses following allogeneic hematopoietic cell transplantation. Blood 2003;101:831–6.

[63] Storek J, Dawson MA, Lim LC-L, et al. Efficacy of donor vaccination before hematopoietic cell transplantation and recipient vaccination before and early after transplantation. Bone Marrow Transplant 2004;33:337–46.

[64] Parkkali T, Käyhty H, Hovi T, et al. A randomized study on donor immunization with tetanus–diphtheria, *Haemophilus influenzae* type b and inactivated poliovirus vaccines to improve the recipient responses to the same vaccines after allogeneic bone marrow transplantation. Bone Marrow Transplant 2007;39(3):179–88.

[65] Vance E, George S, Guinan EC, et al. Comparison of multiple immunization schedules for *Haemophilus influenzae* type b-conjugate and tetanus toxoid vaccines following bone marrow transplantation. Bone Marrow Transplant 1998;22:735–41.

[66] Parkkali T, Ruutu T, Stenvik M, et al. Loss of protective immunity to polio, diphtheria and *Haemophilus influenzae* type b after allogeneic bone marrow transplantation. APMIS 1996; 104:383–8.

[67] Florax A, Ehlert K, Becker K, et al. *Bordetella pertussis* respiratory infection following hematopoietic stem cell transplantation: time for universal vaccination? Bone Marrow Transplant 2006;38(9):639–40.

[68] Engelhard D, Handsher R, Naparstek E, et al. Immune response to polio vaccination in bone marrow transplant recipients. Bone Marrow Transplant 1991;8:295–300.

[69] King SM, Saunders EF, Petric M, et al. Response to measles, mumps and rubella vaccine in paediatric bone marrow transplant recipients. Bone Marrow Transplant 1996;17: 633–6.

[70] Machado CM, Gonçalves FB, Pannuti CS, et al. Measles in bone marrow transplant recipients during an outbreak in São Paulo, Brazil. Blood 2002;99:83–7.

[71] Machado CM, de Souza VA, Sumita LM, et al. Early measles vaccination in bone marrow transplant recipients. Bone Marrow Transplant 2005;35:787–91.

[72] Pauksen K, Duraj V, Ljungman P, et al. Immunity to and immunisation against measles, rubella and mumps in patients after autologous bone marrow transplantation. Bone Marrow Transplant 1992;9:427–32.

[73] Machado CM, Cardoso MR, da Rocha IF, et al. The benefit of influenza vaccination after bone marrow transplantation. Bone Marrow Transplant 2005;36(10):897–900.

[74] Winston DJ, Schiffman G, Wang D, et al. Pneumococcal infections after human bone-marrow transplantation. Ann Intern Med 1979;91:835–41.

[75] Kulkarni S, Powles R, Treleaven J, et al. Chronic graft versus host disease is associated with long-term risk for pneumococcal infections in recipients of bone marrow transplants. Blood 2000;95:3683–6.

[76] Reacher MH, Shah A, Livermore DM, et al. Bacteraemia and antibiotic resistance of its pathogens in England and Wales between 1990 and 1998: trend analysis. BMJ 2000;320: 213–6.

[77] Spoulou V, Victoratos P, Ioannidis JPA, et al. Kinetics of antibody concentration and avidity for the assessment of immune response to pneumococcal vaccine among children with bone marrow transplants. J Infect Dis 2000;182:965–9.

[78] Barra A, Cordonnier C, Preziosi MP, et al. Immunogenecity of *Haemophilus influenzae* type b conjugate vaccine in allogeneic bone marrow recipients. J Infect Dis 1992;166:1021–8.

[79] Avanzini MA, Carra AM, Maccario R, et al. Immunisation with *Haemophilus influenzae* type b conjugate vaccine in children given bone marrow transplantation: comparison with healthy matched controls. J Clin Immunol 1998;18:193–201.

[80] Schutze GE, Mason EO, Wald ER, et al. Pneumococcal infections in children after transplantation. Clin Infect Dis 2001;33:16–21.

[81] Engelhard D, Cordonnier C, Shaw PJ, et al. Infectious Disease Working Party of the European Bone Marrow Transplantation; early and late invasive pneumococcal infection following stem cell transplantation: a European Bone Marrow Transplant survey. Br J Haematol 2002;117:444–50.

[82] Sheridan JF, Tutschka PJ, Sedmak DD, et al. Immunoglobulin G subclass deficiency and pneumococcal infection after allogeneic bone marrow transplantation. Blood 1990;75: 1583–6.

[83] Winston DJ, Ho WG, Schiffman G, et al. Pneumococcal vaccination of recipients of bone marrow transplants. Arch Intern Med 1983;143:1735–7.

[84] Meisel R, Kuypers L, Dirksen U, et al. Pneumococcal conjugate vaccine provides early protective antibody responses in children after related and unrelated allogeneic hematopoietic stem cell transplantation. Blood 2007;109(6):2322–6.

PEDIATRIC CLINICS
OF NORTH AMERICA

Pediatr Clin N Am 55 (2008) 187–209

Good Clinical Practice and the Conduct of Clinical Studies in Pediatric Oncology

Susan Devine, CCRP[a], Ramzi N. Dagher, MD[b],
Karen D. Weiss, MD[b], Victor M. Santana, MD[c],*

[a]Department of Hematology/Oncology, Hospital for Sick Children, Room 8305,
555 University Avenue, Toronto, ON M5G 1X8, Canada
[b]Office of Oncology Drug Products, Center for Drug Evaluation and Research, Food and Drug
Administration, Building 22, 10903 New Hampshire Avenue, Silver Spring, MD 20903, USA
[c]Department of Oncology, St. Jude Children's Research Hospital, 332 North Lauderdale
MS# 260, Memphis, TN, USA

Good clinical practice (GCP) is an international, ethical, and scientific quality standard for trials involving human subjects. The many activities covered by GCP include trial design, definition of scientifically and ethically sound trial objectives, oversight of trial activities, data collection and quality assurance, study analysis, and human subject protections. All of these activities are intended to support clinical research, with the ultimate goals of improving the health and welfare of patients and advancing biomedical science. GCP is fundamentally a system in which responsibilities are shared by clinical investigators, institutions, institutional review boards, industry sponsors, and government regulators. One of the great challenges in applying good clinical practices is defining the roles and responsibilities of those involved and ensuring a dynamic process in which contributions are complementary. This article discusses the principles that guide good clinical practice standards, with particular emphasis on how they to relate to pediatric oncology research and recent efforts at harmonization. The authors also review the clinical trials process and the roles of the participants, highlighting the pivotal role of the clinical investigator and the research team. Finally, the authors briefly review the historical aspects of drug development regulations in the United States and the current regulatory paths for pediatric

This work was supported in part by USPHS awards CA23099, Cancer Center Support Grant CA21765, and by American Lebanese Syrian Associated Charities (ALSAC).

The views expressed do not necessarily represent those of the United States Food and Drug Administration or the United States Government.

* Corresponding author.

E-mail address: victor.santana@stjude.org (V.M. Santana).

oncology drug development. Where relevant, historical events that underlie many of the regulations and their current applications are described, and practical examples are provided.

Overview of good clinical practice and international harmonization

GCP is a roadmap of responsibilities that ensures that clinical research involving human subjects is consistent with appropriate laws, regulations, and ethical principles [1–3]. Compliance with the principles of GCP provides assurance that the rights, confidentiality, and well being of subjects are protected, and that the clinical trial data and reported results are credible. These principles were collaboratively developed by the United States, European Union, and Japan over the past 25 years through the International Conference on Harmonization (ICH), established to develop and harmonize technical requirements for drug development [4]. Working groups, composed of subject matter experts representing the three regions' regulatory agencies and pharmaceutical manufacturers, convene several times a year to develop guidance that reflects the collective current wisdom about how best to develop and test medicinal products. ICH documents also address a broad array of product testing issues, including manufacturing and nonclinical and clinical safety and efficacy evaluation issues. The ICH process is fluid; new working groups are formed as needed, and older documents are updated as new issues arise. For example, an expert working group recently completed guidance on assessment of drugs that have the potential to prolong the QT interval. A list of key ICH documents and their focus is presented in Table 1. Table 2 lists US Federal Drug Administration (FDA) Code of Federal Regulations (CFR) related to good clinical practice and clinical trials.

Conducting clinical trials

Evidence-based medicine is the standard of care for treatment of disease. Through clinical research, health care providers expand on that knowledge to improve evidence-based standards. In the United States, clinical trials have been a standard approach to the care of children with cancer since the 1960s. Because childhood cancer is rare, advances in therapy depend on collaborative clinical trials conducted by cooperative groups and consortia [5,6]. There have been a number of pediatric cooperative groups in the United States, beginning with the Southwest Oncology Group in the 1960s and 70s, followed by the Children's Cancer Group, the Pediatric Oncology Group, the National Wilms Tumor Study Group, the Intergroup Rhabdomyosarcoma Study Group, and more recently, the Children's Oncology Group (COG). COG is presently a National Cancer Institute (NCI)-funded international multicenter, clinical trials organization headquartered in the United States, with more than 200 sites in North America, Australia, the Netherlands, and Switzerland. It brings together specialized professionals to conduct focused clinical investigations in children with cancer.

Table 1
Summary of commonly referenced International Conference on Harmonization clinical efficacy guidelines

Document	Subject	Content
ICH E 2	Adverse event (AE) reporting	Defines terms, timeframes for AE reporting, and formatting of AE reports
ICH E 6	GCP consolidated guidelines	Defines responsibilities of sponsors, investigators, consent process monitoring and auditing procedures, and protection of human subjects
ICH E 9	Statistical principles	Design and conduct of trials intended to support or establish efficacy
ICH E 10	Choice of control groups	Properties and limitations of different kinds of control groups (active control equivalence, noninferiority, etc.)
ICH E 11	Clinical investigations in pediatric population	Principles of clinical investigations in children, including timing of studies and extrapolation of data relative to studies conducted in adults, consent, assent, and interventions
ICH E 14	Evaluation of QT/QTc interval prolongation	Testing the effects of new agents on the QT/QTc interval, as well as cardiovascular adverse events

While clinical trials have become a standard approach to cancer treatment and have improved pediatric cancer outcomes, clinical research introduces additional risks that must be balanced with potential benefits [6]. Consider, for example, a randomized trial in which a subject is assigned to a treatment arm that ultimately is shown to be less effective, or equally effective but with more severe toxicity. It is imperative that clinical researchers follow GCP to ensure the safety of the clinical trial subjects as well as the integrity of the data, which will be used to support changes in evidence-based care and the regulatory approval of new medicines.

Role of the sponsors

GCP defines the sponsor as an individual, company, institution, or organization that takes responsibility for the initiation, management, and/or financing of clinical research. Sponsors oversee the Investigational New Drug

Table 2
United States Food and Drug Administration regulations related to good clinical practice and
clinical trials

21 CFR Part 11	Electronic records; electronic signatures
21 CFR Part 50	Human subject protection (informed consent)
21 CFR Part 50, subpart D	Additional safeguards for children in clinical investigations of FDA-regulated products
21 CFR Part 54	Financial disclosure by clinical investigators
21 CFR Part 56	Institutional review boards
21 CFR Part 312	Investigational new drug application
Forms 1571 and 1572	Investigational new drug application and statement of investigator
21 CFR Part 314	Applications for FDA approval to market a new drug
21 CFR Part 601	Applications for FDA approval of a biologic license
21 CFR Part 812	Investigational device exemptions
21 CFR Part 814	Premarket approval of medical devices

(IND) application and are ultimately responsible for the research and for ensuring the compliance of the investigators. Sponsors must provide investigators with adequate information to support the use of a test product. Sponsors create and update the Investigators Brochure (IB), a document compiling relevant preclinical and clinical information about a new drug, or a new indication for a known drug. It is not unusual in pediatric cancer investigations to have an IND application for the new pediatric use of a commercially available drug. It is the sponsor who ultimately submits a marketing application to the regulatory authorities.

The sponsor is responsible for quality assurance and quality control of the studies. Standard operating procedures define duties to ensure compliance with the protocol at each stage of the trial. The sponsor ensures statistical analyses of the study and, where necessary, designates an independent data monitoring committee [7]. For example, COG has a data safety monitoring committee that meets semiannually (more often if necessary) to ensure that study monitoring plans are followed.

The sponsor is responsible for maintaining essential documents, including the IB, protocol, agreements, regulatory documents, case report forms (CRF) and the records of investigational product accountability. The sponsor also determines subject and investigator compensation and trial financing.

While many of the sponsor's obligations can be delegated to a clinical research organization, the sponsor is ultimately responsible for the IND. In pediatric cancer, sponsors include the Cancer Therapy Evaluation Program of the NCI, the pharmaceutical industry, and in some cases individual investigators or institutions (known as sponsor investigators). Regardless of the sponsor or the funding mechanism, GCP must be followed. Where trials cross international boundaries, additional local sponsor requirements may be necessary. Health Canada, for example, requires that a Canadian senior medical officer be appointed as the Canadian sponsor of all COG studies in that country.

In the cooperative group setting, a physician is designated as the Study Chair of each therapeutic clinical trial to ensure sponsor-required medical expertise. The multidisciplinary study committee (pediatric oncologists, biostatisticians, pharmacologists, surgeons, pathologists, radiation oncologists, radiologists, nurses, and clinical research associates) also collectively ensure quality design. Furthermore, an independent multidisciplinary protocol review committee reviews the scientific merit and other aspects of each COG therapeutic study before final submission. COG, in part, manages its sponsor obligations through its statistics and data center.

Role of the investigator

The investigator—the physician responsible for conduct of the clinical trial at the local site—is expected to be aware of and compliant with GCP and regulatory requirements and with the protocol and its eligibility, testing requirements, treatment plan, therapy modifications, and reporting requirements. GCP defines a subinvestigator as any individual member of a clinical trial team designated and supervised by the investigator to perform critical trial-related procedures and/or make important trial-related decisions (eg, associates, residents, research fellows). Investigators must be qualified by education, training, and experience.

Each investigator provides a curriculum vitae in the form of a "biosketch" to COG, documenting qualifications, and undergoes mandatory human subject protection training as part of the membership application process. Disciplines within COG set standards for membership that ensure adherence to specific professional practice standards. Investigators also file an FDA 1572 Statement of Investigator form annually, affirming investigator responsibilities, which include an agreement to follow the protocol, conduct or supervise the study, obtain informed consent per regulations, report adverse events, understand potential risks and side effects of the test product, ensure the clinical team understands obligations, keep accurate records for inspection, keep the institutional review board (IRB) informed, and comply with all other regulations.

The investigator is responsible for recruiting study subjects at his or her clinical site and for their welfare. The investigator must be a qualified physician, as he or she is responsible for all trial-related medical decisions and must be able to provide medical care for any adverse events. The investigator must obtain informed consent of the study participant (in the case of pediatric research subjects, parental permission and age-appropriate participant assent), collect the protocol-specified evaluations, and report safety information to the IND sponsor. The investigator may delegate the consenting process to other appropriately qualified trial staff based on guidance from the local IRB. The investigator must also account for the investigational medical product, maintain accurate records, and provide interim reports to the IRB. Obligations of clinical investigators are delineated in federal regulations, in the ICH GCP guideline, and within each institution where clinical research is conducted [8].

Institutional review board and research ethics board

The investigator submits all research to the institutional review board or research ethics board (REB) of record for approval before initiating any clinical research study at the local site. The submission includes the sponsor-provided protocol document, study consent forms, IB, and any other written material that will be provided to a subject (questionnaires, information packages, or other forms). During each year of the study the investigator must submit at a minimum a progress report, and request renewal and reapproval of the research by the IRB or REB. The IRB or REB will require an updated IB, as well as a summary of progress. For example, in the COG, the Study Chairs—with the support of biostatisticians—produce study updates based on the monitoring plan and provide them to local investigators for IRB or REB submission.

All changes (amendments) to an ongoing protocol also require approval of the IRB or REB. Of particular importance is new information that might affect a subject's desire to continue participating in a study or that might alter the risk and benefit balance of the research. Additionally, any premature terminations or trial suspensions must be brought to the attention of the local IRB or REB. The investigator is then responsible for performing instructions from the sponsor and the local IRB or REB regarding continuation or discontinuation of the study. The investigator must provide proof to the sponsor that appropriate IRB or REB approvals have been obtained. Many of these processes are performed electronically. The COG, for example, has an on-line tracking system, whereby dates of initial, continuing review, and amendment approvals are entered into a Web-based system. The COG links subject enrollment on a given trial at the local site to this process, thus assuring that protocols meet regulatory review and approval.

Informed consent

Prospective participants cannot be enrolled into a trial without their consent. Elements of the consent form and the consent process are set forth in federal regulations and guidance documents (see Table 2) [9]. Before they consent, study participants must be informed of known and potential risks of participation in the trial, even if the likelihood of risk is remote. The IRB at each participating institution, or a central IRB, must review and approve the consent form and the clinical research protocol before the study can be initiated at that institution. The composition and duties of the IRB are described in the ICH GCP guidelines. Investigators must ensure that the consent process is free of coercion and provide sufficient time for decision-making by the subject. Legal rights of the subject may not be waived, either verbally or in writing, and consent must be personally dated.

Mechanisms exist to strengthen human subject protections for particularly vulnerable study participants, such as children, who cannot give valid consent. The parent or legal guardian gives permission for a child to be enrolled in a research study. The ICH E11 document addresses some of the considerations unique to pediatric clinical trials, including ethical issues. In rare circumstances, when it is not possible to obtain a participant's consent because of the nature of his or her illness or injury, and when obtaining consent from a legally acceptable representative (eg, next of kin) is not feasible, the FDA and other Department of Health and Human Services regulations may permit the clinical trial to proceed with a waiver of consent.

Children are considered a vulnerable population, and additional safeguards are in place to protect them. The age at which a child or legal representative may give consent, and the use of an assent process for minor children, are based on local IRB or REB guidance. If a subject or legal representative is unable to read, an impartial witness must be present during the consent discussion and must sign and date the consent attesting that the information in the consent form is consistent with the discussion, that the subject appears to understand the information, and that consent was given freely.

All subjects enrolled in a clinical trial must first be fully informed about the trial, and each subject (or legal representative) must sign and date the IRB- or REB-approved consent form before participating. If possible, the consent document should have an approval or revision date. This information assures that the correct version is being used. If the consent form is changed during a study and the change affects subjects currently enrolled, those subjects must sign the revised version. In addition, the regulations permit the use of either a written form that embodies the required elements of informed consent (Box 1) or a "short" form, stating that the elements of informed consent have been presented orally. If a short form is used, the oral presentation must be witnessed and the IRB or REB must review and approve a written summary of the information presented.

Participants must be informed which procedures are study-related: that is, those undertaken specifically for study purposes rather than standard-of-care procedures. Taking extra blood or bone marrow samples, as might be the case in leukemia trials, would be considered a study-related procedure requiring prospective consent.

Resources

GCP requires that an investigator have adequate resources to carry out a clinical trial. Resources include the ability to recruit sufficient numbers of research subjects, which is ascertained through careful review of inclusion and exclusion criteria. Resources on-site must also be in place. The investigator must have adequate time to carry out his or her study obligations and oversee delegated study duties. Delegation must be made to appropriately qualified staff, who have sufficient time to carry out the duties and have

---

Box 1. Required elements of an informed consent document

Statements that indicate:
1. Study involves research; purposes, expected duration, description of study procedures, and identification of experimental procedures
2. Description of foreseeable risks or discomforts
3. Description of reasonably expected benefits to subjects or others
4. Disclosure of procedures or treatments
5. Extent of confidentiality of records that can be expected
6. Explanation of availability of treatment or compensation for injuries from the research
7. Contact information for research questions, subject's rights, and research-related injury
8. Statement that participation is voluntary, no penalty or loss of benefits for refusal, ability to discontinue participation at any time

---

adequate information about their specific roles. Delegation logs are used to ensure that all required procedures are undertaken by appropriate individuals.

In the COG example, each site has a principal investigator with ultimate responsibility, plus coinvestigators from a variety of disciplines, such as pathology, surgery, radiation oncology, and nursing. The site also has a research coordinator, called a clinical research associate (CRA), to whom many of the day-to-day tasks are delegated.

Facilities appropriate for the study must also be available. For example, if a study requires radiation therapy, the facility must have access to an approved radiation therapy facility sanctioned by the Quality Assurance Review Center. If a stem cell transplant is a study component, a Foundation for the Accreditation of Cellular Therapy-accredited transplant facility must be available. A careful review of study procedures will reveal requirements and compliance issues that need consideration, such as bed availability to ensure timely treatment, laboratory support for special testing, and diagnostic imaging. Industry sponsors confirm facility compliance through site selection and initiation visits. In the cooperative group model, specific standards are delineated for institutional membership, ensuring availability and access to appropriate quality standards and accreditations.

Compliance

GCP requires that trials be conducted in compliance with the approved protocol, including eligibility criteria, adverse event monitoring, treatment, and modifications. Deviations are permitted only if they are necessary to eliminate an immediate hazard to a subject. If such situations arise, the deviations must be documented in the subject's medical record, and the sponsor and local IRB or REB informed.

Clinicians must recognize that in treating a patient on a therapeutic protocol they are acting both as investigator and as treating physician. The protocol must be followed exactly, adhering to the specified observations and procedures and to their specified timing. This is true at time of entry to the study to determine eligibility, during the delivery of therapy to understand the response and effects of the therapy, and during the protocol-mandated follow-up phase. While it is acceptable to carry out testing additional to that required by protocol, it is not acceptable to disregard the required testing. Furthermore, if a test or procedure is not performed to evaluate an adverse event, that does not signify the absence of an adverse event. Sponsors monitor both the tests and procedures performed and their timing; nonadherence to either is considered a protocol deviation.

The investigator must ensure compliance with study randomization procedures. While the study is ongoing, the randomization code for an individual subject may be broken only as delineated in the protocol: for example, in the case of an adverse event that compromises the health or welfare of the participant. All instances of unblinding must be documented and reported to the sponsor.

Investigational product

Investigators must be familiar with the use of the investigational products in a study. Information is made available through the sponsor-provided IB, which by regulation must be updated annually to include all new information.

The investigator, while responsible for investigational product accountability at the site, may assign these duties to a pharmacist. A key component of successful GCP is excellent communication between the investigator and the pharmacist, often facilitated by the CRA. Records documenting delivery of investigational product to the site, ongoing inventory, disposition to research subjects, and disposition of unused product must be maintained in accordance with the sponsor's requirements, including the ability to track by batch or serial number all investigational products given to individual patients. A common tool used to fulfill these requirements is a Drug or Agent Accountability Record form. Investigational product can be used only by official study patients and must be used in accordance with the approved protocol. In studies of drugs that are commercially available, a common deficiency is the use of incorrect drug supply. GCP also requires the investigator or a designee to explain the correct use of the investigational product to subjects and reconfirm understanding at intervals.

The sponsor will provide drug information for all study medications, including formulation, storage requirements, known toxicities, drug stability, administration information, and the supplier of the medication (which may be the sponsor, as in NCI-held INDs, or a commercial source, if the medication is not investigational).

Recording and reporting of trials

The task of data collection at the sites is generally shared. Investigators produce the source information from which CRAs abstract appropriate information for case report forms. In creating the source information, investigators must ensure that they document not only routine patient care information but also protocol-specific information, such as performance status and toxicity grade and attribution. Important also is the timeliness of alerting the CRA to special circumstances that require reporting, such as disease relapse or progression or serious adverse events.

All documentation must stem from source documents, defined as all information contained in the official medical record or research record, as well as any study-related correspondence. In abstracting data for clinical research, CRAs require a source document. "If it is not written down, it did not happen" is a common creed among CRAs who recognize the importance of source documents.

The investigator must ensure that data submitted to the sponsor are accurate, complete, and timely. If there are discrepancies between the data and the source document, an explanation must be included. If changes are required after data are submitted, modifications should be made without obscuring the initial entry and should be dated, initialed, and explained. Obliterating or destroying data, or back-dating information, could be construed as scientific misconduct.

Adverse events and safety reports

Adverse event recording and reporting is a fundamental aspect of drug development and of human subject protection. The clinical investigator identifies, evaluates, and documents adverse events experienced by study participants at his or her site and informs the sponsor and the IRB or REB. The sponsor is responsible for submitting safety information to the FDA and other regulatory agencies. The NCI uses the Common Terminology Criteria for Adverse Events (CTCAE) version 3.0 [10]. The CTCAE has objective criteria, such as laboratory values, and subjective criteria that require description by investigators using CTCAE-specific language. Adverse event (AE) reporting can require documentation of the event from inception to resolution. One of five grades is assigned to an adverse event. Grades 1 to 3 designate mild, moderate, and severe AE; grade 4, life-threatening, or disabling AE; and grade 5, death. Serious adverse events require or prolong hospitalization, are life threatening, or cause significant disability or incapacity, congenital anomaly, birth defect, or death. It is the investigator's responsibility to assess adverse events, determine their grade, attribution, and relationship to the investigational product, and report in the appropriate manner to the sponsor and the local IRB or REB.

The sponsor reviews serious adverse event reports and shares information about serious, unexpected events with other investigators in the study or investigating the same drug, in the form of a safety report. In pediatrics, it is not uncommon to receive safety reports describing adverse events in elderly patients receiving the same drug on a different study or for a different indication. Safety reports must be submitted by the investigator to the local IRB or REB. The sponsor must also submit a summary of the most frequent and the most serious adverse events in an annual report as part of their IND.

All serious, unexpected adverse events must be reported to regulatory agencies within 15 days of receipt of the information. Any unexpected life-threatening or fatal event must be reported by telephone (or facsimile) within 7 days of receipt. Although causality assessment is integral to reporting, a determination that a given medicinal product caused or was associated with an adverse event is not always possible. Randomized, controlled trials offer the most reliable assessment of the contribution of a test article to an adverse event. Causality is difficult to determine in other settings because of comorbidity and concomitant medications. Regardless of its cause, the event should be reported within the specified time frame unless there is no reasonable possibility that the drug was associated with the adverse event.

For reporting, CRAs abstract the details of adverse events from source documents. Each protocol defines which grades of adverse events require routine versus expedited reporting. Continuous collaboration between investigators and CRAs is imperative to ensure complete, timely adverse event reporting.

Essential documents

GCP defines essential documents as documents that individually and collectively permit evaluation of the conduct of a trial and the quality of the data produced. These documents serve to demonstrate the compliance of the investigator, sponsor and monitor with the standards of GCP and with all applicable regulatory requirements. Essential documents for clinical trials include:

- Investigator's brochure with updates
- Protocol with amendments
- Date-documented IRB approvals
- Curriculum vitae of study investigators
- Normal laboratory ranges
- Investigational agent documentation and accountability
- Monitoring reports
- Signed informed consents

- Source documents
- Complete CRFs with documentation of corrections
- Serious adverse event notifications
- Safety reports and annual reports to IRB or REB

Monitoring and auditing

Although the purposes of monitoring and auditing are similar (to assure appropriate trial conduct and data validity), their approaches differ. The ICH GCP document defines monitoring as the act of overseeing the progress of the clinical trial and ensuring that it is conducted, recorded, and reported in accordance with the protocol, standard operating procedures, GCP, and applicable regulatory requirements. Medical monitors, usually employees of the sponsor, perform on-site (and, if indicated, off-site) evaluations of trial-related activities. The extent and frequency of monitoring should be appropriate for the length, complexity, and other particulars of the trial. Among other duties, the monitor identifies deviations in protocol conduct so that the sponsor may take appropriate corrective steps, such as retraining investigators or closing certain sites.

Auditing is defined in the ICH CGP document as the systematic and independent examination of trial-related activities and documents. The audit is usually conducted at the conclusion of the trial. The sponsor may hire field auditors who document findings in a written report to the sponsor. FDA inspectors also conduct independent study audits. Traditionally, the purpose of FDA audits has been to verify data submitted in support of a marketing application. However, the FDA and the sponsor may conduct "for cause" or directed audits at any stage of investigation if there is reason to suspect a problem with trial conduct or data integrity.

An additional human subject protection is use of a data monitoring committee (DMC) to evaluate accumulating data in a clinical trial [7]. Generally, the sponsor establishes the DMC, selects the members, and devises its charter. DMC members should be independent of the sponsor and clinical investigators. The DMC's role depends on the charter and the nature of the study. The DMC is usually empowered to recommend study modifications to enhance participant safety and, in some cases, may recommend that a study be stopped if accumulating data indicate futility or a major safety concern. DMCs review submitted data but, unlike study monitors, do not visit sites to confirm that the data are accurate, the protocol is followed, consent is documented, and so forth.

Inherent checks and balances exist when the sponsor is not the investigator. When the sponsor is also the investigator, external oversight of the trial is advisable. Individual physicians who assume the role of sponsor, investigator, or both should be familiar with guidance and federal regulations that set out the respective duties.

Considerations in trial design methodology

The key elements of trial design include defining an appropriate patient population; outlining clear objectives; defining the specific treatment plan, including dosing and dose modification parameters; incorporating appropriate safety and efficacy monitoring; and using accepted statistical methods for hypothesis testing. Pediatric oncology trial designs vary depending on the immediate goals, stage of development of the drug if an investigational drug is involved, and the ultimate goal of the drug development plan.

Phases of trials

Three phases of clinical trials are customarily conducted in the development of new treatment approaches for pediatric malignancies. These are also summarized in Table 3.

Phase I

The initial clinical trials of anticancer agents (phase I trials) evaluate doses and schedules appropriate for further development. These are typically open-label, single-arm trials in patients with advanced or refractory malignancies for which there are no known effective therapies.

If no prior human data are available, the starting dose and schedule for such studies is based on nonclinical data derived from toxicology studies, usually in at least two relevant animal species. However, anticancer agents are usually tested in children only after adult studies. Therefore, the starting dose and schedule can often be based on prior human experience; starting doses are typically 80% of the maximum tolerated dose (MTD) in adults with cancer [11,12].

Phase I studies establish the dose-limiting toxicity (DLT) of investigational agents; the DLT is unacceptably severe toxicity that prevents the

Table 3
Phases of clinical development

Phase	Phase I	Phase II	Phase III
Goals	Dose finding, safety	Activity	Safety and efficacy
Population	Refractory	Less refractory, newly diagnosed with high-risk features	Newly diagnosed
Randomization	No	Yes or no	Yes
Typical sample size	Up to 30	20–50	100 or greater
Typical endpoints	Dose-limiting toxicity, maximum tolerated dose, optimal biologic dose, pharmacokinetics	Objective response rate, remission rate	Overall survival, event-free survival, remission rate

use of higher doses. The MTD, usually the dose immediately below that which caused DLT, is used in phase II trials.

This phase I dose-finding model is based on the assumption that the highest safe dose of a cytotoxic agent is the most likely to demonstrate activity and efficacy in later stages of drug development. However, a different endpoint may be appropriate for biologically targeted therapies, such as the effect of a given dose on a biologic disease parameter. This dose is referred to as the optimal biologic dose and may be lower than the MTD [13,14].

Phase II

After an appropriate dose and schedule are identified, antitumor activity is assessed in phase II trials. These are usually open-label, single-arm trials. For solid tumors, the primary endpoint of interest is objective tumor response as measured by radiologic criteria [15]. For hematologic malignancies, remission induction or re-induction is a common goal.

The two-stage design is widely used for phase II trials. The sample size in the first stage is designed to confirm a minimum response rate, and the second stage is conducted only if this level of activity is observed. This method limits the number of patients exposed to drugs with poor activity. From a broader perspective, it allows the re-distribution of resources to other agents with greater promise [16].

Randomized phase II trials are increasingly being conducted. One rationale is to define an optimal dose for further development. A randomized phase II trial comparing the activity and toxicity of two doses of a single drug can be helpful. As targeted drugs with noncytotoxic effects are developed, radiologic tumor response criteria may be of limited value. If these agents stabilize disease rather than significantly reduce tumor size, evaluation of the time to progression or of progression-free survival is more informative. Such an endpoint, even in preliminary studies, is best assessed in a randomized setting, where bias can be minimized.

Phase III

Randomized phase III trials are usually undertaken to demonstrate the efficacy and safety of a specific drug or treatment approach. Although the primary focus may be a new agent, multimodality therapy regimens (including combination chemotherapy) are often investigated. Therefore, advances in treatment often require randomized trials that explore additions or substitutions to regimens that may improve efficacy or reduce toxicity. Important elements of phase III trial design are discussed below.

Trial objectives

It is important to clearly specify trial objectives that address relevant clinical and scientific questions appropriate to the stage of clinical development and patient population. It is also important to distinguish primary objectives (eg, defining the MTD in phase I studies or evaluating objective tumor responses in phase II trials) from secondary objectives, such as assessing the role of a biomarker in predicting outcome. This distinction is important in all stages of development for several reasons, including the relationship of the primary objectives to the statistical components of trial design (eg, sample size, which is based on the primary objective) and the allocation of resources to priority endpoints.

Prioritization of resources is a significant concern in designing pediatric oncology trials because the number of patients available for enrollment is often inadequate to test multiple hypotheses. Only about 13,000 new pediatric malignancies are diagnosed in the United States each year, in contrast to more than 1.2 million new adult malignancies, excluding skin cancers. Several pediatric solid tumors (neuroblastoma, osteosarcoma) are diagnosed in only a few hundred patients per year.

Common efficacy endpoints in pediatric oncology trials include survival, event-free survival, time to progression or progression-free survival, and objective tumor response rate. A more detailed discussion of these endpoints and of safety endpoints follows later in this section.

Subject selection

The intended patient population for any clinical trial must be clearly defined through eligibility inclusion and exclusion criteria. In pediatric oncology trials, documentation of the histologic diagnosis is usually required. When tumor tissue cannot be obtained without great risk to the patient, other diagnostic tools can be used. One example is brainstem gliomas, diagnosis of which is usually based on a combination of clinical and radiologic findings. Additional pathologic evaluation is playing an increasing role in cancer diagnosis in general, especially in eligibility for pediatric oncology studies. Immunohistochemistry for cytogenetics and cell surface markers is a routine component of the diagnosis and staging of pediatric leukemias and lymphomas. The distinction between small, round, blue cell tumors of childhood (neuroblastoma, rhabdomyosarcoma, non-Hodgkin's lymphoma, Ewing tumors) relies on immunohistochemical testing and, more recently, cDNA expression profiling as well as clinical findings [17].

Eligibility criteria should include clinical parameters that define the patient population. These may include age, disease stage, and extent of prior therapy. Laboratory parameters for defining adequate organ function often focus on bone marrow, renal, and liver function, which are affected by many chemotherapy regimens. Some regimens require additional attention to baseline organ function. For example, children who will receive anthracyclines should have evidence of adequate ventricular ejection fraction as measured by a multiple gated acquisition scan or echocardiogram. Some baseline eligibility requirements require pediatric-specific tools. The performance status of children can be evaluated by using a play-performance scale commonly known as the Lansky scale, which is concise and uses parents as observer-reporters [18]. Some of the baseline assessment tools are also used to monitor children with cancer during the course of a clinical trial.

Randomization

Single-arm trials that use historical controls for comparison can be misleading if there are differences in patient characteristics (age, performance status, prior therapy, staging, supportive care, follow-up). Even when matched historical or concurrent controls can be selected, unknown factors may be unevenly distributed between two groups. Randomization can help to minimize potential bias caused by such factors. When prognostic factors are known, these must be taken into consideration when comparing outcomes between study arms. A stratification process at the time of randomization can distribute prognostic factors evenly between treatment arms. The categories used to define a stratification factor must be mutually exclusive (eg, age greater than or equal to 5 years versus age less than 5 years) and must be known at the time of diagnosis [19].

Randomized trials offer other advantages. For example, efficacy can be evaluated on the basis of time-to-event endpoints, such as overall or event-free survival, and safety is evaluated most thoroughly by randomization to placebo and active comparator arms.

Blinding

Blinding of subject assignment in a randomized trial is used to minimize bias. Cancer clinical trials, including those conducted in children, have not routinely used this strategy. The toxicity profile of many cancer drugs and the different schedules and routes of administration used make blinding difficult. Orally administered forms of several new drugs with limited toxicity have allowed blinding in some cases [20].

Upfront investigational window studies

When existing data support the evaluation of drug activity in a population not eligible for a phase I dose-finding study (eg, when therapy that provides a benefit is available), an upfront window study design may be appropriate. The agent's activity can be assessed in the "upfront window" before standard therapy in newly diagnosed patients with high-risk disease, if mechanisms are in place to assure safety and to ensure that the benefits of standard therapy are not compromised. Patients who respond can then receive the newer agent, along with the standard combination chemotherapy, to evaluate the effect on survival or disease-free survival. This approach has been used to evaluate the introduction of topotecan and irinotecan into treatment regimens for metastatic neuroblastoma and rhabdomyosarcoma [21–23].

Efficacy assessment

Assessment of clinical efficacy in pediatric oncology trials may involve a number of endpoints, depending on the diagnosis, stage of development of the drug, and nature of the expected drug effect. Endpoints commonly used include those related to direct tumor kill, such as the radiologically measured objective response rate, or time-to-event endpoints such as progression-free survival. The most commonly examined endpoints are discussed below.

Overall survival

Overall survival, defined as time from randomization to death from any cause, is often measured in randomized phase III trials. Survival can be continuously assessed through contact during hospitalizations or office visits or by telephone. The date of death can easily be confirmed and is independent of causality. However, this endpoint has some limitations, including the need for a relatively larger sample size, potential confounding by cross-over treatments, and a relatively long period of follow-up. In pediatric oncology, limitations of sample size and follow-up can be problematic, especially given the small number of patients available for enrollment. In addition, dramatic improvement of survival of some diseases over the past several decades has altered their natural history, and many years of follow-up would be required for a mature analysis of overall survival.

Event-free survival

Event-free survival is an endpoint often used in pediatric cancer trials. It is defined as the time from randomization to occurrence of a major adverse clinical event, such as failure to achieve remission, relapse, and death during remission. This endpoint has been used in studies of pediatric leukemias and solid tumors to overcome some of the limitations of an overall survival endpoint [14].

Objective tumor response

Objective tumor response, defined as a reduction in solid tumor size, is usually evaluated in the phase II setting. This endpoint provides initial evidence of a treatment's biologic activity. Tumor response is also a secondary endpoint in many phase III trials, allowing evaluation of response in a more homogeneous, less treatment-refractory population. Unlike time-to-event endpoints, which are affected by both the treatment and the natural history of the disease, tumor response can usually be attributed entirely to treatment in single-agent studies, or in randomized studies comparing a standard regimen to the standard regimen plus the new treatment.

Safety assessment

In trials with a primary objective of assessing efficacy, secondary objectives may include evaluation of safety parameters. Regardless of stated primary and secondary objectives, pediatric oncology trials routinely include elements of safety monitoring. These focus primarily on laboratory and clinical monitoring of bone marrow, hepatic, renal, and when appropriate, pulmonary and cardiac function. The frequency and nature of monitoring depends on the treatment regimen being evaluated.

Pediatric cancer trials often use NCI criteria for grading of adverse reactions. The original criteria were developed in 1982 for use in adverse drug experience reporting, study adverse events summaries, reports to the FDA, and publications. The criteria have undergone several revisions. Version 3.0, the Common Terminology Criteria for Adverse Events, published in 2003 [24], reflects feedback from the pharmaceutical industry, regulatory agencies, and cancer cooperative groups. Version 3.0 includes new guidelines for late effects, surgical and pediatric effects, and multimodality issues, and for reporting duration of an effect [10]. The occurrence, frequency, and severity of these effects are considered in treatment decisions, with clear criteria prespecified for dose interruption, dose modification, or treatment cessation.

Safety endpoints are increasingly an integral part of pediatric cancer trials, especially when current treatments provide significant benefit. The goal has shifted to maintaining the efficacy of existing therapies while minimizing short-term and long-term toxicity. For example, the National Wilms Tumor Study Group has demonstrated that radiation therapy can be safely eliminated for stage I and II Wilms tumor [6]. Endpoints for evaluating long-term toxicity include neurocognitive, immune, and cardiac function, occurrence of second malignancies, fertility, and psycho-social factors.

A regulatory perspective: the Investigational New Drug, new drug application, and biological license application process

The path from drug discovery to marketing takes many years and many dollars. The FDA's involvement usually begins after the research and discovery phase and before the first human studies ("first-in-man" studies). The sponsor of the investigational drug or biologic commonly requests a pre-IND meeting. During the meeting, the FDA provides feedback about the manufacturing process (chemistry/manufacturing/controls), in vitro and animal studies, and the proposed clinical trial. The sponsor must submit an IND application to conduct clinical studies of the drug or biologic. The agency reviews the application and determines within 30 days whether the study can proceed. The FDA may impose a clinical hold (halt or delay the start of a clinical study). In that event, the FDA must provide the sponsor written communication of the IND deficiencies within a specified period. The FDA lifts the clinical hold when (or if) the sponsor satisfactorily addresses the deficiencies. INDs generally undergo numerous amendments covering manufacturing, nonclinical, and clinical aspects of the product testing, including safety reports and an annual summary of activity.

The initial IND submission for the first human studies of a product usu-ally contains a clinical phase I protocol. After phase II and III studies, the sponsor generally submits an application to market the drug (a new drug ap-plication or a biological license application). The FDA must review the com-plete marketing application within 6 months for a priority application, and 10 months for a standard application. Agency personnel may conclude that the product it is safe and effective for its intended use and grant market ap-proval or may identify deficiencies that require submission of additional data. Phase IV studies are those conducted after marketing approval. While the FDA tracks the progress of these postmarketing commitment (PMC) studies, most are not required by law [25] and there is no penalty for failure to comply. The two exceptions where these studies are required are the PMCs for drugs and biologics granted accelerated approval, and PMCs to study the drug or biologic under the Pediatric Research Equity Act.

Accelerated approval may be granted for drugs or biologics intended to treat a serious disease for which there is no existing or comparable therapy. In such cases, the FDA may approve the product on the basis of data on a surrogate endpoint that predict "reasonably likely" clinical benefit. The sponsor must complete a clinical study or studies to verify and describe the clinical benefit. The FDA may, after a hearing, take the product of the market if the sponsor fails to complete the required PMC study or if the study fails to confirm benefit.

History and present status of drug development regulations

The FDA's statutory authority began with the 1906 Pure Food and Drugs Act prohibiting interstate commerce of misbranded food and drugs. Over the years, often as the result of medical mishaps, Congress has passed additional reform legislation. In the mid-1930s several children died after being given elixir of sulfanilamide, and Congress passed the 1938 Food, Drug and Cosmetic Act requiring proof of safety before marketing. After thalidomide caused birth defects, Congress passed the 1962 Kefauver-Harris amendment requiring proof of efficacy; this legislation gave rise to new reg-ulations governing investigational products (the IND regulations). Biologic product legislation developed in parallel. After the deaths of several children who received contaminated diphtheria antitoxin, the 1902 Biologics Control Act imposed conditions on the manufacture of vaccines, toxins, and anti-toxins. Biologics facility inspections were required starting in 1955, after more than 200 cases of polio and 11 deaths from inappropriate poliovirus inactivation during vaccine manufacture. Biologic products were initially regulated by the National Institutes of Health. In 1972, oversight was trans-ferred to the FDA. New statutes and regulations during and after the 1990s specifically addressed and encouraged pediatric studies. Box 2 summarizes important milestones in pediatric drug development.

Box 2. Milestones in pediatric drug development

- 1977 – American Academy of Pediatrics Committee on Drugs—Report on study of drugs in children
- 1979 – FDA articulates how to provide information on labeling
- 1997 – FDA Modernization Act/Exclusivity Provision
- 1998 – Pediatric Rule Regulation (enjoined 2002)
- 2001 – Subpart D regulations (adoption by FDA)
- 2002 – Best Pharmaceuticals for Children Act (BPCA)
- 2003 – Pediatric Research Equity Act (PREA)
- 2007 – BPCA and PREA re-authorized by Congress

The 1997 FDA Modernization Act (FDAMA) added a pediatric exclusivity provision to the regulations [18] that provided drug manufacturers an economic incentive of 6-months marketing exclusivity in return for conducting studies in pediatric populations. The pediatric studies had to be consistent with an FDA legal document, the "written request," which stipulates study requirements. Data from the studies must be submitted before the existing patent expires [26]. New regulations also specified that every new drug or biologic product (or any new indication or dosage) must be studied in children. This regulation, "the Pediatric Rule," became final in 1998 [27]. Unlike the exclusivity provision, it required studies and did not provide financial incentives.

The exclusivity provision and the Pediatric Rule increased the number of pediatric studies. Exclusivity was supposed to expire in 2002 [28], but its positive results led to the 2002 Best Pharmaceuticals for Children Act (BPCA) [29]. BPCA renewed exclusivity for an additional 5 years, provided a mechanism for study of drugs no longer under patent, and established the Pediatric Subcommittee of the Oncology Drugs Advisory Committee (ODAC). This Subcommittee is composed of experts in pediatric oncology and other fields (eg, statisticians), and patient, consumer, and industry representatives. The ODAC is a forum for discussion of pediatric oncology drug development. It has recently discussed such topics as endpoints for trials of new drugs to treat pediatric brain tumors, the FDA process for handling drug shortages, off-patent oncology drugs for which pediatric studies are needed, safety monitoring of clinical studies enrolling children, and age-appropriate formulations for use in pediatric oncology.

The Pediatric Rule, understandably less popular than exclusivity in the regulated industry, underwent legal challenge, and the US District Court enjoined FDA from enforcing the rule. However, in 2003, Congress passed the PREA, which reiterates many of the Pediatric Rule principles [30]. Table 4 compares the two laws. Pediatric studies required under PREA, if not

Table 4
Comparison of the Best Pharmaceuticals for Children Act and the Pediatric Research Equity Act

BPCA	PREA
Voluntary, financial incentives	Required, no financial incentive
Includes orphan indication	Orphan indications exempt
Studies: whole moiety, other indications	Only drug/indication under development
Applies only to drugs	Applies to drugs and biologicals
Trigger: written request	Trigger: marketing application
Results posted regardless of approval	Results confidential if not approved
Safety data reviewed 1 year later	Standard safety reporting

completed when the product comes to market, become required PMCs. Failure to conduct or complete these studies can result in economic penalties.

Today, BPCA and its predecessor (pediatric exclusivity provisions under FDAMA) and PREA and its predecessor (the Pediatric Rule) are the stimuli (the carrot in the case of BPCA, the stick in the case of PREA) for pediatric studies. Since their inception, the FDA has seen hundreds of pediatric studies enrolling thousands of patients and, more importantly, more than 100 drug labels contain new prescribing information for children [31,32].

With the exception of supportive care and some forms of leukemia, most drugs approved for adult cancer are not relevant to pediatric patients, and required studies under PREA are waived. Although pediatric patients with cancer gain little from PREA, new insights into oncogenesis may one day allow a molecular grouping of cancers (eg, epidermal growth factor receptor-expressing tumors) that will show whether certain pediatric and adult malignancies are sufficiently similar that PREA may be applicable.

During the early years of exclusivity, there was little rationale for pediatric research with drugs approved for adults. However, because BPCA is voluntary and is associated with incentives, many manufacturers were interested in evaluating their adult-cancer drugs in pediatric cancers. In 2000, the FDA issued guidance on studies that could lead to exclusivity for pediatric oncology settings [33]. Since 2000, the FDA has issued written requests to manufacturers to study pediatric malignancies. To date, 11 drugs studied in pediatric malignancies have received exclusivity, and in nine, the information was included in the drug labeling. These data were presented at the June 2007 meeting of the Pediatric Oncology Subcommittee to the Oncology Drugs Advisory Committee (Transcripts of the June 27, 2007 Pediatric Oncology Subcommittee of the Oncology Drugs Advisory Committee, Rockville, MD). BPCA also included provisions for the study of certain older, off-patent drugs, which are identified and prioritized by an expert panel of pediatric subspecialists. At present, the five off-patent oncology drugs on the priority list are vincristine, daunomycin, actinomycin D, methotrexate and isotretinoin.

In January 2007 new legislation governing the development and authorization of medicines for use in children was introduced in the European Union. Regulation No. 1901/2006 as amended (the "Pediatric Regulation") introduces sweeping changes into the regulatory environment for pediatric medicines to better protect the health of children in the European Union. The Pediatric Regulation also brings many new tasks and responsibilities to the European Medicines Agency, chief of which is the creation and operation of a Pediatric Committee within the European Medicines Agency to provide objective scientific opinions on any development plan for medicines for use in children [34].

Summary

Pediatric oncologists have a duty and responsibility to advance the care of their patients through scientifically and ethically valid clinical research. Such research has been a cornerstone of the dramatic progress in curing childhood cancer. Central to this success is the conduct of clinical investigations adhering to principles of good clinical practice. Ultimately, this is an activity sanctioned by laws, regulations, and guidance that carries with it the responsibility of public trust.

References

[1] Federal Food, Drug, and Cosmetic Act (FD&C Act), 21 USC Chapter 9. http://www.fda.gov/opacom/laws/fdcact/fdctoc.htm and Amendments. Available at: http://www.fda.gov/opacom/laws/default.htm#amendments. Accessed September 17, 2007.
[2] Code of Federal Regulations – Title 21, parts 50 and 56; Title 45, part 46.
[3] National Comission for the Protection of Human Subjects of Biomedical and Behavioral Research. The Belmont report: ethical principles and guidelines for the protection of human subjects of research. Washington DC: US Goverment Printing Office; 1979.
[4] International Conference on Harmonization. Available at: http://www.ich.org. Accessed September 17, 2007.
[5] Murphy SB. The national impact of clinical cooperative group trials for pediatric cancer. Med Pediatr Oncol 1995;24:279–80.
[6] McGregor LM, Metzger ML, Sanders R, et al. Pediatric cancers in the new millennium: dramatic progress, new challenges. Oncology 2007;21(7):809–20.
[7] Guidance for clinical trial sponsors: establishment and operation of clinical trial data monitoring committees. Available at: http://www.fda.gov/cder/guidance/index.htm. Accessed November 27, 2007.
[8] Obligations of clinical investigators: 21 CFR, part 312.
[9] Elements of Informed Consent. 21 CFR, 50.25; 45 CFR, 46.116. Available at: http://www.fda.gov/oc/ohrt/irbs/informedconsent.html. Accessed September 17, 2007.
[10] Trotti A, Colevas AD, Setser A, et al. CTCAE v3.0: development of a comprehensive system for the adverse effects of cancer treatment. Semin Radiat Oncol 2003;13(3):176–81.
[11] Shah S, Weitman S, Langevin AM, et al. Phase I therapy trials in children with cancer. J Pediatr Hematol Oncol 1998;20(5):431–8.
[12] Smith M, Bernstein M, Bleyer WA, et al. Conduct of phase I trials in children with cancer. J Clin Oncol 1998;16:966–78.
[13] Lee DP, Skolnik JM, Adamson PC. Pediatric phase I trials in oncology: an analysis of study conduct efficiency. J Clin Oncol 2005;23(33):8431–41.
[14] Ungerleider RS, Ellenberg S, Berg S. Cancer clinical trials: design, conduct, analysis, and reporting. In: Pizzo P, Poplack D, editors. Principles and practice of pediatric oncology. 4th edition. Philadelphia: Lippincott, Williams and Wilkins; 2002. p. 385.

[15] Weitman S, Ochoa S, Sullivan J, et al. Pediatric phase II cancer chemotherapy trials: a Pediatric Oncology Group study. J Pediatr Hematol Oncol 1997;19(3):187–91.

[16] Simon R. Optimal two-stage designs for phase II clinical trials. Control Clin Trials 1989; 10(1):1–10.

[17] Chen QR, Vansant G, Oades K, et al. Diagnosis of the small round blue cell tumors using multiplex polymerase chain reaction. J Mol Diagn 2007;9(1):80–8.

[18] Lansky SB, List MA, Lansky LL, et al. The measurement of performance in childhood cancer patients. Cancer 1987;60(7):1651–6.

[19] Dagher R, Pazdur R. The phase III clinical cancer trial. In: Anticancer drug development guide: preclinical screening, clinical trials and approval. Andrews P, Teicher B, editors. Totowa (NJ): Humana Press, 2004.

[20] Dagher RN, Pazdur R. Clinical trial design and regulatory issues. In: Antiangiogenic cancer therapy. Abbruzzese JL, Davis D, Herbst R, editors. Boca Raton (FL): Taylor and Francis, 2007.

[21] Kretchmar CS, Kletzel M, Murray K, et al. Response to paclitaxel, topotecan and topotecan-cyclophosphamide in children with untreated disseminated neuroblastoma treated in an upfront phase II investigational window: a Pediatric Oncology Group study. J Clin Oncol 2004;22(20):4119–26.

[22] Pappo AS, Lyden E, Breitfeld P, et al. Two consecutive phase II window trials of irinotecan alone or in combination with vincristine for the treatment of metastatic rhabdomyosarcoma: the Children's Oncology Group. J Clin Oncol 2007;25(4):362–9.

[23] Walterhouse DO, Lyden ER, Breitfeld PP, et al. Efficacy of topotecan and cyclophosphamide given in a phase II window trial in children with newly diagnosed metastatic rhabdomyosarcoma: a Children's Oncology Group study. J Clin Oncol 2004;22(8):1398–403.

[24] Common Terminology Criteria for Adverse Events (CTCAE) version 3.0. National Cancer Institute; 2003. Available at: http://ctep.cancer.gov/forms/CTCAEv3.pdf. Accessed November 27, 2007.

[25] Guidance for industry: reports on the status of postmarketing study commitments—implementation of section 130 of the Food and Drug Administration Modernization Act of 1997. 2006. Available at: http://www.fda.gov/ohrms/dockets/98fr/99n-1852-gdl0002.pdf. Accessed September 17, 2007.

[26] Guidance for industry: qualifying for pediatric exclusivity under section 303A of the FD&C Act 1999. Available at: http://www.fda.gov/cder/guidance/2891fnl.htm. Accessed September 17, 2007.

[27] Regulations Requiring Manufacturers to Assess the Safety and Effectiveness of New Drugs and Biological Products in Pediatric patients. 63 Federal Register 66631, 1998.

[28] Pediatric exclusivity provision: status report to Congress. US Food and Drug Administration; 2001. Available at: http://www.fda.gov/cder/pediatric/reportcong01.pdf. Accessed November 27, 2007.

[29] Best Pharmaceutical for Children Act, January 4, 2002 (Public Law No. 107–9; S-1789, 107th Congress).

[30] Guidance for industry: how to comply with the Pediatric Research Equity Act. US Food and Drug Administration; 2005. Available at: http://www.fda.gov/cder/guidance/6215dft.pdf. Accessed September 17, 2007.

[31] Hirschfeld S, Ho PT, Smith M, et al. Regulatory approvals of pediatric oncology drugs: previous experience and new initiatives. J Clin Oncol 2003;21(6):1066–73.

[32] Benjamin DK, Smith PB, Murphy D, et al. Peer-reviewed publication of clinical trials completed for pediatric exclusivity. JAMA 2006;296(10):1266–73.

[33] Guidance for industry: pediatric oncology studies in response to a written request. US Food and Drug Administration; 2000. Available at: http://www.fda.gov/cder/guidance/3756dft.htm. Accessed September 17, 2007.

[34] European Medicines Agency. Medicines for children. 2007. Available at: http://www.emea.europa.eu/htms/human/paediatrics/introduction.htm. Accessed September 17, 2007.

ELSEVIER
SAUNDERS

PEDIATRIC CLINICS
OF NORTH AMERICA

Pediatr Clin N Am 55 (2008) 211–222

Rethinking Pediatric Assent: From Requirement to Ideal

Yoram Unguru, MD, MS, MA[a,b,*],
Max J. Coppes, MD, PhD, MBA[a,c,d,e],
Naynesh Kamani, MD[f,g,h]

[a]*Division of Hematology/Oncology, Center for Cancer and Blood Disorders, Children's
National Medical Center, 111 Michigan Avenue NW, Washington, DC 20010-2970, USA*
[b]*Berman Bioethics Institute, Johns Hopkins University, Hampton House 348,
624 N. Broadway, Baltimore, MD 21205, USA*
[c]*Department of Medicine, Georgetown University, 3800 Reservoir Road NW,
Washington, DC 20007, USA*
[d]*Department of Oncology, Georgetown University, Research Building, Suite E501,
3970 Reservoir Road NW, Washington, DC 20007, USA*
[e]*Department of Pediatrics, Georgetown University, 3800 Reservoir Road NW,
2PHC, Washington, DC 20007, USA*
[f]*Department of Pediatrics, George Washington University, 2300 Eye Street NW,
Suite 713W, Washington, DC 20037, USA*
[g]*Department of Immunology, George Washington University, 2300 Eye Street NW,
Suite 713W, Washington, DC 20037, USA*
[h]*Institutional Review Board, Children's National Medical Center, 111 Michigan Avenue NW,
Washington, DC 20010-2970, USA*

*Assent of the child is indeed an idea before its time. It is a fragile idea that can
easily be crushed amidst the boulders of consent, autonomy, rights, and competence. It's an idea that is so foreign to adult reality that its central thrust is
missed even by astute minds.*

Intentional or not, this powerful and telling statement, written a quarter
of a century ago by William Bartholome [1], a pediatrician and ethicist, has
challenged professionals from a wide array of disciplines to elucidate, define,
and provide a meaningful understanding of the concept of assent: one that
can be applied practically in both clinical and research settings. Perhaps no
profession has been more challenged than pediatric oncology.

* Corresponding author. Center for Cancer and Blood Disorders, Division of
Hematology/Oncology, Children's National Medical Center, 111 Michigan Avenue NW,
Washington, DC 20010-2970.
E-mail address: yunguru@cnmc.org (Y. Unguru).

Much has been written about assent in the past 25 years [2–28]. Despite significant progress there is still considerable disagreement surrounding many fundamental components of assent. No consensus exists in guidelines, as disseminated by the federal government [29–32], professional associations [33–35], or by the "assent community" [2,6,7,9,14,15,18,19,21,22,24–27,36–48]. Controversies include the definition of assent, the age at which investigators should solicit assent from children, who should be involved in the assent process, how to resolve disputes between children and their parents, the relationship between assent and consent, the quantity and quality of information to disclose to children and their families, how much and what information children desire and need, the necessity and methods for assessing both children's understanding of disclosed information and of the assent process itself, and what constitutes an effective, practical, and realistically applicable decision-making model. The unresolved issues have become so complex that some key contributors to the discussion suggest a transformation in the way assent is contemplated. Bluebond-Langer and colleagues [49], and Joffe [10] offer particularly insightful arguments supporting such an approach, with the former asserting that under certain conditions, assent far too easily "can become a sham," while Joffe has called for abandoning the term assent altogether.

In this article, we present a critical review of the current assent literature. Consideration is devoted to guidelines proposed by federal regulators and professional medical associations and to various decision-making models. We then discuss obstacles that make obtaining adequate assent difficult, and conclude by offering suggestions for improvement.

The birth of assent

The assent requirement [50] emerged in a 1977 report by The National Commission for the Protection of Human Subjects of Biomedical and Behavioral Research [29] and created a protectionist set of guidelines for overseeing research. The assent requirement, traced to the concept of respecting children as individuals, calls for the need to recognize and respect the wishes of children as they develop cognitively and mature. The Commission suggested that assent be solicited from all potential research subjects aged 7 years and older.

The Belmont Report [30] subsequently established the three pillars that continue to govern ethically sound research involving human subjects: (1) respect for persons, (2) beneficence, and (3) justice. Respecting a person means helping them to make choices that are as informed as possible. From an ethical perspective, it is not sufficient simply to provide information to research subjects; the researcher must also ensure that the subject comprehends the information as part of the informed consent process. Hence, the Report states that understanding is dependent on the subject's "maturity," and that "investigators are responsible for ascertaining that the subject has comprehended the information" [30].

The discussion has become especially impassioned following passage of federal regulations in 1983 that govern children's research as articulated in Subpart D of Title 45, Code of Federal Regulations, Part 46 (45 CFR 46) [31]. Federal regulations define assent as "a child's affirmative agreement to participate in research. Mere failure to object should not, absent affirmative agreement, be construed as assent." Unlike the National Commission recommendation that investigators obtain assent of all children 7 and older, federal regulations do not set a specific age limit, and they leave this decision to local institutional review boards (IRBs). Factors to be considered by IRBs in assessing capacity to assent include "ages, maturity, and psychological state of the children" [31]. Federal regulations can thus be viewed as unrestrictive and vague. They give IRBs free rein in their interpretation, yet they fail to enumerate what is exactly required for assent. In adopting such a minimalist definition, current federal regulations offer far too little guidance as to a meaningful concept of assent. Evidence of this is seen in how IRBs substantially differ in operationally defining assent and in their interpretation of the regulations as they relate to individual protocols [36,51,52].

While federal regulations do not adopt the National Commission's age requirement (rightfully so, we contend), they also fail to institute the Belmont Report's recommendation that investigators assess the research subject's understanding of research-related information. This serious omission has the potential for preventing assent from being meaningful.

Elements of assent

We suggest that meaningful assent is built upon several fundamental concepts. First and foremost, assent must be viewed independently of consent. Equating them does a disservice to both principles. Viewing assent as a corollary of consent [27,36,38] overemphasizes the importance that a child understands risks and benefits. Many IRBs and investigators are comfortable with this approach, and in doing so essentially adhere to adult research regulations, using it as a default when examining assent [51]. Equating assent and consent holds children to an unfair standard [53,54], with the potential for limiting their ability to participate in research at all. Second, for assent to be valid, it must be inclusive and contextual. The spectrum of a child's individual life experiences must be taken into account within the context of larger familial relationships. Third, respect for an individual child's decision-making capacity and those of his or her parents makes sense intuitively and should serve as a practical paradigm for assent. Finally, as understood in the Belmont Report [30], a truly meaningful notion of assent requires that clinicians and investigators assess both the quality and adequacy of children's understanding (ie, what do they comprehend and appreciate) about the assent process itself. Only by commitment to these principles will assent become the important ethical ideal it was meant to be.

The child's role in the assent process

Children constitute a vulnerable population and require additional protections when included in research. Children's vulnerability relates directly to their limited decision-making capacity. This does not mean, however, that children are incapable of participating in decisions. Compared with adults, a less exacting capacity for decision-making is necessary for a child to meaningfully assent to research participation [21,26,29,32,55]. Children need not appreciate all eight components of informed consent as mandated by CFR46.116 [56] when assenting to partake in research [53]. Decision-making capacity by children requires that the child's choice is voluntary, their choice must be both reasonable and rational, and especially important, the child must understand information relevant to their choice. Thus, before soliciting assent from a child, it is crucial that investigators assess the child's level of understanding. In addition to giving a child information that he or she needs to know, a second important aspect to consider is what children want to know. Few studies have examined the extent of a child's desire to be included in research-related decisions, and most of these have studied healthy children using hypothetical cases [8,21,41,42,57].

Twenty-five years ago, one of the few surveys of adolescent cancer patients found that pediatric oncologists largely failed to appreciate what adolescents considered most important about their cancer [40]. Physicians emphasized social and psychologic aspects, while adolescent patients focused more on factual information related to prognosis and long-term outcome. Moreover, 85% of adolescents felt that "new facts about cancer research" was either an extremely important or an important topic, compared with less than 50% of physicians who shared this view. Combined with the finding that more than 95% of adolescents considered it extremely important or important to know how cancer can be prevented, this suggests that adolescents with cancer may be more interested in research participation than previously thought. The above findings have significant implications for assent in pediatric oncology.

Because a child's understanding of research is central to the assent process, improving methods of assessing children's understanding of research is imperative. One way of doing this is by talking to them and by taking them seriously. Determining what children need to understand is the logical result of talking to them. A mechanism for accomplishing this is to borrow from what has already been done in adult medicine. We are currently embarking on an age-adjusted questionnaire survey to assess the quality of assent among children enrolled in pediatric oncology research protocols. Borrowing a term from Joffe [58], the survey is called a "quality of assent questionnaire (QuAs)." The two-part questionnaire assesses what children enrolled in research protocols understand about the research endeavor and what they want to know. We hope that the questionnaire will address some of the impediments in achieving a more meaningful assent. After completing the survey, investigators will be able to clarify topics that children themselves describe as poorly understood, and be better equipped to include children as active participants in research, rather than as mere subjects. This will allow investigators to isolate areas of deficiency as selected by children, rather than assume what a particular child may or may not understand. This meets the Belmont Report's requirement that investigators ascertain comprehension. Equally important, this guarantees that due diligence has taken place and that children have been equipped with the necessary tools to meaningfully participate in research.

Assent in pediatric oncology

Assent has particular relevance to pediatric oncology because over two-thirds of children with cancer are treated according to a clinical research trial sometime during the course of their illness [59].

In 2005, the Children's Oncology Group (COG) Assent Task Force published a position paper focused on children's role in decision-making about research participation, with the goal of establishing guidelines for pediatric oncology practice [35]. This three-pronged schema for reviewing "particular cases" provides children with (1) greater decision-making roles as their autonomy develops, during which they are (2) supported by their parents (thereby recognizing that each child and family is unique and bring their own experiences to the table, which may not be accounted for by a universal guideline), and that (3) policies and decisions relating to specific protocols should be flexible and contextually based. Where the COG guidelines stand out is in the role they ascribe to oncologists, who must "encourage parents to weigh children's views in their decision-making." This idea resonates with that proposed by the American Academy of Pediatrics [33], namely, that physicians' first priority is to represent the patient's best interests.

In contrast to CFR46.408(a), which establishes IRBs as responsible for evaluating a child's capacity for assent, COG guidelines give greater weight to the investigator. Intuitively this makes sense. Investigators are in a position to know the child-subject more intimately than IRB members. However, when assent is solicited within 1 to 2 days of a diagnosis, as is often the case, how well can an investigator really know a child? Moreover, physicians must balance sensibly the ever-present tension resulting from their combined role as physician and investigator (each with different goals and responsibilities). These are real barriers, with the potential for creating an ethically uneasy situation, but they should not impact on the investigator's ability to determine if a child is capable of assent.

Decision-making models

Numerous decision-making models attempt to provide a template for assent [3,7–9,12,16–18,21,43,49,60,61], including models specific for pediatric oncology [19,28,35]. While each contributes something toward creating a comprehensive standard for assent, each views assent and the roles of the parties who participate in it differently. Some place parents at the center, with children in a more peripheral role, while others adopt the opposite approach. Finally, a third group strives for a more balanced distribution of responsibilities. Each approach places physician-investigators at a different point along the same axis. Some argue that developmental concerns play a primary role, with another group advocating that psychologic or social concerns dominate. Others propose that the principle of autonomy serves as the basis for meaningful assent, while still another group favors a best-interest design. Best-interests models seek to secure the most favorable outcome for the child by focusing on many factors, including a child's preference for participation, their emotions, and the advantages and disadvantages to research participation. They go beyond autonomy-based models, many of which are based on (adult) informed consent and which focus on competence, a legal term, rather than capacity, a developmental one.

What is important to appreciate is that a multidimensional conceptual model that views assent as a process, establishing appropriate roles for children, parents, and physicians, and which accounts for developmental, individual, and contextual factors is a lofty, yet fitting paradigm for assent. Realizing such an ideal requires much effort by all parties and may not be possible in all cases. However, even attempts to fulfill these principles will bring us closer to respecting the assent requirement, as we believe it was meant to be understood.

Evidence-based medicine is the sine qua non of modern medical practice. Unfortunately, this standard has not been applied to pediatric assent. Because no express criteria exist to assist physician-investigators in assessing a child's decision-making capacity and abilities, the final determination is often based on individual physicians' subjective opinions [62]. Empirical based studies into children's understanding of what it means to assent to research and their preference for involvement are needed.

Discussion

Pediatric assent is a complex construct that has been mired in controversy since its inception. It is amorphous. Assent is not easily situated within the confines of a single discipline. Practitioners across an array of professions lay claim to it as their own. Each addresses assent according to their own language and set of rules [2,3,6–9,12,14–18,21,26,27,36–38,43,49,60,63]. As a result, assent is in the midst of an identity crisis. Assent has become such a loaded and charged concept that some do not refer to it by name [10], while others refuse to acknowledge its purpose [63]. Fundamental elements of assent, such as an appropriate definition, are contentiously deliberated, while more complicated issues relating to the moral authority of a child's decision and the ethical tension surrounding the dual role of physician-investigator are met with skepticism. This has resulted in the creation of two camps.

In the first are those for whom assent is best understood as a requirement. For them, assent is a dictate, mandated by an IRB. Within this camp is a group that views assent as a burden; making their important task of improving the health of sick children more difficult. For others however, assent is an ideal and though elusive, is an important component in their attempts to improve the health of children and worthy of their efforts. We believe that assent should be viewed as an ideal and not as a requirement. There are ways to simplify the transition from requirement to ideal and make assent more meaningful in the process. Accomplishing this requires a paradigm shift in how the pediatric assent community interprets assent.

As a vulnerable group, children are in need of protection. By giving children a voice, assent is one way of ensuring some protection. Beyond protecting children, assent is also about respecting a child's personal dignity and promoting what is best for them. Ideally, to respect a person it is best to know something about them. Current approaches to assent focus on knowing a child's cognitive abilities and their capacity for making decisions. These are important and necessary parts of assent, but do not allow for truly knowing a child. To know a child demands an appreciation for what they understand and for their preferences. Physician-investigators primarily rely on a child's parents to help them know a child. Therefore, the minimal standard for assent should include appropriate roles for the child-subject, parent-surrogate, and physician-investigator.

In most instances however, inclusion alone is not enough. Including a child in decisions without allowing them to actually participate in them is pointless. Moreover, to know someone it is not enough to depend on their surrogates. Parents may not realize that it is acceptable to include a child in decisions [42] or they may not want their child to be included in decisions [49]. Children also vary in how they see their role [22,24]. Some children are comfortable having a limited decision-making role and this should be respected. Other children however, want to be included in decisions and expect their parents and caregivers to listen to them and to weigh their choices; this too should be respected. Physician-investigators are therefore in a unique position as both educators and arbiters. They must educate families about a child's condition and options and establish that both parents and children understand their, as well as each other's role and responsibilities. Parents need to know that their authority will be honored, but that they must consider their child's opinions. Parents should be provided with the tools to promote children's independent thinking while continuing to support them. Children must be given a range of choices. This will enable them to be involved in the assent process and provide them with a sense of control and empowerment. Children also need to know that while they will be allowed to participate in the process, their decisions may sometimes be vetoed and the reasons for this should be revealed to them; in other cases, physician-investigators may acknowledge a priori that children's decisions will be respected. Effective communication is a prerequisite for shared decision-making, a strong foundation on which to base assent.

Just as each child's condition is unique, each child and family has distinctive experiences and values that mandate an assent process malleable enough to accommodate their situation. While a perfect system for soliciting meaningful assent may be unachievable, a workable model is necessary and feasible. Guidelines are not meant to be universally applicable. Rather, they should provide a general framework and counsel. The assent community must be willing to compromise, rather than have an all-or-nothing approach. There must be agreement on key areas of assent while other and less crucial aspects need not be as strictly enforced. At the very least, consensus is required concerning: (1) the need to appreciate assent from a child's point of view; (2) the importance of a child's understanding and preference for involvement; (3) the acknowledgment by physician-investigators that their dual role creates the potential for a very real ethical tension, necessitating honest and frank disclosure to children and parents; and (4) a sound model of assent is practical and applicable only if it is multifaceted and flexible in its approach toward families.

Summary

Important strides have been made in elucidating the concept of assent since Bartholome's challenge in 1982. Nevertheless, assent is in a state of disrepair. We disagree with those in the assent community who believe that it should be abandoned. Meaningful assent requires that physician-investigators assess both the quality and adequacy of the assent process by focusing on children's understanding, as called for by the Belmont Report. Similar endeavors have taken place in adult medicine [58,64–66], but unfortunately are lacking in pediatrics, despite numerous calls for exactly such an undertaking [3,12,19,24,26,30,32,35,46,67–72]. While it is impossible to guarantee that every child (or adult) will understand all disclosed information, giving research subjects information without making certain that they understand it not only violates the intent of the Belmont Report [73], it is tantamount to not giving information at all. This is especially true when research subjects have a diminished ability to understand, as children might.

While informed consent has its detractors, it is largely accepted as an important and worthwhile principle in adult medicine. Assent deserves an equal footing in pediatrics. The assent community must commit to taking the necessary steps for assent to occupy the place it deserves as an important pediatric ethical ideal.

References

[1] Bartholome WG. In defense of a child's right to assent. Hastings Cent Rep 1982;12: 44–5.

[2] Bartholome WG. Ethical issues in pediatric research. In: Vanderpool HY, editor. The ethics of research involving human subjects. Frederick (MD): University Publishing Group; 1996. p. 339–70.

[3] Baylis F, Downie J, Kenny N. Children and decision making in health research. Health Law Review 2000;8:3 9.

[4] Bluebond-Langer M. Decision-making for children with cancer: what are the cultural and moral factors? Anthropology News 2005;46:36.

[5] Brody H, Miller FG. The clinician-investigator: unavoidable but manageable tension. Kennedy Inst Ethics J 2003;13:329 46.

[6] Burke TM, Abramovitch R, Zlotkin S. Children's understanding of the risks and benefits associated with research. J Med Ethics 2005;31:715–20.

[7] Erlen JA. The child's choice: an essential component in treatment decisions. Child Health Care 1987;15:156–60.

[8] Geller G, Tambor ES, Bernhardt BA, et al. Informed consent for enrolling minors in genetic susceptibility research: a qualitative study of at-risk children's and parent's views about children's role in decision-making. J Adolesc Health 2003;32:260–71.

[9] Goodenough T, Williamson E, Kent J, et al. "What did you think about that?" Researching children's perceptions of participation in a longitudinal genetic epidemiological study. Children and Society 2006;17:113–25.

[10] Joffe Steven. Rethink "affirmative agreement," but abandon "assent." Am J Bioeth 2003;3: 9–11.

[11] Kamps WA, Akkerboom JC, Nitschke R, et al. Altruism and informed consent in chemotherapy trials of childhood cancer. In: DeBellis R, Hyman GA, Seeland IB, et al, editors. Psychosocial aspects of chemotherapy in cancer care: the patient, family, and staff. New York: Hawthorn Press; 1987. p. 93–110.

[12] King N, Cross A. Children as decision makers: guidelines for pediatricians. J Pediatr 1989; 115:10–6.

[13] Kodish Eric. Informed consent for pediatric research: is it really possible? J Pediatr 2003;142: 89–90.

[14] Kodish E, editor. Ethics and research with children: a case-based approach. New York: Oxford University Press; 2005. p. 361.

[15] Leiken S. Minors assent, consent, or dissent to medical research. IRB 1993;15:1–7.

[16] Leiken SL. An ethical issue in biomedical research: the involvement of minors in informed and third party consent. Clin Res 1983;31:34–40.

[17] Levine R. Adolescents as research subjects without permission of their parents or guardians: ethical considerations. J Adolesc Health 1995;17:287–97.

[18] Miller VA, Drotar D, Kodish E. Children's competence for assent and consent: a review of empirical findings. Ethics Behav 2004;14:255–95.

[19] Olechnowicz JQ, Eder M, Simon C, et al. Assent observed: children's involvement in leukemia treatment and research discussions. Pediatrics 2002;109:806–14.

[20] Pyke-Grimm K, Degner L, Small A, et al. Preferences for participation in treatment decision making and information needs of parents of children with cancer: a pilot study. J Pediatr Oncol Nurs 1999;16:13–24.

[21] Rossi WC, Reynolds W, Nelson RM. Child assent and parental permission in pediatric research. Theor Med 2003;24:131–48.

[22] Scherer D. The capacities of minors to exercise voluntariness in medical treatment decisions. Law Hum Behav 1991;15:431–49.

[23] Simon C, Eder M, Raiz P, et al. Informed consent for pediatric leukemia research: clinician perspectives. Cancer 2001;92:691–700.

[24] Susman EJ, Dorn LD, Fletcher JC. Participation in biomedical research: the consent process as viewed by children, adolescents, young adults, and physicians. J Pediatr 1992;121:547–52.

[25] Weithorn LA, Campbell SR. The competency of children and adolescents to make informed treatment decisions. Child Dev 1982;53:1589–98.

[26] Weithorn LA, Scherer DG. Children's involvement in research participation decisions: psychological consideration. In: Grodin MA, Glantz LH, editors. Children as research subjects: science, ethics, and law. New York: Oxford University Press; 1994. p. 133–79.

[27] Wendler DS. Assent in paediatric research: theoretical and practical considerations. J Med Ethics 2006;32:229–34.

[28] Whitney SN, Ethier AM, Fruge E, et al. Decision making in pediatric oncology: who should take the lead? The decisional priority in pediatric oncology model. J Clin Oncol 2006;24:160–5.

[29] National Commission for the Protection of Human Subjects of Biomedical and Behavioral Research. Research involving children: report and recommendations. Washington, DC: DHEW; Publication No. (OS) 77-0044, 1977.

[30] National Commission for the Protection of Human Subjects of Biomedical and Behavioral Research. The Belmont Report: ethical principles and guidelines for the protection of human subjects of research. Washington, DC: US Government Printing Office; 1979.

[31] U.S. Department of Health and Human Services. 45 CFR 46. Subpart D—additional protections for children involved as subjects in research. Federal Registrar 1983;48:9818.

[32] Institute of Medicine Committee on Clinical Research Involving Children. Ethical conduct of clinical research involving children. Washington, DC: National Academies Press; 2004.

[33] Committee on Bioethics, American Academy of Pediatrics. Informed consent, parental permission, and assent in pediatric practice. Pediatrics 1995;95:314–7.

[34] Society for Adolescent Medicine. Position paper of the Society of Adolescent Medicine, guidelines for adolescent health research. J Adolesc Health 2003;33:396–409.

[35] The Assent Task Force, Children's Oncology Group. Guidelines for involving children in decision-making about research participation. 2005. Available at: https://members.childrensoncologygroup.org/Disc/bioethics/default.asp,cogassentguidelines.pdf. Accessed February 5, 2007.

[36] Kimberly MB, Hoehn KS, Feudtner C, et al. Variation in standards of research compensation and child assent practices: a comparison of 69 Institutional Review Board-approved informed permission and assent forms for 3 multicenter pediatric clinical trials. Pediatrics 2006;117:1706–11.

[37] Ross LF. Informed consent in pediatric research. Camb Q Healthc Ethics 2004;13:346–58.

[38] Tait AR, Voepel-Lewis T, Shobba M. Do they understand? (Part II): assent of children participating in clinical anesthesia and surgery research. Anesthesiology 2003;98:609–14.

[39] Ondrusek N, Abramovitch R, Pencharz P, et al. Empirical examination of the ability of children to consent to clinical research. J Med Ethics 1998;24:158–65.

[40] Pfefferbaum B, Levenson P. Adolescent cancer patient and physician response to a questionnaire on patient concerns. Am J Psychiatry 1982;139:348–51.

[41] Bradlyn AS, Kao PM, Beale IL, et al. Pediatric oncology professionals' perceptions of information needs of adolescent patients with cancer. J Pediatr Oncol Nurs 2004;21:335–42.

[42] Angst DB, Deatrick JA. Involvement in health care decisions: parents and children with chronic illness. J Fam Nurs 1996;2:174–94.

[43] Sourkes B. The medical encounter: A child's eye view. In: Sourkes B, editor. Armfuls of time: the psychological experience of the child with a life-threatening illness. Pittsburgh (PA): Pittsburgh University Press; 1995. p. 31–44 and 53–60.

[44] Applebaum PS, Roth LH, Lidz CW, et al. False hopes and best data: consent to research and the therapeutic misconception. Hastings Cent Rep 1987;17:20–4.

[45] Dixon-Woods M, Young B, Heney D. Partnerships with children. BMJ 1999;319:778–80.

[46] Joffe S, Truog RD, Shurin SB, et al. Ethical considerations in pediatric oncology. In: Pizzo PA, Poplack DG, editors. Principles and practice of pediatric oncology. 5th edition. Philadelphia: Lippincott Williams and Wilkins; 2006. p. 1466–75.

[47] Lantos J. Informed consent: the whole truth for patients? Cancer Supplement 1993;72:2811–5.

[48] Leiken SL. Beyond proforma consent for childhood cancer research. J Clin Oncol 1985;3:420–8.

[49] Bluebond-Langer M, DeCicco A, Belasco J. Involving children with life-shortening illnesses in decisions about participation in clinical research: a proposal for shuttle diplomacy and negotiation. In: Kodish E, editor. Ethics and research with children: a case-based approach. New York: Oxford University Press; 2005. p. 336.

[50] National Commission for the Protection of Human Subjects of Biomedical and Behavioral Research. Research involving children: report and recommendations of the national commission for human subjects of biomedical and behavioral research. Federal Registrar 1978;43(9):2084–114.

[51] Whittle A, Shah S, Wilfond B, et al. Institutional Review Board practices regarding assent in pediatric research. Pediatrics 2004;113:1747–52.

[52] Erb TO, Schulman SR, Sugarman J. Permission and assent for clinical research in pediatric anesthesia. Anesth Analg 2002;94:1155–60.

[53] Miller VA, Nelson RM. A developmental approach to child assent for nontherapeutic research. J Pediatr 2006;149:S25–30.

[54] Kim E. Protection of child human subjects. J Wound Ostomy Continence Nurs 2004;31: 161–7.

[55] Canadian Institutes of Health Research, Natural Sciences and Engineering Research Council of Canada, Social Sciences and Humanities Research Council of Canada. Tri-Council Policy Statement: ethical conduct for research involving humans. 1998 (with 2000, 2002, 2005 amendments).

[56] U.S. Department of Health and Human Services. 45 CFR 46. Subpart A-Basic HHS policy for protection of human research subjects. 46.116. Available at: http://www.hhs.gov/ohrp/humansubjects/guidance/45cfr46.htm#46.116. Accessed October 24, 2007.

[57] Broome ME, Kodish E, Geller G, et al. Children in research: new perspectives and practices for informed consent. IRB 2003;25:S20–5.

[58] Joffe S, Cook F, Cleary PD, et al. Quality of informed consent: a new measure of understanding among research subjects. J Natl Cancer Inst 2001;93:139–47.

[59] Tejeda HA, Green SB, Trimble EL, et al. Representation of African-Americans, Hispanics, and whites in National Cancer Institute cancer treatment trials. J Natl Cancer Inst 1996;88: 812–6.

[60] Ross LF. Children, families, and health care decision-making. Oxford: Oxford University Press; 1998. p. 216.

[61] Ross LF. Children in medical research: access versus protection. New York: Oxford University Press; 2006. p. 304.

[62] Kuther TL. Medical decision-making and minors: issues of consent and assent. Adolescence 2003;38:343–58.

[63] Lee KJ, Havens PL, Sato TT, et al. Assent for treatment: clinician knowledge, attitudes, and practice. Pediatrics 2006;118:723–30.

[64] Joffe S, Cook F, Cleary PD, et al. Quality of informed consent: a cross-sectional survey. Lancet 2001;358:1772–7.

[65] Miller CK, O'Donnell DC, Searight HR, et al. The Deaconess informed consent comprehension test: an assessment tool for clinical research subjects. Pharmacotherapy 1996;16:872–8.

[66] Janofsky JS, McCarthy RJ, Folstein MF. The Hopkins competency assessment test: a brief method for evaluating patients' capacity to give informed consent. Hosp Community Psychiatry 1992;43:132–6.

[67] Nelson RM, Reynolds WW. Child assent and parental permission: a comment on Tait's "do they understand?" Anesthesiology 2003;98:597–8.

[68] McIntosh N, Bates P, Brykczynka G, et al. Royal College of Paediatrics and Child Health: Ethics Advisory Committee. Guidelines for the ethical conduct of medical research involving children. Arch Dis Child 2000;82:177–82.

[69] Kon A. Assent in pediatric research. Pediatrics 2006;117:1806–10.

[70] Wasson K. Altruism and pediatric oncology trials: it does not tip the decision-making scales. Am J Bioeth 2006;6:48.

[71] Kon AA, Klug M. Methods and practices of investigators for determining participants' decisional capacity and comprehension of protocols. J Empir Res Hum Res Ethics 2006; 1:61–8.
[72] Ungar D, Joffe S, Kodish E. Children are not small adults: documentation of assent for research involving children. J Pediatr 2006;149:S31–3.
[73] Beauchamp TL. The Belmont Report. In: Emanuel EJ, Grady C, Lie R, et al, editors. Oxford textbook of clinical research ethics. New York: Oxford University Press; 2008 [in press].

ELSEVIER
SAUNDERS

PEDIATRIC CLINICS
OF NORTH AMERICA

Pediatr Clin N Am 55 (2008) 223–250

Integration of Palliative Care Practices into the Ongoing Care of Children with Cancer: Individualized Care Planning and Coordination

Justin N. Baker, MD[a,b,f,h],
Pamela S. Hinds, RN, PhD, FAAN[c],
Sheri L. Spunt, MD[a,d],
Raymond C. Barfield, MD, PhD[a,e,f],
Caitlin Allen, PhD[c],
Brent C. Powell, M Div[g], Lisa H. Anderson, M Div[g],
Javier R. Kane, MD[a,b,f,h],*

[a]Department of Oncology, St. Jude Children's Research Hospital,
332 North Lauderdale Street, Mail Stop 260, Memphis, TN 38105-2794, USA
[b]Quality of Life Service, St. Jude Children's Research Hospital, 332 N. Lauderdale,
Mail Stop 260, Memphis, TN 38105, USA
[c]Division of Nursing Research, St. Jude Children's Research Hospital,
332 N. Lauderdale, Mail Stop 738, Memphis, TN 38105, USA
[d]Solid Tumor Division, St. Jude Children's Research Hospital, 332 N. Lauderdale,
Mail Stop 260, Memphis, TN 38105, USA
[e]Stem Cell Transplant Division, St. Jude Children's Research Hospital, 332 N. Lauderdale,
Mail Stop 260, Memphis, TN 38105, USA
[f]Ethics Committee, St. Jude Children's Research Hospital, 332 N. Lauderdale,
Mail Stop 260, Memphis, TN 38105, USA
[g]Division of Behavioral Medicine, Chaplain Services St. Jude Children's Research Hospital,
332 N. Lauderdale, Mail Stop 101, Memphis, TN 38105, USA
[h]Palliative and End-of-Life Care, St. Jude Children's Research Hospital, 332 N. Lauderdale,
Mail Stop 101, Memphis, TN 38105, USA

To cure sometimes, to relieve often, to comfort always – this is our work.
—Author unknown

This work was supported in part by National Institutes of Health Cancer Center Support Core Grant CA-21765 and the American Lebanese Syrian Associated Charities.
* Corresponding author. Department of Oncology, St. Jude Children's Research Hospital, 332 North Lauderdale Street, Mail Stop 260, Memphis, TN 38105-2794.
 E-mail address: javier.kane@stjude.org (J.R. Kane).

Suffering is nearly universal in pediatric cancer patients and their families. Addressing this suffering is an ethical imperative. High-quality palliative care is now an expected standard during the treatment of children with life-threatening illnesses. An American Academy of Pediatrics policy statement recommends that "all general and subspecialty pediatricians, family physicians, pain specialists, and pediatric surgeons need to become familiar and comfortable with the provision of palliative care to children" [1]. The goal of palliative care is the best quality of life for patients and their families that is consistent with their values and priorities. Pediatric palliative medicine may be further defined as "the art and science of patient- and family-centered care aimed at enhancing quality of life, promoting healing and attending to suffering" [2]. Inherent in these definitions is the need to integrate quality palliative care into the mainstream of medical treatment of all children suffering from chronic, life-threatening, and life-limiting illnesses, regardless of the curative intent of therapy.

Improving the quality of palliative and end-of-life care through individualized care planning and coordination

Most parents of children with cancer have dual primary goals: a primary cancer-directed goal of cure and a primary comfort-related goal of lessening suffering [3]. Early introduction of palliative care principles and practices into their child's treatment is respectful and supportive of these goals. The individualized care planning and coordination (ICPC) model (Fig. 1) is designed to facilitate this integration [4]. Individualized care planning emphasizes the value of subjective experiences in the context of meaningful personal relationships and uses a patient- and family-centered approach to information delivery, needs assessment, and understanding of the patient's and family's illness experience. It aims to enhance communication about difficult issues by discerning patient and family values and priorities before critical decision points are reached. Application of the ICPC model helps patients, families, and their clinicians negotiate care options in the presence of uncertainty by assessing the patient's and family's understanding of prognosis, elucidating their goals of care, and allowing them to choose from available goal-directed treatment alternatives. A comprehensive, individualized care plan that balances medical and personal goals, based on the relationship that has been established and the treatment options chosen, can then be generated.

Individualized care coordination, the process of implementing the individualized care plan, is detailed here. The authors' purpose is to address specific clinical gaps in the care of children with cancer. They highlight the deficiencies in the current provision of care, identify the national standards of care, recommend specific processes that should be integrated into pediatric oncology to fulfill the national standards, and identify research and education needs. The specific individualized care coordination processes that are the subject of palliative and end-of-life care quality improvement efforts

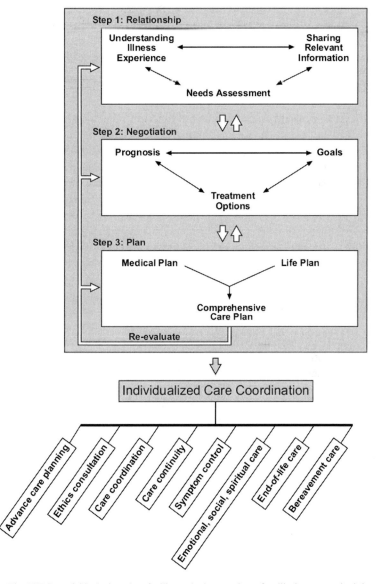

Fig. 1. The ICPC model is designed to facilitate the integration of palliative care principles and practices into the ongoing care of children with cancer. The individualized care plan is implemented through individualized care coordination.

and are discussed here include advance care planning; ethics consultation; care coordination; care continuity; symptom control; emotional, social, and spiritual care; end-of-life care; and bereavement care.

The further integration of palliative care into pediatric oncology practice can harness the inherent "healer" nature of cancer clinicians to enhance the quality of patients' and families' lives. Clinicians' strong desire to provide compassionate, competent, and quality care to the seriously ill child and the child's family can be effectively translated into clinical practice through individualized care planning and individualized care coordination processes, allowing the primary care team as a unit and the health care system as a whole to address their specific palliative and end-of-life care needs. The National Quality Forum, the Institute of Medicine, and the National Institutes of Health have identified palliative and end-of-life care as national priorities and have proposed that palliative care be a key component of high-quality medical care for children with advanced illness. The National Quality Forum has outlined preferred practices for ensuring the provision of high-quality palliative care. These practices are integrated into pediatric oncology programs at present with varying degrees of adequacy, but application of the individualized care coordination processes is likely to fill many of the gaps (Box 1). Obtaining reimbursement for these processes is currently difficult, but codes to facilitate billing can be found in Tables 2 and 3.

Attention to the relational aspects of the ICPC model is of utmost importance because parents' perceptions of the quality of care emphasize caring and communication themselves more than any specific interventions or biomedical parameters [5,6]. These care processes must be evaluated in regards to the impact on the quality of palliative care delivered (eg, quality indicators for comfort care, interdisciplinary collaboration, enhanced health care provider communication, care of the imminently dying child, and so forth), and on patient and family outcomes (eg, coping, family cohesion, satisfaction with care, improved symptom control, greater patient and family participation in decision making, optimal physical and psychosocial functioning, optimal quality of life for patient and family, or uncomplicated bereavement) [7].

To improve palliative care competence and improve quality, several approaches have been used to reduce the palliative care educational gap [8]. Important needs include curricula to "educate the educators" and faculty guidelines for teaching palliative medicine at the bedside and during rounds; both must be supported by standardization of didactic learning opportunities [9]. Several tools are now available, including education in palliative and end-of-life care (EPEC), end-of-life nursing education curriculum (ELNEC), and initiative for pediatric palliative care (IPPC). However, none of these curricula have been assessed for improvement of the quality of care. Another example is the Harvard Medical School program in palliative care education and practice curriculum for palliative care faculty, which integrates clinical content with educational methods to enhance the clinical faculty's capacity to model and teach [9,10]. Although these interventions have not yet been linked to quality improvement outcomes, any effort to improve the quality of palliative and end-of-life care in pediatric oncology must be accompanied by an educational strategy to enhance the level of competence among health care providers with regard to palliative and end-of-life care skills and understanding of individualized care planning and individualized care coordination processes [11].

Advance care planning

Decision making is a challenge for everyone involved in the care of pediatric cancer patients. Parents surveyed 6 months to 2 years after their child died of cancer reported few opportunities to participate in treatment decisions until near the end of their child's life. The four most common difficult decisions they identified were whether to pursue more chemotherapy or to discontinue disease-directed treatment; whether to choose a phase I therapy versus no cancer treatment; whether to maintain or withdraw life support; and whether to adopt a "do not resuscitate" (DNR) order [12]. Like adult cancer patients, pediatric cancer patients and their parents identify hope for a cure or for longer survival as a major factor in the decision to receive phase I chemotherapy versus comfort care only [13–18]. Not only are each of these decisions emotionally laden, but the ways in which they are approached by patients, families, and care providers often differ.

Evidence suggests that avoiding or delaying discussions about end-of-life decisions may influence the type and quality of care. A survey of bereaved parents and their child's former physician showed that when both the parent and the physician recognized that no realistic chance existed for cure 50 days or more before the child's death, there was a statistically significantly earlier discussion of hospice care, better parental ratings of the quality of care delivered by the home care team, earlier institution of a DNR order, and less cancer-directed treatment during the last month of life [3]. The advance care planning process can facilitate end-of-life care decisions by improving parents' emotional support, quality of information, and medical understanding, and by enhancing the listening skills and sensitivity of health care providers [19,20]. Further, as stated earlier, parents value communication and relationships over biomedical measures of success [5]. Therefore, the advance care planning process supports what parents value and is likely to enhance satisfaction by addressing parents' perceptions of good quality.

An environment conducive to optimal advance care planning enhances decision making. As described by the American Society of Clinical Oncology, communication should be "both family centered and child focused" [21]. Optimally, end-of-life decisions should flow naturally from an ongoing conversation among the patient, family, and medical care team about care priorities. Essential to this process is a trusting relationship established through individualized care planning in which information can be shared nonjudgmentally [4,21]. Parents value emotional expression and support

Box 1. Preferred practices for quality palliative and hospice care categorized by individualized care coordination processes

General
- Provide palliative and hospice care by an interdisciplinary team of skilled palliative care professionals.
- Provide access to palliative and hospice care that is responsive to the patient and family 24 hours a day, 7 days a week.

Education
- Provide continuing education to all health care professionals on the domains of palliative care and hospice care.
- Provide adequate training support to ensure that health care providers are competent in palliative care.
- Ensure that hospice care and specialized palliative care professionals are appropriately trained, credentialed, or certified in their area of expertise.

Advance care planning
- Formulate, use, and regularly review a timely care plan based on a comprehensive, interdisciplinary assessment of the values, preferences, goals, and needs of the patient and family.
- Present hospice as an option to all patients and families when death within a year would not be surprising; reintroduce the hospice option as the patient declines.
- Assess physicians' or health care professionals' ability to discuss hospice as an option.
- Enable patients to make informed decisions about their care by educating them on the process of their disease, prognosis, and the benefits and burdens of potential interventions.
- Determine the primary decision maker or makers within the family unit. If the child is able to participate, determine the degree of his or her participation.
- Document the designated surrogate or decision maker in accordance with state law for every patient in primary, acute, and long-term care and in palliative and hospice care.
- Document the patient's, parent's, and surrogate's preferences for goals of care, treatment options, and setting of care at first assessment and at frequent intervals as conditions change.
- Convert the patient treatment goals into medical orders such as the Physician Orders for Life-Sustaining Treatment (POLST).
- Document advance directives and surrogacy designations.
- For minors with decision-making capacity, document the child's views and preferences for medical care, including assent for treatment, and give them appropriate weight in decision making.
- Make appropriate professional staff members available to the child and the adult decision maker for consultation and intervention when the child's wishes differ from those of the adult decision maker.

Ethics consultation
- Establish or have access to ethics committees or ethics consultation across care settings to address ethical conflicts at the end of life.

Care coordination
- Provide education and support to families and unlicensed caregivers, based on the patient's individualized care plan, to ensure safe and appropriate care for the patient.
- Conduct and document regular patient and family care conferences with physicians and other appropriate members of the interdisciplinary team to provide information; to discuss goals of care, disease prognosis, and advance care planning; and to offer support.

Care continuity
- To the extent that existing privacy laws permit, ensure that the plan is broadly disseminated internally and externally to all professionals involved in the patient's care.
- Ensure that medical orders such as the POLST are transferable and applicable across care settings, including long-term care, emergency medical services, and hospital care.
- Make advance directives and surrogacy designations available across care settings, while protecting patient privacy and adherence to Health Insurant Portability and Accountability Act regulations (eg, by using Internet-based registries or electronic personal health records).
- Ensure that, on transfer between health care settings, communication of the patient's goals, preferences, values, and clinical information is timely and thorough, so that continuity of care and seamless follow-up are assured.

- Develop health care and community collaborations to promote advance care planning and the completion of advance directives for all individuals (eg, the Respecting Choices and Community Conversations on Compassionate Care programs).

Symptom control
- Measure and document pain, dyspnea, constipation, and other symptoms using available standardized scales.
- Assess and manage symptoms and side effects in a timely, safe, and effective manner to a level that is acceptable to the patient and family.
- Measure and document anxiety, depression, delirium, behavioral disturbances, and other common psychologic symptoms using available standardized scales.
- Manage anxiety, depression, delirium, behavioral disturbances, and other common psychologic symptoms in a timely, safe, and effective manner to a level that is acceptable to the patient and family.

Emotional, social, and spiritual care
- Assess and manage the psychologic reactions of patients and families (including stress, anticipatory grief, and coping) in a regular, ongoing fashion to address emotional and functional impairment and loss.
- Develop and implement a comprehensive social care plan that addresses the social, practical, and legal needs of the patient and caregivers, including, but not limited to, relationships, communication, existing social and cultural networks, decision making, work and school settings, finances, sexuality/intimacy, caregiver availability/stress, and access to medicines and equipment.
- Develop and document a plan based on an assessment of religious, spiritual, and existential concerns using a structured instrument, and integrate the information obtained from the assessment into a comprehensive care plan.
- Provide information and make spiritual care available, either through organizational spiritual care counseling or through the patient's own clergy relationships.
- Include spiritual care professionals who are appropriately trained and certified in palliative care.
- Build partnerships with community clergy and provide education and counseling related to end-of-life care.
- Incorporate cultural assessment, including, but not limited to, locus of decision making; preferences regarding disclosure of information, truth telling, and decision making; dietary preferences; language; family communication; desire for palliative therapies and complementary and alternative medicine; perspectives on death, suffering, and grieving; and funeral and burial rituals.
- Provide professional interpreter services and culturally sensitive materials in the patient's and family's preferred language.

End-of-life care
- Recognize and document the transition to the active dying phase, and communicate to the patient, family, and staff the expectation of imminent death.
- Educate the family on a timely basis regarding the signs and symptoms of imminent death in an age-appropriate, developmentally appropriate, and culturally appropriate manner.
- As part of the ongoing care planning process, routinely ascertain and document patient and family wishes about the care setting for the site of death, and fulfill patient and family preferences when possible.
- Provide adequate dosage of analgesics and sedatives as appropriate to achieve patient comfort during the active dying phase, and address concerns and fears about using opioids and analgesics hastening death.
- Treat the body after death with respect according to the cultural and religious practices of the family and in accordance with local law.

Bereavement care
- Develop and offer a grief and bereavement care plan to provide services to patients and families before, and for at least 13 months after, death of the patient.
- Facilitate effective grieving by implementing, in a timely manner, a bereavement care plan after the patient's death, when the family becomes the focus of care.

Adapted from National Quality Forum. A national framework and preferred practices for palliative and hospice care quality: a consensus report. Washington DC: National Quality Forum; 2006. Available at: http://www.qualityforum.org/publications/reports/palliative.asp. Accessed September 15, 2007; with permission.

from care providers, and "being supported by staff" was among the factors most frequently identified as influencing their decision making [22]. Also, parents indicate that they prefer to know at the time of diagnosis that their child may not survive and want the treating team to alert them to changes in their child's clinical status and to available care options [12].

Adults identify a sense of control over decisions as an element of quality end-of-life care, and patient involvement in decision making is key [21,23–27]. Less clear is how and at what age pediatric patients should participate in end-of-life decisions. Engaging the child recognizes his or her stake in the decisions being made and respects his or her capacity for informed decision making. Eighty-nine percent of parents of childhood cancer survivors reported that they would allow a child as young as 4 to be involved in a decision to pursue experimental chemotherapy [28]. Also, in a study of end-of-life care preferences, children as young as 10 recognized that they were involved in an end-of-life decision, understood its consequences, and demonstrated the capacity to weigh complex issues, including potential risks to themselves and others [29]. Parents of children with cancer also identify "making decisions with my child" as a major factor in their own decision making [12]. Parents, surrogates, and health care providers must recognize the subjective nature of suffering and must respect the child's autonomy and capacity to make decisions, particularly if the patient is an emancipated or mature minor [30]. If possible and indicated, caregivers should invite children to participate in decisions about their own care and honor their wishes, recognizing the personal context in which the illness unfolds [26]. Recognition of the unique contributions of the parents and the child to the discussion and integration of their input into the decision process ensures a truly family-centered approach to care.

As a facilitator of decision making, the clinician must understand the child's and family's perspective on the illness and its impact on their lives. Beliefs, values, hopes, and fears shape their perspective and must be understood, to guide them through the process. Patients and families also need clear, accurate information about prognosis to weigh the benefits and burdens of treatment options and prepare to make difficult decisions about their care, particularly at the end of life. However, physicians report providing a frank estimate of survival likelihood only 37% of the time, and discrepancies frequently exit; 70% of discrepant survival estimates were overly optimistic [31]. Despite the evident underdisclosure of prognosis, "information from health care professionals" was the factor most frequently reported by parents of children with cancer to influence their decision making [12].

Effective communication of the prognosis is the foundation for establishing realistic goals of care. Over time, goals may shift as prognosis changes or as the patient's and family's priorities change. The goals of medical treatment must be integrated with personal goals to ensure holistic decision making. Neglect of the emotional and social aspects of care goals can lead to medical decisions that increase patient and family suffering

[32]. After care goals are established, treatment options can be weighed in terms of their benefits, burdens, and contribution to achieving the identified goals.

The advance care planning process must be documented in the medical record where it can be easily shared with members of the interdisciplinary care team and across health care settings. The authors have found the four-box method for clinical ethics developed by Jonsen and colleagues [33] to be a particularly useful tool for organizing and documenting the rationale behind the decisions made (see Table 1) [20].

Ethics consultation

Generally, clear and open communication throughout the illness trajectory yields a consensus about care. Conflict may occur when the patient or family receives inadequate information about prognosis and treatment options or has limited opportunity to process this information and consider their goals and priorities. In pediatric oncology, some families have unrealistic expectations and, even with the best communication (eg, use of the advance care planning process), demand treatments that are medically inappropriate on the basis of existing standards. In these cases, frequent weighing of the benefits and burdens of medical interventions with the help of a patient advocate and the involvement of an ethics committee is recommended to allow deliberation about medical decisions in a safe atmosphere.

In palliative and end-of-life care, the ethics consultation process should function as the back-up of the advance care planning process, because the primary responsibility for medical care and resolution of ethical problems in patient management lies with the physician, the health care team, the patient, and the patient's parents, family, or guardian. An ethics committee should be available, particularly at times of conflict, to provide consultation about ethical dilemmas related to patient care, facilitate physician–family–patient communication, and assist in the resolution of complex situations. This process should be confidential and aimed at facilitating communication, conflict resolution, and support of relationships rather than making specific treatment recommendations.

The ethics committee also plays a palliative care role with regard to the development and implementation of care policies that support the decision-making process, enhance symptom control, promote care coordination and continuity, and facilitate care of the child and family throughout the illness trajectory, including bereavement and across multiple care settings.

Care coordination

The care coordination process involves interdisciplinary communication and collaboration that link children with special health care needs to the appropriate services and resources throughout the disease trajectory. The

Table 1
Advance care planning documentation tool incorporating key components of the individualized care planning process

97 Demographic Information	
Name: Date: Medical Record number:	
Medical Issues	**Quality of Life Issues**

1. From the medical team's perspective:
  • *List summary of patient's medical problems. History? Diagnosis? Is the problem acute? Chronic? Critical? Emergent?*
  • *Is the patient's condition considered potentially curable? Is it incurable?*
  • *What is the primary goal of care? Curative? Life-prolongation? Comfort?*
  • *What are the secondary goals of medical care?*
  • *What are the probabilities of success?*
  • *What are the plans in case of therapeutic failure?*
2. From the patient's and family's perspective:
  • *What are the patient and family's perceptions about prognosis for survival? Life expectancy? Suffering?*
  • *What are the patient and family's perceptions about the medical goals and available goal-directed treatment options?*
  • *Are there any particular medical decisions that the patient and/or family must make? (e.g. withholding cancer-directed therapy, participating in clinical trial, withholding or withdrawing treatment with curative intent, DNR)*
3. In sum, how can this patient and family be benefited by medical care, and how can harm be avoided?
	1. From the medical team's perspective:
	  • *What are the prospects, with or without treatment, for a return to normal life?*
	  • *What physical, mental, and social deficits is the patient likely to experience during and after treatment?*
	  • *Are there biases that might prejudice the provider's evaluation of the patient's quality of life?*
	  • *Is there any consideration to forgo treatment in order to maximize quality of life?*
	  • *Are there plans for comfort and palliative care?*
	2. From the patient's and family's perspective:
	  • *How has being sick been for the child? Family?*
	  • *What are their needs, hopes, beliefs, values, expectations, fears, preferences?*
	  • *What does good quality of life mean for the child? Family?*
	  • *What are the most concerning or distressing symptoms that interfere with good quality of life?*
	  • *Is the patient's present or future condition such that his or her continued life might be judged undesirable?*
	3. In sum, how can this patient and family be benefited by greater emphasis on quality of life, and how can suffering be minimized?

Patient and family's preferences	**Contextual features**

1. Who is(are) the primary decision maker(s)?
  • *What are the information needs of the primary decision maker(s)?*
  • *Has the primary decision maker(s) been informed of benefits and risks, understood this information, and given assent or consent?*
  • *Is there evidence of incapacity of the primary decision maker(s) (e.g., age, cognitive or developmental status, mental illness?)*
  • *Is the primary decision maker(s) using appropriate standards for decision making?*
  • *Has the patient expressed prior preferences, e.g., Advance Directives?*
  • *Is the patient, parent or surrogate unwilling or unable to cooperate with medical treatment?*
2. If the child-patient is capable of participating in the decision-making process:
  • *What is the extent of that participation?*
  • *What is he or she stating about preferences for medical treatment?*
  • *What is he or she stating about preferences for quality of life?*
3. If the child-patient is unable to participate in the decision-making process and someone else is making decisions on his or her behalf:
  • *What is the extent of their participation?*
  • *What is the parent or surrogate decision-maker stating about preferences for medical treatment?*
  • *What is the parent or surrogate decision-maker stating about preferences for quality of life?*
4. In sum, is the patient and family's right to choose being respected to the extent possible in ethics and law?
	1. What are the rights of the child relative to the rights of the family?
	2. Are there family issues that might influence treatment decisions? (e.g., language barriers, psychosocial issues, place of residence in rural area?)
	3. Are there health care provider issues that might influence treatment decisions? (e.g., no open research protocol)
	4. Are there health care system issues that might influence treatment decisions? (e.g., limited resources, availability of treatment)
	5. Are there financial and economic factors? (e.g., unfunded patient, illegal immigrant)
	6. Are there religious or cultural factors? (e.g., end-of-life rituals, care of the body)
	7. Are there limits on confidentiality? (e.g., divorced parents, extended family)
	8. Are there problems of allocation of resources? (e.g., critical care, expensive technologies of limited benefit, home health and hospice care)
	9. How does the law affect treatment decisions?
	10. Is clinical research or teaching involved?
	11. Is there any conflict of interest on the part of the providers or the institution?

Discussion	
Document discussion points	
Plan	
Document advance care plan	

Data from Hays RM, Valentine J, Haynes G, et al. The Seattle Palliative Care Project: effects on family satisfaction and health-related quality of life. J Palliat Med 2006;9(3):716–28; and Jonsen A, Siegler M, Winslade WJ. Clinical ethics: a practical approach to ethical decisions in clinical medicine. 6th edition. New York: McGraw-Hill; 2006.

goal is to limit fragmentation of care by orchestrating the delivery of medical services while advocating for comfort and quality of life. Children with cancer, and their families, must navigate an extremely complex modern health care system involving multiple caregivers from various backgrounds and disciplines. Pediatric oncology has long functioned as the model for multidisciplinary care, but, in reality, care is extremely fragmented. Families must become experts in inpatient care, outpatient clinics, and the home health system and, to keep their child's life as "normal" as possible, they must stay connected with community resources, including school, church, and so forth. This process is complicated by economic and sociocultural barriers, because the multiple systems of care do not have a single point of entry [34,35]. The Institute of Medicine has identified care coordination and care of children with special health care needs as priority areas for quality improvement and has recognized the "medical home" as the optimal venue for care coordination and family-centered care [36,37].

Pediatric oncology programs are considered the medical home for children with cancer. The American Academy of Pediatrics describes the medical home as a means of delivering primary care that is accessible, continuous, comprehensive, family-centered, coordinated, compassionate, and culturally effective [34,35]. The goals of the medical home are therefore process-oriented rather than static. They include an integrated plan of care; documentation and database management; sharing of information across disciplines, providers and settings; patient and family education and support; and ongoing evaluation.

Barriers to pediatric oncology programs' achievement of these goals include the use of resources that do not fall under the umbrella of the medical home; inadequate reimbursement for additional administrative responsibilities, including documentation and counseling; lack of continuity in care across multiple service providers; lack of communication and collaboration between the oncologist and other specialists; lack of communication between the care team and community agencies; undefined roles of the care team and community agencies; time considerations; and cultural and language barriers.

Collaboration has been identified as the central principle of care coordination by the American Academy of Pediatrics [35]. The National Institutes of Health also notes that effective communication among disciplines is a particularly important aspect of palliative care in pediatrics [27,38]. Multiple disciplines are well represented in current clinical settings, but they often provide their services in isolation from one another and with limited communication. Interdisciplinary teams share information, and their work is guided by the individual patient's needs. The medical home is best served by integrating elements of a transdisciplinary approach into an interdisciplinary framework, in which roles and responsibilities are shared, with few seams between the members' functions [39]. Although this approach is limited in specialized medical procedures and interventions, it is valuable in the exchange of general planning, and psychosocial and spiritual information.

The interdisciplinary team meeting is at the center of the care coordination process and the promotion of an interdisciplinary and transdisciplinary approach to the patient and family. Although pediatric oncology centers often meet to discuss patients (eg, tumor board, psychosocial rounds, and so forth), the interdisciplinary team meeting seeks active participation of members from various disciplines to discuss specific patient and family care issues. A summary of these meetings is usually documented as part of a comprehensive care plan. Participation of the patient or family in these meetings may be recommended in some circumstances. Their purpose is to come to a common understanding of the patient's clinical condition and treatment goals. They are the perfect opportunity to communicate as a team about specific decisions made during the advance care planning process and the important physical, social, emotional, and spiritual aspects of care while enhancing interdisciplinary collaboration to implement a comprehensive care plan for the child and family. For better integration of care coordination into the mainstream of pediatric oncology care, interdisciplinary partnership should be promoted, a transdisciplinary approach should be taken, and interdisciplinary team meetings should be implemented as part of routine care, particularly for patients with poor prognosis or those with advanced cancer.

Care continuity

The benefits of early integration of palliative care and the many needs of pediatric oncology patients and their families underscore the importance of a coordinated, interdisciplinary approach that links hospital, home health, and hospice settings [40,41]. An increasing number of children with complex chronic conditions in the United States are dying at home, possibly as the result of shifting attitudes and decisions about palliative and end-of-life care and the greater capacity of the health care system to provide home-based services [42]. The care continuity process allows access to coordinated, high-quality palliative care in which key therapeutic interpersonal relationships are maintained throughout the illness and across various settings, which can help the child and family regain a sense of personal control over their care.

The development of partnerships among pediatric oncology programs and local home health and hospice agencies is a key strategy for enhancing the quality of palliative care throughout the patient's illness. From a hospital perspective, integration of palliative care principles and practices into the continuum of care (ie, elaboration of a comprehensive care plan) and the creation of bridging programs between cancer center care and services provided in the community would be most beneficial. From a community perspective, pediatric hospice programs that are established within or in partnership with a home health agency and that collaborate with the cancer center would allow a more effective response to the patient's and family's needs from the point of diagnosis onward.

Until a national health policy is implemented to compensate providers for individualized care coordination processes including advance care planning, care coordination, and care continuity, individual pediatric oncology centers and home health and hospice programs must find creative solutions to overcome the many structural, financial, professional, regulatory, institutional, and organizational barriers to these partnerships [43]. Possible strategies include identifying local advocates from various disciplines, teaching interdisciplinary palliative and end-of-life care, providing medical leadership, and establishing a liaison nurse to represent palliative and hospice care within the hospital setting [44]. Integrating the palliative care physician consultant and a hospital-based individualized care coordinator into complex pediatric oncology cases is also useful. The value of interdisciplinary care planning and coordination and the use of patient care conferences to promote communication and collaboration among hospital, home health, and hospice providers cannot be overemphasized [4].

Working toward positive partnerships in the palliative and end-of-life care of pediatric oncology patients through the care continuity process also involves critical evaluation of strengths and weaknesses. Useful principles to guide the evaluation process include acknowledgment of the need for partnership, clarity, and realism of purpose; commitment and ownership; development and maintenance of trust; establishing robust care plan arrangements; and organizational monitoring, review, and learning [45].

Symptom control

Few things are more heartrending than the suffering of a young patient ravaged by cancer and its treatment. Timely and skilled management of pain and symptoms is the cornerstone of palliating suffering [46]. Integrating palliative care principles and practices into the mainstream of pediatric oncology programs requires appropriate attention to expected and unexpected symptoms, from the point of diagnosis onward, through a specific symptom control process. The patients themselves have told us that distressing symptoms are highly prevalent and of a high intensity during cancer treatment [47,48]. The pediatric pain literature now clearly demonstrates that "there is no such thing as a little stick" and that the effects of underdiagnosed and undertreated pain and unrelieved procedural pain are long lasting [49,50]]. The same may apply to many other symptoms yet to be studied in this manner. Symptom management and attention to the suffering of children experiencing a cancer-related death must be comprehensive [51,52].

Children and adolescents who die of cancer experience many physical symptoms, including pain, fatigue, behavior changes, breathing changes and dyspnea, reduced mobility, nausea and vomiting, anemia and bleeding, loss of appetite, and many others [51–56]. Pain, poor appetite, and fatigue are usually cited as the most common symptoms. Many of these symptoms are widely reported to be untreated or unsuccessfully treated [51,52]. This deficiency is at odds with the main goals of parents, which include both cure or life-prolongation and relief of suffering [3].

These children and their families suffer not only physically but psychologically. Patients are reported to experience sadness, difficulty in discussing their feelings about dying with their parents, and fear of being alone. Parents most frequently experience fear of the child's death and fear of the child's physical symptoms [57]. Other psychologic symptoms frequently encountered in pediatric oncology include anxiety, excessive worry, depression, and irritability [52,58].

Effective symptom control is essential to provide high-quality palliative care. However, few instruments for measuring symptoms in children are reliable, valid, and developmentally appropriate, and the symptoms that are most concerning to the child at end of life have not been identified [46]. Appropriate instruments to measure these symptoms and the distress they cause in children dying a cancer-related death should be developed and researched. In children with cancer, the presence, or even the severity, of a symptom may not predict the distress it causes to the dying child, family, and health care providers [47,58]. The authors' experience suggests the need for a specific symptom control process to provide a more systematic approach to symptom assessment. An interdisciplinary approach is crucial because significant spiritual, emotional, and existential distress is frequently identified.

Conscientious symptom assessment and management must be incorporated into mainstream pediatric oncology in a more systematic way. In fact, distressing symptoms should be treated as a medical emergency and monitored at regular intervals. Although the cancer-related death of a child can frequently be anticipated and the symptomatology is well described, many issues interfere with optimal symptom management at the end of life. The literature suggests that palliative care specialists are consulted mainly for children with unmanageable symptoms or for children in the home setting who have complex symptom management needs. Parents indicate that their dying child's symptoms at the end of life were better controlled or less problematic when a provider with a specialized level of training in palliative care was available [52,59,60]. Clinicians with expertise in symptom management should be integrated into the primary oncology team to allow an ongoing therapeutic relationship with the child and family and to promote symptom control education.

The National Comprehensive Cancer Network has developed clinical practice guidelines for the management of cancer- and treatment-related emesis, anemia, fatigue, distress, and pediatric pain. These guidelines and other appropriate symptom management techniques should be integrated into pediatric oncology programs so that distressing symptoms are managed from the point of diagnosis onward. Evidence-based symptom control practices should be properly implemented and evaluated, including effective nonpharmacologic approaches (eg, hypnosis, acupuncture, relaxation techniques), and continuity of services across settings should be emphasized. Because clinical care providers for children at the end of life report being unfamiliar or uneasy with identifying and treating symptoms, provider education about symptom management must be promoted [59,61,62]. In addition, pediatric oncology programs must be better equipped for symptom management in the home setting, where parents often choose to have their child die [63,64].

Emotional, social, and spiritual care

Compassionate, competent, and sensitive care of the seriously ill child and the child's family requires ongoing, interdisciplinary patient- and family-centered assessment of emotional, social, and spiritual needs. This assessment identifies the values and priorities of the parent or parents and the ill child (when possible) and provides an indicator of the effectiveness of the comprehensive care plan [65–67]. Family culture (values, beliefs, attitudes, and dynamics) defines what a family perceives to be medically appropriate care in different situations [68]. Clinicians collaborate with the child and the family to incorporate their values and priorities into care planning and care goals [4,69]. Ongoing, regular assessment of patient- and family-centered needs allows the family and the clinical care team to formulate jointly a care plan to deal appropriately with the immediate clinical situation and lays the foundation for future collaboration in the formulation of comprehensive care plans [70].

An ongoing emotional, social, and spiritual assessment requires that clinicians listen intensely and respectfully to gain an understanding of the child's and family's relationships, preferences, and priorities [71]. Such care priorities may shift rapidly with the child's clinical condition or treatment options. As a result, clinician assessment of patient and family needs must be an ongoing combination of formal and less formal assessment queries. Informal assessments can be brief (eg, a single query to revisit care priorities after a clinical change). Formal assessments tend to be documented on care planning forms that become a part of the child's medical record.

A limited number of instruments are available for the formal assessment of emotional, social, and spiritual needs of the child or family. Clinically useful palliative care instruments (which include emotional, social, and spiritual parameters) are developmentally appropriate for children, brief, and clearly worded; use a limited time frame (such as the past 24 hours or current week) because of the likelihood of rapidly changing conditions; and are sensitive to change. Few comprehensive instruments exist and none has been validated in the pediatric oncology setting at the end of life. More such instruments are needed to prevent underassessment and the undertreatment of suffering in children with cancer and their families [72].

Clinically, it is useful to apply a generalist and a specialist approach to the provision of emotional, social, and spiritual care. Physicians, for example, can aim to be psychosocial generalists and medical specialists, whereas social workers and psychologists can aim to be psychosocial specialists and have a general understanding of disease management and assessment of physical comfort. As another example, doctors and nurses can assess the broad spiritual concerns of patients and families to refer them to appropriate spiritual advisors, whereas chaplains must take into account the medical issues, plan of care, and prognosis to understand the context of spiritual needs and to anticipate impending spiritual crises. All team members, given training, experience, and motivation, have the capacity to provide a generalist level of social, emotional, and spiritual care [73,74]. It is crucial that these assessments be free of judgment and free of the clinician's own agenda. Collaborative working relationships, interdisciplinary team meetings, care coordination, and patient care conferences are essential in the emotional, social, and spiritual care of children with cancer and their families.

End-of-life care

The principles and practices of palliative care can best be incorporated into the care of children dying a cancer-related death if specific processes are implemented. Parents report that end-of-life decisions are among the most difficult they face on behalf of their seriously ill child [12]. However, parents also state that they want to be involved in care decisions during their child's final days and they appreciate the opportunity to do so. They want to be kept informed of changes in the child's condition and to participate in adjustments to the care plan. The end-of-life care process includes advance care planning that focuses on the preferences of the patient and family, including desired location of death, potential care interventions, and other decisions such as DNR status or withholding or withdrawing artificial life-sustaining therapies. We do not fully understand the parental decision process or what factors influence it. Neither do we know the appropriate age at which children should be included in end-of-life decision making. Study findings indicate that many seriously ill children and adolescents can navigate a complex decision process in which risk is considered [29]. The advanced care planning process should be used to support and understand decision making in the care of the imminently dying child by ascertaining the patient's and family's priorities, values, and goals. Patient and family preferences may help to determine referral to hospice care, the desired location of death, plans for funeral arrangements, and DNR status.

The end-of-life care process also includes enhanced care coordination to facilitate an interdisciplinary approach to the patient and family. A coordinated interdisciplinary effort is crucial in working with the child and family near the end of life. As death becomes imminent, many parents notice less interaction with the medical team. Certain members of the care team may become less visible as curative efforts are replaced by comfort measures, but this change is difficult for families to comprehend, and parents report feeling abandoned [75]. These feelings of abandonment may complicate grief issues after the child's death. A change in caregivers during the last, and often the most intense, days of illness can be stressful for the patient and family. Maintaining open communication is essential for this reason. Parents report that receiving consistent information from a consistent team is helpful at these times [59]. Team members, however, frequently report not knowing the patient's current clinical status, what decisions have been made, or the content of discussions between other clinicians and the family. A focus on care coordination, including patient care conferences and interdisciplinary team meetings, is essential to effectively maintain the lines of communication and provide the support needed by patients' families.

The end-of-life care process includes care of the imminently dying patient and the patient's family but should be implemented well before death is imminent. Cancer patients near death have symptoms that are often not treated or are treated unsuccessfully, despite parents' great concern that their child not suffer at the end of life [51–57]. Bereaved parents who report unrelieved pain in their dying child have been found to experience long-term distress [76]. Comprehensive, systematic symptom assessment should be ongoing for all children dying a cancer-related death. Aggressive symptom control is crucial during this time because many patients suffer at the end of life, and their suffering also leads to poor family and caretaker outcomes.

Aside from physical symptoms, psychosocial and spiritual needs are consistently identified as very important to patients and their families [22]. Psychologic concerns are frequently underaddressed but should be managed as aggressively as physical symptoms. Many clinicians are not trained to address the spiritual concerns of patients and families so this aspect of care is also frequently unattended. Clinicians may understand and care about the spiritual and religious needs of the patient and family but may not know how to help [77]. Parents and children, however, state that they feel a connection to a religious or spiritual domain at end of life and belief in a "Greater Being" is very important for parents at the time of end-of-life decision making and care [12,78].

Communication is of utmost importance at all times, but its significance is heightened during the final days and hours of a child's life. Caregivers find it extremely difficult to shift from the "doing" mode to one in which they are willing to sit and "be" with the patient and family, witnessing the mysteries of suffering and death. Open, honest, thoughtful, and caring communication at this time can provide emotional comfort in a situation filled with uncertainty and fear. Finally, conducting end-of-life debriefing sessions can also help the staff cope with the tragedy of losing a patient who is at the dawn of his or her life.

Bereavement care

Although survival rates for pediatric cancer are improving, many patients still die, leaving bereaved families trying to cope. Adults experience a higher intensity of grief after their child's death than after a spouse's or parent's death [79–81]. Support for bereaved families must be a priority in pediatric oncology because bereaved parents have an elevated risk of psychiatric hospitalization even 5 or more years after their child's death and have a higher risk of early death and poorer health outcomes [82,83].

The treatment of pediatric cancer places many burdens on families. Children receiving treatment for cancer are often hospitalized far from home for lengthy periods, geographically separating family members and reducing access to social support from friends and extended family. Parents often come to depend on the hospital staff for their psychosocial needs. When a child dies and these services are no longer available, families may feel abandoned by hospital staff [84]. Most families desire some continued contact with members of their child's care team and report that the contact is meaningful to them [59,75,85,86].

Approximately 45% to 59% of pediatric cancer deaths occur while the child is hospitalized [19,80,87]. Unlike hospice, which has clearly established guidelines for the care of bereaved families, many hospitals do not provide formal bereavement care [88]. The bereavement care process should include an interdisciplinary and appropriately trained team; bereavement follow-up services should be offered for at least 12 months; and family members should be clinically assessed to identify those at risk of complicated grief [40].

A practical approach for providing care for bereaved families begins when the child is first admitted for treatment. The foundation is laid for future relationships during the early stages of the child's treatment. Using a "hope for the best, plan for the worst" approach enables care teams to help prepare a family for loss, which, in turn, may lower the risk of psychologic disturbance after the death. The goal of integrating bereavement care into the mainstream of the child's care also suggests the need to develop and implement effective evaluation tools that permit the team to identify families at risk of complicated bereavement. Initial assessments by chaplaincy and social work can alert the team to families whose coping may be less than adaptive. The individuals most at risk are often those most reluctant to seek help; this factor can complicate attempts at intervention [89]. Individuals who lack a good social support network and those with a childhood history of neglect and abuse are at highest risk of complicated bereavement.

The eight warning signs of complicated grief are trouble accepting the death; inability to trust others; excessive bitterness toward the death; uneasiness about moving on with life; detachment from other people to whom the person was previously close; the feeling that life is now meaningless, the view that the future holds no prospect for fulfillment; and agitation since the death. These signs must be persistent and disruptive to the bereaved person, and must have lasted more than 6 months [90]. In addition, family members displaying disbelief, yearning, anger, or depression 6 months after the death of the child may need further evaluation [91].

Thus, to identify and help people who may be suffering from complicated bereavement, the bereavement care process should be programmatic and must include regular contact between trained staff and family members over an extended period, which requires financial commitment to fund such support. A minimal, hospital-based program for families whose child has died might include the following: the creation of a memento of the child, often a hand print or lock of hair, for the family; attendance at the funeral or memorial service by members of the primary care team, when possible; a personalized condolence card sent by the team and telephone or written contact periodically, especially around the child's birthday, holidays, and the anniversary of the child's death [59,92–94]. It is important that parents know they have "permission" to contact team members if they are experiencing problems, and that team members have the appropriate resources to make referrals to services in the parent's community. Many programs send appropriate books and other literature to families. Some hospitals hold annual events to honor the memory of children who have died and invite families to attend. Although all these efforts attempt to meet the needs of bereaved families, little outcomes-based research exists to support their continued existence and justify their expense. Evidence-based practices should be developed and evaluated to improve interventions for bereaved parents. Expert opinion can be a useful starting point, but only formal assessment and outcomes measures can demonstrate that we are truly helping families and justify the expense of bereavement intervention.

Coding and reimbursement for hospice and palliative care services

Reimbursement practices for many of the care processes described in the ICPC model may be possible using existing coding and reimbursement mechanisms [95]. The process used for billing and reimbursement depends on the role of the provider, the relationship of the health care professional with the agency providing the care, and whether or not the patient is hospitalized or receiving home health or hospice services. Billing and reimbursement processes differ between public and private insurers and across states. In general, claims for services provided by health care professionals are submitted by using the *Current Procedural Terminology* (*CPT*) evaluation and management code system [96]. *CPT* codes may be used by physicians and other health care providers for outpatient and inpatient visits for the advance care planning, care coordination, and symptom control processes, and for other psychosocial care processes. Useful *CPT* codes for qualified physicians are outlined in Table 2. In addition to *CPT* codes, physicians may describe the reasons for their services by using one of the *International Classification of Disease, Ninth Revision, Clinical Modification* (*ICD-9-CM*) codes produced by the National Center for Health Statistics [97]. When the palliative care consultant is also a pediatric oncologist, claims submitted for palliative care services must have a different diagnosis to minimize the risk of having the claim denied. *ICD-9* codes commonly used in palliative care are listed in Table 3.

Table 2
Evaluation and management codes for palliative care

Attending/managing physician

New office	Established office	Initial hospital	Subsequent hospital	Prolonged services[a]	
				Office/home[b]	Inpatient[c]
99201 10 min	99211 5 min	99221 30 min	99231 15 min	99354 30 min	99356 30 min
99202 20 min	99212 10 min	99222 50 min	99232 25 min	For each subsequent 30 minutes:	99357
99203 30 min	99213 15 min	99223 70 min	99233 35 min	99355	
99204 45 min	99214 25 min				
99205 50 min	99215 40 min				

New home	Established home	Interdisciplinary team meetings
99324 20 min	99334 15 min	99361 30 min
99325 30 min	99335 25 min	99362 60 min
99326 45 min	99336 40 min	
99327 60 min	99337 60 min	
99328 75 min		

Consult physician

Office/home	Initial hospital	Subsequent hospital
99241 15 min	99251 20 min	99231 15 min
99242 30 min	99252 40 min	99232 25 min
99243 40 min	99253 55 min	99233 35 min

Health and behavior assessment[d]

Assessment	Reassessment	Individual therapy	Group therapy	Without patient present	With patient present
96150 15 min	96151 15 min	96152 15 min	96153 15 min	96154 15 min	96155 15 min

Psychiatric therapeutic procedures[e]

Diagnostic interview	Developmental assessment	Psychologic testing	Neuropsychologic testing	Mental status examination
90801 15 min	96111 1 hour	96102 1 hour	96118 1 hour	96116 1 hour

Office/home	Inpatient	Interactive[f] visit/office	Interactive visit/inpatient
90804 20–30 min	90816 20–30 min	90810 20–30 min	90823 20–30 min
90806 45–50 min	90818 45–50 min	90812 45–50 min	90826 45–50 min
90808 75–80 min	90821 75–80 min	90814 75–80 min	90828 75–80 min

Group therapy	Family therapy without patient present	Family therapy with patient present
90853 15 min	90846 15 min	90847 15 min

[a] These add-on codes are used if the time spent in counseling or information giving is more than 50% of the visit. Proper documentation is required.

[b] Total time the physician spends face to face with a patient. In pediatrics, some but not all payers recognize time spent face to face with the primary decision maker within the family unit. The time spent on activities related to the visit but not face to face with the patient or family is not to be added to the visit.

[c] Total time the physician spends in the hospital unit, including the time spent in face-to-face contact with the patient and family, chart review, documentation, and care coordination.

[d] Used by qualified mental health providers (ie, physician, clinical psychologist, clinical social worker, nurse practitioner, clinical nurse specialist, or physician assistant) in the absence of psychiatric illness (ie, coping, self-care, poor family cohesion, when they interfere with the care of the patient). Each 15 minutes of visit is claimed as a unit; a 60-minute visit is claimed as four units.

[e] Used by qualified mental health providers (ie, psychiatrist, clinical psychologist) for the treatment of a psychiatric condition (ie, anxiety disorders, depression, individual or family dysfunction during complicated bereavement).

[f] Interactive visit codes are used when the health care professional uses equipment and other resources to provide care (ie, rehabilitation unit).

Table 3
Palliative care diagnoses: *ICD-9* codes and descriptions

263.9: Inanition	780.01: Coma	780.96: Generalized pain
286.6: Dyspnea	780.09: Unconscious state	789.00: Abdominal pain, unspecified site
298.9: Confusion	780.39: Convulsions	789.01: Abdominal pain, right upper quadrant
783.0: Anorexia	780.4: Dizziness	789.02: Abdominal pain, left upper quadrant
300.00: Anxiety state	780.52: Insomnia, unspecified	789.03: Abdominal pain, right lower quadrant
300.20: Phobia	780.54: Hypersomnia	789.04: Abdominal pain, left lower quadrant
307.9: Agitation	780.55: Disrupted 24-h sleep–wake cycle	789.05: Abdominal pain, periumbilic
308.3: Acute reaction to stress	780.6: Fever	789.06: Abdominal pain, epigastric
309.0: Maladjustment, depressed mood	780.79: Malaise and fatigue	789.07: Abdominal pain, generalized
309.28: Maladjustment, anxiety, depressed mood	780.9: Mental status change	789.09: Abdominal pain, multiple sites
309.83: Maladjustment, withdrawal	782.1: Rash	724.5: Backache, unspecified
309.9: Unspecified adjustment reaction	782.3: Edema	724.1: Pain in thoracic spine
311: Depressive disorder	783.0: Anorexia	724.2: Lumbago
313.0: Overanxious disorder	783.1: Abnormal weight gain	729.5: Pain in limb
338.3: Neoplasm-related pain	783.21: Loss of weight	733.90: Pain in bone
459.0: Hemorrhage, unspecified	784.0: Headache	786.50: Chest pain
527.7: Disturbance of salivary secretion	785.1: Palpitations	719.45: Pain in hip
528.01: Mucositis due to antineoplastic therapy	786.05: Shortness of breath	729.1: Muscle pain
528.09: Stomatitis and mucositis	786.2: Cough	724.60: Sacroiliac pain
558.9: Diarrhea	787.01: Nausea with vomiting	784.1: Throat pain
564.00: Constipation	787.02: Nausea alone	723.1: Neck pain
698.9: Unspecified pruritic disorder	787.03: Vomiting alone	799.3: Debility
707.00: Decubitus ulcer, unspecified site	787.2: Dysphagia	V61.8: Other specified family circumstances
728.85: Spasm of muscle	787.91: Diarrhea	V62.82: Encounter for bereavement
	799.2: Nervousness	V66.7: Encounter for palliative care
	780.97: Altered mental status, delirium	

Attending physicians caring for hospice patients who are not employed by the hospice may use *CPT* and *ICD-9* codes to submit claims directly to Medicaid. Physicians employed by the hospice agency must submit patient care claims directly to the hospice agency. The hospice agency then submits these claims for reimbursement as part of their claims for the care of the patient. Consulting physicians who are asked to see a hospice patient must also submit their claims to the hospice agency, which then reimburses the consultant directly based on preexisting contractual arrangements.

Under the hospice benefit, the per diem payment to the hospice covers all services provided by nonphysician health care professionals. For patients who are not enrolled in hospice, nonphysician professionals may be able to access fee-for-service reimbursement mechanisms through either Medicaid or private insurers. Useful *CPT* codes that can be used by nonphysician providers are listed in Table 2. Health and behavior assessment codes may be used by qualified health care professionals for grief assessment and counseling (ie, stress, coping, self-care, family cohesion). Neither evaluation and management codes for child life and spiritual care services nor procedure and service codes for care of bereaved family members of the ill child are available. Health and behavior, and psychiatric therapeutic procedure codes may be used for the evaluation of bereavement or management of pathologic bereavement but claims must be submitted to the insurer of the bereaved family member. Billing and reimbursement for physician and nonphysician providers of palliative care services using these billing and coding mechanisms may not be optimal and payment remains a challenge, particularly for bereavement care and when patients are not enrolled in hospice.

Summary

The goal of pediatric oncology and pediatric palliative care involves curing as many children as possible while actively and effectively addressing suffering. According to the World Health Organization, "palliative care for children is the active total care of the child's body, mind and spirit, and also involves giving support to the family. It begins when illness is diagnosed, and continues regardless of whether or not a child receives treatment directed at the disease" [98]. An integrated palliative care approach to these children and their families requires that we acknowledge the current gaps in the structure of pediatric oncology programs and develop processes to fill these gaps. Implementation of the ICPC model will help meet these needs and facilitate the further integration of palliative care principles into the care of children with cancer. Through these processes, the therapeutic relationships established in the context of the medical home can best address the suffering of pediatric cancer patients and their families. Patient and family values, preferences, goals, and needs will also be elucidated earlier in the course of illness so that appropriate goal-directed treatment options can be offered in times of uncertainty and emotional duress.

References

[1] American Academy of Pediatrics. Committee on Bioethics and Committee on Hospital Care. Palliative care for children. Pediatrics 2000;106(2 Pt 1):351–7.

[2] Kane JR, Himelstein BP. Palliative care for children. In: Berger AM, Shuster JL, Von Roenn JH, editors. Principles and practice of palliative medicine and supportive oncology. 3rd edition. Philadelphia: Lippincott Williams & Wilkins; 2007.

[3] Wolfe J, Klar N, Grier HE, et al. Understanding of prognosis among parents of children who died of cancer: impact on treatment goals and integration of palliative care. JAMA 2000; 284(19):2469–75.

[4] Baker JN, Barfield R, Hinds PS, et al. A process to facilitate decision making in pediatric stem cell transplantation: the individualized care planning and coordination model. Biol Blood Marrow Transplant 2007;13(3):245–54.

[5] Mack JW, Cook EF, Wolfe J, et al. Understanding of prognosis among parents of children with cancer: parental optimism and the parent-physician interaction. J Clin Oncol 2007; 25(11):1357–62.

[6] Kane JR, Hellsten MB, Coldsmith A. Human suffering: the need for relationship-based research in pediatric end-of-life care. J Pediatr Oncol Nurs 2004;21(3):180–5.

[7] A national framework and preferred practices for palliative and hospice care quality. National Quality Forum. 2006. Available at: www.qualityforum.org. Accessed September 15, 2007.

[8] Bagatell R, Meyer R, Herron S, et al. When children die: a seminar series for pediatric residents. Pediatrics 2002;110(2 Pt 1):348–53.

[9] Sullivan AM, Warren AG, Lakoma MD, et al. End-of-life care in the curriculum: a national study of medical education deans. Acad Med 2004;79(8):760–8.

[10] Sullivan AM, Lakoma MD, Billings JA, et al. Teaching and learning end-of-life care: evaluation of a faculty development program in palliative care. Acad Med 2005;80(7):657–68.

[11] Greiner A, Knebel E, editors. Health professions education. A bridge to quality. Washington, DC: The National Academies Press; 2003.

[12] Hinds PS, Oakes L, Furman W, et al. End-of-life decision making by adolescents, parents, and healthcare providers in pediatric oncology: research to evidence-based practice guidelines. Cancer Nurs 2001;24(2):122–34.

[13] Agrawal M, Grady C, Fairclough DL, et al. Patients' decision-making process regarding participation in phase I oncology research. J Clin Oncol 2006;24(27):4479–84.

[14] Barrera M, D'Agostino N, Gammon J, et al. Health-related quality of life and enrollment in phase 1 trials in children with incurable cancer. Palliat Support Care 2005;3(3):191–6.

[15] Grunfeld EA, Maher EJ, Browne S, et al. Advanced breast cancer patients' perceptions of decision making for palliative chemotherapy. J Clin Oncol 2006;24(7):1090–8.

[16] Matsuyama R, Reddy S, Smith TJ. Why do patients choose chemotherapy near the end of life? A review of the perspective of those facing death from cancer. J Clin Oncol 2006; 24(21):3490–6.

[17] Slevin ML, Stubbs L, Plant HJ, et al. Attitudes to chemotherapy: comparing views of patients with cancer with those of doctors, nurses, and general public. BMJ 1990; 300(6737):1458–60.

[18] Tomlinson D, Capra M, Gammon J, et al. Parental decision making in pediatric cancer end-of-life care: using focus group methodology as a prephase to seek participant design input. Eur J Oncol Nurs 2006;10(3):198–206.

[19] Klopfenstein KJ, Hutchison C, Clark C, et al. Variables influencing end-of-life care in children and adolescents with cancer. J Pediatr Hematol Oncol 2001;23(8):481–6.

[20] Hays RM, Valentine J, Haynes G, et al. The Seattle Pediatric Palliative Care Project: effects on family satisfaction and health-related quality of life. J Palliat Med 2006;9(3):716–28.

[21] Cancer care during the last phase of life. J Clin Oncol 1998;16(5):1986–96.

[22] Meyer EC, Ritholz MD, Burns JP, et al. Improving the quality of end-of-life care in the pediatric intensive care unit: parents' priorities and recommendations. Pediatrics 2006;117(3): 649–57.

[23] Rietjens JA, van der HA, Onwuteaka-Philipsen BD, et al. Preferences of the Dutch general public for a good death and associations with attitudes towards end-of-life decision-making. Palliat Med 2006;20(7):685–92.

[24] Singer PA, Martin DK, Kelner M. Quality end-of-life care: patients' perspectives. JAMA 1999;281(2):163–8.

[25] Steinhauser KE, Clipp EC, McNeilly M, et al. In search of a good death: observations of patients, families, and providers. Ann Intern Med 2000;132(10):825–32.

[26] American Academy of Pediatrics Committee on Bioethics: guidelines on foregoing life-sustaining medical treatment. Pediatrics 1994;93(3):532–6.

[27] NIH State-of-the-Science Conference. statement on improving end-of-life care. 2004. p. 1–28.

[28] Kamps WA, Akkerboom JC, Kingma A, et al. Experimental chemotherapy in children with cancer–a parent's view. Pediatr Hematol Oncol 1987;4(2):117–24.

[29] Hinds PS, Drew D, Oakes LL, et al. End-of-life care preferences of pediatric patients with cancer. J Clin Oncol 2005;23(36):9146–54.

[30] Freyer DR. Children with cancer: special considerations in the discontinuation of life-sustaining treatment. Med Pediatr Oncol 1992;20(2):136–42.

[31] Lamont EB, Christakis NA. Prognostic disclosure to patients with cancer near the end of life. Ann Intern Med 2001;134(12):1096–105.

[32] Weiner JS, Roth J. Avoiding iatrogenic harm to patient and family while discussing goals of care near the end of life. J Palliat Med 2006;9(2):451–63.

[33] Jonsen A, Siegler M, Winslade WJ. Clinical ethics: a practical approach to ethical decisions in clinical medicine. 6th edition. New York: McGraw-Hill; 2006.

[34] Council on Children with Disabilities. Care coordination in the medical home: integrating health and related systems of care for children with special health care needs. Pediatrics 2005;116(5):1238–44.

[35] Ziring PR, Brazdziunas D, Cooley WC, et al. American Academy of Pediatrics. Committee on Children with Disabilities. Care coordination: integrating health and related systems of care for children with special health care needs. Pediatrics 1999;104(4 Pt 1):978–81.

[36] Adams K, Corrigan J, editors. Priority areas for national action: transforming health care quality. Washington, DC: The National Academies Press; 2001.

[37] Committee on Palliative and End-of-Life Care for Children and Their Families Board on Health Sciences Policy. When children die: improving palliative and end-of-life care for children and their families. Washington, DC: The National Academies Press; 2003.

[38] Kane JR, Primomo M. Alleviating the suffering of seriously ill children. Am J Hosp Palliat Care 2001;18(3):161–9.

[39] Parker GM. Cross-functional teams: working with allies, enemies and other strangers. San Francisco (CA): Jossey-Bass Publishers; 2004.

[40] National Consensus Project for Quality Palliative Care. Clinical practice guidelines for quality palliative care. Pittsburg (PA): National Consensus Project for Quality Palliative Care; 2004.

[41] National Institute of Clinical Excellence. Improving supportive and palliative care for adults with cancer: the manual. London: National Institute for Clinical Excellence; 2004.

[42] Feudtner C, Feinstein JA, Satchell M, et al. Shifting place of death among children with complex chronic conditions in the United States, 1989–2003. JAMA 2007;297(24):2725–32.

[43] Walshe C, Caress A, Chew-Graham C, et al. Evaluating partnership working: lessons for palliative care. Eur J Cancer Care (Engl) 2007;16(1):48–54.

[44] Baresford L. Hospital-hospice partnerships in palliative care. Creating a continuum of service. National Hospice and Palliative Care Organization and the Center to Advance Palliative Care; 2007. Available at: http://www.capc.org/palliative-care-across-the-continuum/Hospital-Hospice-Partnerships.pdf. Accessed September 2007.

[45] Hudson B, Hardy B. What is a successful partnership and how can it be measured? In: Glendinning C, Powell M, Rummery K, editors. Partnerships, new labour and the governance of welfare. Bristol (UK): The Policy Press; 2002. p. 51–65.

[46] Himelstein BP, Hilden JM, Boldt AM, et al. Pediatric palliative care. N Engl J Med 2004; 350(17):1752–62.

[47] Collins JJ, Byrnes ME, Dunkel IJ, et al. The measurement of symptoms in children with cancer. J Pain Symptom Manage 2000;19(5):363–77.

[48] Collins JJ, Devine TD, Dick GS, et al. The measurement of symptoms in young children with cancer: the validation of the Memorial Symptom Assessment Scale in children aged 7–12. J Pain Symptom Manage 2002;23(1):10–6.

[49] Weisman SJ, Bernstein B, Schechter NL. Consequences of inadequate analgesia during painful procedures in children. Arch Pediatr Adolesc Med 1998;152(2):147–9.

[50] Berde CB, Sethna NF. Analgesics for the treatment of pain in children. N Engl J Med 2002; 347(14):1094–103.

[51] Goldman A, Hewitt M, Collins GS, et al. Symptoms in children/young people with progressive malignant disease: United Kingdom Children's Cancer Study Group/Paediatric Oncology Nurses Forum survey. Pediatrics 2006;117(6):e1179–86.

[52] Wolfe J, Grier HE, Klar N, et al. Symptoms and suffering at the end of life in children with cancer. N Engl J Med 2000;342(5):326–33.

[53] McCallum DE, Byrne P, Bruera E. How children die in hospital. J Pain Symptom Manage 2000;20(6):417–23.

[54] Stevens MM, Dalla PL, Cavalletto B, et al. Pain and symptom control in paediatric palliative care. Cancer Surv 1994;21:211–31.

[55] Wolfe J, Friebert S, Hilden J. Caring for children with advanced cancer integrating palliative care. Pediatr Clin North Am 2002;49(5):1043–62.

[56] Jalmsell L, Kreicbergs U, Onelov E, et al. Symptoms affecting children with malignancies during the last month of life: a nationwide follow-up. Pediatrics 2006;117(4):1314–20.

[57] Theunissen JM, Hoogerbrugge PM, van AT, et al. Symptoms in the palliative phase of children with cancer. Pediatr Blood Cancer 2007;49(2):160–5.

[58] Drake R, Frost J, Collins JJ. The symptoms of dying children. J Pain Symptom Manage 2003;26(1):594–603.

[59] Contro NA, Larson J, Scofield S, et al. Hospital staff and family perspectives regarding quality of pediatric palliative care. Pediatrics 2004;114(5):1248–52.

[60] Nitschke R, Meyer WH, Sexauer CL, et al. Care of terminally ill children with cancer. Med Pediatr Oncol 2000;34(4):268–70.

[61] McCluggage HL. Symptoms suffered by life-limited children that cause anxiety to UK children's hospice staff. Int J Palliat Nurs 2006;12(6):254–8.

[62] Hilden JM, Emanuel EJ, Fairclough DL, et al. Attitudes and practices among pediatric oncologists regarding end-of-life care: results of the 1998 American Society of Clinical Oncology survey. J Clin Oncol 2001;19(1):205–12.

[63] Kurashima AY, Latorre MR, Teixeira SA, et al. Factors associated with location of death of children with cancer in palliative care. Palliat Support Care 2005;3(2):115–9.

[64] Davies B, Deveau E, deVeber B, et al. Experiences of mothers in five countries whose child died of cancer. Cancer Nurs 1998;21(5):301–11.

[65] Freyer DR, Kuperberg A, Sterken DJ, et al. Multidisciplinary care of the dying adolescent. Child Adolesc Psychiatr Clin N Am 2006;15(3):693–715.

[66] Levetown M, Frager G. UNIPAC eight: the hospice/palliative medicine approach to caring for pediatric patients. Glenview (IL): American Academy of Hospice and Palliative Medicine; 2003.

[67] Robinson MR, Thiel MM, Backus MM, et al. Matters of spirituality at the end of life in the pediatric intensive care unit. Pediatrics 2006;118(3):e719–29.

[68] De TM, Kovalcik R. The child with cancer. Influence of culture on truth-telling and patient care. Ann N Y Acad Sci 1997;809:197–210.

[69] Kane JR, Barber RG, Jordan M, et al. Supportive/palliative care of children suffering from life-threatening and terminal illness. Am J Hosp Palliat Care 2000;17(3):165–72.

[70] Sharman M, Meert KL, Sarnaik AP. What influences parents' decisions to limit or withdraw life support? Pediatr Crit Care Med 2005;6(5):513–8.

[71] Rushton CH. A framework for integrated pediatric palliative care: being with dying. J Pediatr Nurs 2005;20(5):311–25.

[72] Harris MB. Palliative care in children with cancer: which child and when? J Natl Cancer Inst Monogr 2004;(32):144–9.

[73] Meyer EC, Burns JP, Griffith JL, et al. Parental perspectives on end-of-life care in the pediatric intensive care unit. Crit Care Med 2002;30(1):226–31.

[74] Handzo G, Koenig HG. Spiritual care: whose job is it anyway? South Med J 2004;97(12): 1242–4.

[75] Hinds PS, Schum L, Baker JN, et al. Key factors affecting dying children and their families. J Palliat Med 2005;8(Suppl 1):S70–8.

[76] Kreicbergs U, Valdimarsdottir U, Onelov E, et al. Care-related distress: a nationwide study of parents who lost their child to cancer. J Clin Oncol 2005;23(36):9162–71.

[77] Grossoehme DH, Ragsdale JR, McHenry CL, et al. Pediatrician characteristics associated with attention to spirituality and religion in clinical practice. Pediatrics 2007;119(1):e117–23.

[78] Balboni TA, Vanderwerker LC, Block SD, et al. Religiousness and spiritual support among advanced cancer patients and associations with end-of-life treatment preferences and quality of life. J Clin Oncol 2007;25(5):555–60.

[79] National Comprehensive Cancer Network. The palliative care clinical practice guidelines in oncology (version 1.2007). National Comprehensive Cancer Network, Inc.; 2007. Available at: http://www.nccn.org/professionals/physician_gls/PDF/palliative.pdf. Accessed September 15, 2007.

[80] Bradshaw G, Hinds PS, Lensing S, et al. Cancer-related deaths in children and adolescents. J Palliat Med 2005;8(1):86–95.

[81] Sanders C. A comparison of adult bereavement in the death of a spouse, child and parent. Omega 1979;10(4):302–32.

[82] Li J, Laursen TM, Precht DH, et al. Hospitalization for mental illness among parents after the death of a child. N Engl J Med 2005;352(12):1190–6.

[83] Li J, Precht DH, Mortensen PB, et al. Mortality in parents after death of a child in Denmark: a nationwide follow-up study. Lancet 2003;361(9355):363–7.

[84] Truog RD, Meyer EC, Burns JP. Toward interventions to improve end-of-life care in the pediatric intensive care unit. Crit Care Med 2006;34(11 Suppl):S373–9.

[85] deCinque N, Monterosso L, Dadd G, et al. Bereavement support for families following the death of a child from cancer: practice characteristics of Australian and New Zealand paediatric oncology units. J Paediatr Child Health 2004;40(3):131–5.

[86] deCinque N, Monterosso L, Dadd G, et al. Bereavement support for families following the death of a child from cancer: experience of bereaved parents. J Psychosoc Oncol 2006;24(2): 65–83.

[87] Feudtner C, Christakis DA, Zimmerman FJ, et al. Characteristics of deaths occurring in children's hospitals: implications for supportive care services. Pediatrics 2002;109(5):887–93.

[88] Billings JA, Pantilat S. Survey of palliative care programs in United States teaching hospitals. J Palliat Med 2001;4(3):309–14.

[89] Zhang B, El-Jawahri A, Prigerson HG. Update on bereavement research: evidence-based guidelines for the diagnosis and treatment of complicated bereavement. J Palliat Med 2006;9(5):1188–203.

[90] Hawton K. Complicated grief after bereavement. BMJ 2007;334(7601):962–3.

[91] Maciejewski PK, Zhang B, Block SD, et al. An empirical examination of the stage theory of grief. JAMA 2007;297(7):716–23.

[92] Jong-Berg MA, deVlaming D. Bereavement care for families part 1: a review of a paediatric follow-up programme. Int J Palliat Nurs 2005;11(10):533–9.

[93] Jong-Berg MA, Kane L. Bereavement care for families part 2: evaluation of a paediatric follow-up programme. Int J Palliat Nurs 2006;12(10):484–94.

[94] Russo C, Wong AF. The bereaved parent. J Clin Oncol 2005;23(31):8109–11.

[95] von Gunten CF, Ferris FD, Kirschner C, et al. Coding and reimbursement mechanisms for physician services in hospice and palliative care. J Palliat Med 2000;3(2):157–64.

[96] American Medical Association. CPT 2008. Chicago: American Medical Association; 2007.

[97] American Medical Association. ICD-9-CM official guidelines for coding and reporting. Chicago: American Medical Association; 2006.

[98] World Health Organization. 2007. WHO definition of palliative care for children. Available at: http://www.whoint/cancer/palliative/definition/en/. Accessed August 23, 2007.

PEDIATRIC CLINICS
OF NORTH AMERICA

Pediatr Clin N Am 55 (2008) 251–273

Challenges After Curative Treatment for Childhood Cancer and Long-Term Follow up of Survivors

Kevin C. Oeffinger, MD[a,*], Paul C. Nathan, MD, MSc[b], Leontien C.M. Kremer, MD, PhD[c]

[a]Department of Pediatrics, Memorial Sloan-Kettering Cancer Center, 1275 York Avenue,
New York, NY 10021, USA
[b]Division of Haematology/Oncology, The Hospital for Sick Children, 555 University Avenue,
Toronto, ON M5G 1X8, Canada
[c]Department of Paediatric Oncology, Emma Children's Hospital/Academic Medical Center,
Meibergdreef 9, 1105 AZ Amsterdam, the Netherlands

Cancer in childhood or adolescence is rare. Each year, for every 100,000 persons under the age of 21 years, 16 are diagnosed with cancer. Today, more than 80% of those diagnosed with a childhood cancer will become a long-term survivor [1]. Many cancer survivors will develop serious morbidity, die at a young age from noncancer causes, and experience diminished health status. Among children treated in the 1970s to 1990s, about 75% will develop a chronic disease by 40 years of age, and over 40% will develop a serious health problem [2,3]. The absolute excess risk of premature death from a second cancer, cardiovascular disease, or pulmonary disease is significantly elevated beyond 30 years after the cancer diagnosis [4,5]. Almost half of long-term survivors will have moderate to extremely diminished health status, including limitations in activity and functional impairment [6,7]. Although some serious problems occur during the cancer therapy or soon thereafter (long-term effects), the majority do not become clinically apparent until many years after the cancer has been cured (late effects) [3]. Contemporary therapy has evolved with a primary aim of not only improving cure but also decreasing the risk of long-term sequelae. It is anticipated that children treated in the 21st century will not experience the frequency and severity of morbidity of those treated in the late 1900s. Furthermore, with proactive and anticipatory risk-based care and healthy lifestyles, the

* Corresponding author.
E-mail address: oeffingk@mskcc.org (K.C. Oeffinger).

0031-3955/08/$ - see front matter © 2008 Elsevier Inc. All rights reserved.
doi:10.1016/j.pcl.2007.10.009
pediatric.theclinics.com

frequency and severity of many late effects of cancer therapy can be significantly reduced [8,9].

Most childhood cancer survivors in North America and Europe are not
followed at a cancer center [10,11]. Instead, over time, they generally drift
back to the care of a primary care physician without a formal transition
from the cancer center, generally unaware of their risks, without a summary
of their cancer or cancer treatment, and with an inadequate understanding
of their previous therapy [11,12]. In a routine year in a typical primary care
practice, a clinician is likely to see fewer than five childhood cancer survivors, each with a different cancer treated with a different regimen. Recognizing the competing demands of a busy primary care practice and the relative
infrequency of seeing a childhood cancer survivor, it can be difficult to stay
up-to-date with the health risks associated with different types of cancer
therapy, much less with the recommendations for surveillance. However,
the primary care physician can play a pivotal role in the health and well
being of a childhood cancer survivor by delivering risk-based health care.

This article is intended to assist the primary care physician in this role.
With a focus on contemporary therapy, the authors begin by providing
a brief discussion of four major types of late effects about which survivors
and their families commonly have questions, including neurocognitive dysfunction, cardiovascular disease, infertility and gonadal dysfunction, and
psychosocial problems. While these questions are often directed to the oncologist during therapy, families may seek further input from their primary
care physician. In the authors' experience, these are also the most common
questions that survivors or their families will ask years after the cancer therapy, often when they are no longer followed by the oncologist. Following
these four topics, the authors discuss the concept of risk-based care, promote the use of recently developed evidence-based guidelines, describe current care in the United States, Canada, and the Netherlands, and articulate
a model for shared survivor care that aims to optimize life-long health of
survivors and improve two-way communication between the cancer center
and the primary care physician. It is not the intent of this article to provide
an exhaustive review of late effects, as recent publications have provided this
information based upon treatment exposure [13] or affected organ system
[14,15]. Two excellent books also provide much detail regarding late effects
and the care of this population [16,17]. Rather, the goal of this article is
to orient the reader regarding the key problems, highlight ways that a primary care physician can positively influence the health of childhood cancer
survivors, and point toward reliable resources for further inquiry.

Neurocognitive dysfunction

The potential for neurocognitive dysfunction is perhaps the most worri-
some outcome to survivors and parents alike. When neurocognitive

problems occur, children commonly present with school difficulties. Primary care physicians that deliver care for survivors should be aware of those at greatest risk, recognize the school difficulties associated with prior cancer therapy, and have an approach to screening, intervention and advocacy. Often this will involve helping the child and the family obtain the legally mandated supports required from the school system [18]. Survivors of central nervous system (CNS) tumors and acute lymphoblastic leukemia (ALL) are at particular risk of neurocognitive late effects, but difficulties have been observed in patients treated with a stem cell transplant [19] or with radiation for tumors of the head or neck. Cranial radiotherapy, particularly higher doses, is the major risk factor for adverse neurocognitive functioning [20–22], and survivors of CNS tumors treated with radiation at a young age are at considerable risk of global neurocognitive difficulties. Fortunately, neurocognitive dysfunction is much less common and severe with contemporary ALL therapy, where cranial radiotherapy is no longer used in patients at low or standard risk of CNS relapse [23]. However, two-thirds of studies of children treated for ALL with chemotherapy alone demonstrate some degree of neurocognitive decline [24], with methotrexate [24–27], corticosteroids [28], and high-dose cytarabine [29] most frequently associated with neurocognitive late effects. Female gender [30–32], younger age at therapy (particularly children less than 3 years) [21,32–39], and increasing time from treatment increase the risk of these sequelae. Worsening academic performance is usually related to a reduced rate of skill acquisition rather than to loss of previously learned information [40], and is independent of the number of days of school missed because of therapy.

Survivors may have impairment in any area of neurocognitive function, but problems with attention and concentration [24,41,42], processing speed, visual perceptual skills [43], executive function [41], and memory [24] are most common. Deficits in attention often manifest without hyperactivity, and can be misinterpreted as disinterest or bad behavior. Careless errors, incomplete assignments, and inconsistent academic performance are common [44], and these survivors often need extra time to complete their schoolwork. This can be compounded by difficulties with planning and organization [41]. Mathematics, reading, and spelling are the most frequently impacted academic areas, [24] and many survivors of ALL and CNS tumors require special education services [45]. School difficulties may not manifest during the primary grades when rote-learning (memorization by repetition) may be relatively intact, but become evident as children transition to middle or high school where organizational, reasoning, and time management skills become essential to successful school performance [18].

When following a childhood cancer survivor, a primary care physician should assess school performance annually. Many pediatric cancer survivor programs obtain detailed neuropsychologic assessments in survivors at higher risk of difficulties, but in some circumstances these tests must be arranged by the survivor's primary care physician. Unfortunately, many insurance providers do not cover this service, and test results may be available only from evaluations performed through the school system. While school-based testing can be helpful in developing an individualized education program, some important, subtle late effects may be missed. The primary care physician can assist parents by educating school personnel about the academic challenges faced by survivors. Several United States federal laws protect the rights of children with mental and physical limitations to receive special education, accommodation, and related services within the school system, and in many cases, these statutes can be applied to cancer survivors with learning difficulties [18].

Once completed, information from neuropsychologic assessments should be shared with the school. Simple educational accommodations include locating the child in the front of the classroom where there is less distraction, reducing the number of items on multiple choice tests, breaking assignments into discrete steps, and allowing more time for the completion of examinations [46]. Other interventions, such as cognitive remediation [42] and pharmacotherapy [47], are currently undergoing investigation with multicenter trials. Even if no specific educational intervention is identified after an initial assessment, it is important to continually reassess a survivor's needs, because deficits may develop over time.

Cardiovascular disease

The developing cardiovascular system of a child or adolescent is very vulnerable to cancer therapy. A cardiomyopathy may develop following exposure to anthracyclines. Mantle radiotherapy promotes the development of coronary and carotid artery disease. In addition, perhaps most commonly, premature cardiovascular disease may result from alterations in multiple organ systems. The following sections describe each of these outcomes and emphasize the role of surveillance and prevention.

Anthracycline-induced cardiomyopathy

Anthracyclines, including doxorubicin and daunorubicin, are an important class of chemotherapeutic agents in the treatment of children with cancer. About half of those treated with contemporary therapy receive an anthracycline. Unfortunately, anthracycline cardiotoxicity is a major and generally unavoidable complication of childhood cancer therapy. The consequences of anthracycline cardiotoxicity for survivors are extensive. Late effects, resulting from myocardial damage, can manifest as left ventricular dysfunction, clinical heart failure, or as cardiac death. Anthracycline cardiotoxicity can be divided in asymptomatic (subclinical) and symptomatic (clinical) cardiotoxicity. Asymptomatic cardiotoxicity is defined as various cardiac abnormalities diagnosed with different diagnostic methods in asymptomatic patients; symptomatic cardiotoxicity is defined as clinical heart failure (CHF). Anthracycline-induced left ventricular dysfunction develops via two mechanisms: depressed contractility and an increased afterload [48]. Late-onset anthracycline cardiotoxicity, occurring after the first year of survivorship, is the direct result of damage done during therapy, and is progressive [48].

Numerous studies have evaluated the cardiotoxic effects of anthracycline therapy in survivors of childhood cancer. As described in previous systematic reviews [49,50], some studies have methodologic limitations: only a selected subgroup of survivors have been evaluated, follow-up is incomplete, or nonstandardized diagnostic measurements have been used. For asymptomatic cardiotoxicity in childhood cancer survivors, a wide variation in the prevalence, from 0% to 56%, has been described [50–53]. Differences in the selection of study groups, cumulative anthracycline dose, outcome definitions, and follow-up period could explain a part of this wide range. The risk of anthracycline-induced (A-) CHF in childhood cancer survivors has been evaluated in several cohort studies [49]. In a cohort study of 831 subjects treated with anthracyclines for childhood cancer, the estimated risk of A-CHF, 20 years after the first dose of anthracyclines, was 9.8% for subjects who received a cumulative dose of greater than or equal to 300 mg/m^2 [54]. Risk factors for anthracycline cardiotoxicity include higher cumulative dose of anthracyclines, radiotherapy involving the heart region, and a few studies suggest younger age at treatment and the female sex [49,50].

The risk of developing clinical heart failure for survivors treated with anthracyclines remains a life-long threat, and guidelines for long-term follow-up advise life-long cardiac monitoring for survivors treated with anthracycline [55,56]. However, management of childhood cancer survivors with asymptomatic cardiotoxicity is unclear [57]. Two studies have investigated the effect of angiotensin converting enzyme inhibitors in childhood cancer survivors [58,59]. Although the results were promising, the noncontrolled trial suggested that enalapril treatment could delay, but not completely prevent, progression of subclinical and clinical cardiotoxicity in survivors [59]. So primary prevention during treatment is essential, such as reducing the cumulative dose of anthracyclines, the use of possible less cardiotoxic anthracycline analogs, and reducing the peak dose or the use of cardioprotective agents [60,61].

Coronary and carotid artery disease following mantle radiotherapy

Moderate dose mantle irradiation (3,500 centigray or cGy–4,500 cGy) was the mainstay for treatment of early stage supradiaphragmatic Hodgkin's disease from the 1960s to the 1980s. The mantle field encompasses the primary lymph node regions of the neck, supraclavicular, infraclavicular, axillary, and mediastinal areas. In a British cohort of 7,003 Hodgkin's survivors with an average of 11.2 years of follow-up, the standardized mortality risk secondary to myocardial infarction was 3.2 for those who were treated with mantle irradiation [62]. The absolute excess risk was 125.8 per 100,000 person-years. Aleman and colleagues [63] reported that by 30 years after mediastinal irradiation, the cumulative incidence of myocardial infarction was 12.9%. They reported a standardized incidence ratio of 3.6 for myocardial infarction, with 357 excess cases per 100,000 person-years. Traditional risk factors (smoking, hypercholesterolemia, diabetes) increased risk. In Dutch Hodgkin's survivors treated with moderate dose mediastinal irradiation (median, 3,720 cGy), Reinders and colleagues [64] reported an actuarial risk of symptomatic ischemic coronary artery disease of 21.2% by 20 years after irradiation. This increased risk of premature coronary artery disease and myocardial infarction following mediastinal irradiation has been consistently reported in several other well-designed studies [65–70]. Carotid artery disease has also been reported following mantle radiotherapy [71,72].

In the past 15 years, modified mantle radiotherapy with a lower total dose (2,000 cGy–2,500 cGy) to involved fields has been used in combination with multiagent therapy. More recent methods, of shielding the heart and equally weighting the anterior and posterior fields, appear to decrease the risk of cardiac disease. However, even with current shielding techniques, the proximal coronary arteries are within the modified mantle fields. So, despite modifications in therapy aimed at reducing risk, children and adolescents treated on contemporary Hodgkin's disease protocols likely still face an increased risk of coronary and carotid artery disease. Longitudinal studies of survivors treated with contemporary therapy are needed to delineate the frequency, onset, and modifying factors of this risk. Aggressive risk reduction of traditional coronary artery disease risk factors (tobacco avoidance and cessation; optimum management of lipid disorders, diabetes mellitus, and hypertension; promotion of physical activity) should also reduce morbidity.

Cardiovascular disease following childhood acute lymphoblastic leukemia a model for multifactorial cardiovascular disease

Children who have survived ALL are more likely to be physically inactive [73,74] and obese [75,76], have increased visceral adiposity [77], develop insulin resistance [78,79] and dyslipidemia [75,80] at a young age, and have poor cardiorespiratory fitness [81]. These outcomes are in part related to cranial radiation, a therapy that is currently used in about 5% to 15% of children with ALL. However, children treated with chemotherapy alone also develop these outcomes, although the risk appears to be somewhat attenuated and possibly later in onset. This constellation of risk factors can be expected to lead to an increased incidence of cardiovascular disease, likely at a relatively young age. Similar outcomes have also been reported in brain tumor survivors [82] and in those treated with a stem cell transplant [83,84]. Research aimed at better understanding these relationships and the mechanisms leading to these outcomes is under way. In addition, the primary care physician should promote healthy behaviors (tobacco avoidance, healthy diet, and physical activity), screen for lipid disorders and insulin resistance, and closely monitor these survivors.

Fertility and gonadal dysfunction

When a child or adolescent is diagnosed with cancer, the discussion of cancer therapy is difficult and complicated, as the oncologist describes the response rates of various protocols, the associated acute toxicities of therapy, and the potential for future health problems related to the therapy. During this stress laden period when therapeutic decisions are made, as a parent faces the potential of losing a child, details regarding the potential for infertility and gonadal dysfunction are often not understood or remembered by families, and sometimes are not adequately provided by the cancer treating team [85]. Later, as the cancer is cured and the interval from completion of the cancer therapy lengthens, questions regarding fertility and gonadal function become more prevalent. The loss of fertility (or even the fear of impaired fertility) and alterations in gonadal function influence the survivor's developing body image, dating relationships, and marriage patterns [86].

Fertility is the most difficult outcome to study in survivors, as the primary endpoint is pregnancy, an outcome that is influenced by many physical and societal factors beyond the direct effect of the cancer therapy on ovarian or testicular function. Fertility is particularly difficult to study in males, as many men are not willing to have a semen analysis and self-reporting a successful impregnation is subject to both over- and under-reporting biases. Further compounding the investigation of fertility in both genders are the often overlapping effects of different cancer therapies on the reproductive system, and the sometimes late recovery of function. Recognizing the complexity of this subject, a detailed description is beyond the scope of this article. Following is a brief overview; for the clinician interested in better understanding these outcomes, two excellent articles written by leading researchers in this area are helpful resources [87,88].

Female survivors, acute ovarian failure, premature menopause, and fertility preservation

Though the ovaries during childhood and adolescence are relatively resistant to chemotherapy-induced damage, they are sensitive to radiation. Among 3,390 women in the Childhood Cancer Survivor Study (CCSS), loss of ovarian function during or shortly following completion of therapy (acute ovarian failure) was reported in 6.3% [89]. More than 70% of women who had been treated with 2,000 cGy or more of ovarian irradiation had acute ovarian failure. Doses of ovarian irradiation below 1,000 cGy were

capable of inducing acute ovarian failure in women who received concomitant alkylating agents (eg, cyclophosphamide) or were older at exposure.
Survivors at greatest risk for acute ovarian failure are those treated with
total body irradiation (TBI) in preparation for a stem cell transplant. Virtually all women treated with TBI after age 10 years will develop acute ovarian
failure [90,91]. In contrast, only 50% of those treated before 10 years of age
will develop this outcome. In addition, women treated with high dose myeloablative therapy (eg, busulfan, melphalan, thiotepa), rather than TBI,
before a stem cell transplant are at high risk of developing acute ovarian
failure [92,93].

Female survivors who do not develop acute ovarian failure are potentially at risk of developing premature menopause (ie, menopause before
age 40 years) and having reduced ovarian reserve. Among 2,819 women
in the CCSS cohort who did not have acute ovarian failure, Sklar and colleagues [94] reported a relative risk of nonsurgical premature menopause of
13.2, when compared with 1,065 siblings. Risk factors for premature menopause among survivors included older attained age, exposure to increasing
dose of radiation to the ovaries, increasing dose of alkylating agents, and
a diagnosis of Hodgkin's disease. For women treated with an alkylating
agent plus abdominopelvic radiation, the cumulative incidence of nonsurgical menopause approached 30% by 40 years of age.

In an assessment of 100 Danish childhood cancer survivors with a median
age of 26 years, Larsen and colleagues [95] reported that women with preserved menstrual cycles had sonographic and endocrine changes suggestive
of diminished ovarian reserve. Decreased number of antral follicles per
ovary was associated with treatment that included ovarian irradiation or
use of alkylating agents, older age at diagnosis, and increasing years of therapy. With cranial radiation doses of 3,000 cGy or higher to the hypothalamic-pituitary axis, women may develop gonadotropin deficiency
affecting fertility and sex hormone production [96–98]. The consequences
of ovarian failure and premature menopause extend beyond the issue of
fertility and may include alterations in bone metabolism, leading to osteoporosis, sexual dysfunction, and body image changes.

In recent years, much attention has been directed toward preserving fertility in females undergoing cancer therapy during their childhood years.
When radiation fields include the pelvis, the ovaries can be surgically trans-
posed to a more protected location [99,100]. However, even after transposi-
tion of the ovaries, some women will develop premature menopause
secondary to their chemotherapy. Hormonal protection of the ovaries with
a gonadotropin-releasing hormone analog has been attempted, with varying
success, in small uncontrolled trials in patients undergoing therapy with moderate to high dose alkylating agents [101]. Because the success rate of cryopreservation of unfertilized oocytes is very low, and the necessary ovarian
hormonal stimulation before removal of the oocytes may delay cancer therapy, this approach is used infrequently in adolescents with cancer [102].

Lastly, ovarian tissue cryopreservation is an investigational method of fertility preservation that has the advantage of requiring neither a sperm donor nor ovarian stimulation [85]. The American Society of Clinical Oncology recommends that oncologists discuss fertility preservation options as appropriate, and to refer interested patients and their families to reproductive specialists [85].

Encouragingly, women who become pregnant following childhood cancer generally have favorable outcomes. Among 1,953 women in the CCSS, 4,029 live births were reported and no association was found between chemotherapy and an adverse pregnancy outcome [103]. Previous pelvic irradiation was associated with lower birth weight.

Male survivors, infertility, fertility preservation, and androgen deficiency

The germinal epithelium of the testis is sensitive to radiation. Even low-dose testicular irradiation is associated with decreased spermatogenesis, with doses above 200 cGy invariably causing oligospermia or azoospermia [87]. Thus, males treated TBI, with a fractionated dose of 1,200 cGy to 1500 cGy, are often rendered infertile [104]. Similarly, males with ALL who are treated with irradiation of the testis for a testicular relapse will almost always be azoospermic. Though the testes are shielded with modern techniques, scatter radiation from high-dose radiation can result in oligospermia or azoospermia. Examples include pelvic, inguinal, or spinal radiation for a sarcoma, Hodgkin's disease, or CNS tumor, respectively [105,106]. Lastly, radiation to the hypothalamic-pituitary axis may result in a gonadotropin deficiency, thus indirectly affecting spermatogenesis and reproductive potential.

Spermatogenesis is also quite affected by several chemotherapeutic drugs, including alkylating agents (eg, cyclophosphamide and ifosfamide), procarbazine, and cisplatin. Outcomes are agent specific and dose-dependent. Treatment with moderate to high-dose cyclophosphamide or ifosfamide often results in azoospermia. The combination of these two agents, used in the treatment of patients with Ewing sarcoma, causes infertility in virtually all males [107]. Similarly, the combination of cisplatin with either ifosfamide or cyclophosphamide, used in the contemporary treatment of osteosarcoma, results in oligospermia or azoospermia in over 90% of males [107]. High-dose melphalan or busulfan, used in some preconditioning regimens before a stem cell transplant, also causes impaired spermatogenesis in the vast majority of males [87]. Early chemotherapeutic regimens used for Hodgkin's disease, including six courses of mechlorethamine, vincristine, procarbazine, and prednisone, generally resulted in a high incidence of azoospermia. To preserve fertility, contemporary multimodality therapy of Hodgkin's disease and non-Hodgkin lymphoma generally includes only three courses of an alkylating agent or procarbazine, alternating with another group of agents with a different set of toxicities.

Sperm cryopreservation is an effective method of fertility preservation in males [85,108]. Unfortunately, spermarche does not occur until about 13 to 14 years of age, thus limiting sperm banking to adolescent males. In general, methods to preserve fertility in younger males, including testicular tissue cryopreservation, have not been successful [85]. While it is recommended that the oncologist discuss sperm banking with all appropriate patients, it is also important for the primary care physician to be aware of this option if the patient or the family has any questions.

In comparison with the germinal epithelium, the Leydig cells are less affected by chemotherapy and radiotherapy. Testicular irradiation with doses of greater than 2,000 cGy and 3,000 cGy are associated with Leydig cell dysfunction in prepubertal and sexually mature males, respectively [87]. Even with high dose cyclophosphamide, frankly subnormal levels of testosterone are rare, though Leydig cell dysfunction may be evidenced by an elevated luteinizing hormone level [109]. Whether or not mild Leydig cell dysfunction will lead to premature androgen deficiency as this population ages is not known. Androgen deficiency can also result from hypogonadotropic hypogonadism following cranial radiotherapy.

Psychosocial issues in survivors and their families

The experience of being diagnosed and treated for cancer during childhood exerts considerable psychologic strain on both the patient and the family. Despite this, many survivors report normal psychologic health, and some even demonstrate psychologic growth as a result of their cancer experience. Additionally, most studies suggest that survivors are less likely to exhibit risky behaviors, such as cigarette smoking or drug use [110–112]. However, on average, childhood cancer survivors are more likely to present with mental health disorders and to complain of chronic pain or fatigue than the general population. Hudson and colleagues [6] reported that 17% of 9,535 young adult survivors of childhood cancer in the CCSS had depressive, somatic, or anxiety symptoms, and 10% reported moderate to extreme pain as a result of their cancer. Approximately one out five young adult survivors of childhood cancer reports symptoms of posttraumatic stress disorder (PTSD) [113,114], characterized by re-experiencing elements of their prior cancer experience or its associated emotions, avoidance of people or places that remind them of their previous cancer, and increased anxiety or arousal. Avoidant behaviors may inhibit survivors from seeking appropriate follow-up care, particularly if care is delivered in the hospital where they received their cancer therapy. Additionally, both parents [115,116] and siblings [117] of survivors may develop symptoms of PTSD, and thus the primary care physician must extend their assessment of mental health to survivors' families. Rather than developing PTSD, some survivors demonstrate posttraumatic growth [118] and psychosocial thriving [119] as a result of their cancer experience. Many rate themselves highly on their ability to cope as a result of their prior cancer, suggesting that this life-altering event promotes resiliency [120]. When survivors do report psychologic distress, it is associated frequently with poorer health status, lower levels of income, and poorer social functioning [121,122].

Physicians need to be sensitive to the concerns expressed by survivors who often worry about fertility and parenthood, obtaining health and life insurance, educational difficulties, job availability after completing school, and their risk for future health problems, including second cancers [123,124]. Although most survivors become socially independent and leave home at a similar age to the general population, rates of marriage are slightly lower [125–127]. Survivors of CNS tumors are at particular risk of not marrying, and many are unable to live independently [128]. Additionally, survivors of CNS tumors (but not other cancers) may be at increased risk of hospitalization for a psychiatric disorder [129]. Primary care physicians can support these patients by providing interventions that improve health, support educational or occupational advancement to improve income potential, and promote social interaction [121]. In particular, the development of a social network has been shown to enhance quality of life in survivors [130].

Several organizations provide services that can assist survivors, their parents, and their health care providers in dealing with the various challenges that may arise as these children and adolescents move beyond their primary cancer (Table 1). Two books written for survivors or their families provide quality information and address the specific challenges of the cancer experience and survivorship [131,132].

Risk-based health care and shared care of cancer survivors

Because the risk and severity of many late effects is modifiable, and some are preventable, life long health care is recommended for all childhood cancer survivors [9]. A systematic plan for longitudinal screening, surveillance, and prevention that incorporates risks based on the previous cancer, cancer therapy, genetic predispositions, lifestyle behaviors, and comorbid health conditions should be developed for all childhood cancer survivors.

To facilitate and standardize risk-based care of childhood cancer survivors, several evidence-based guidelines have been developed [55,56, 133,134]. In the development of these guidelines, the evidence of the association between a therapeutic exposure and a late effect is generally of high quality. However, with a relatively small population of childhood cancer survivors limiting prospective study design, there are no studies that have estimated the reduction in morbidity or mortality with surveillance. Thus, principles of screening in the general population and other high-risk groups have been applied, in addition to the collective clinical experience of expert panels, in the development of surveillance recommendations [55].

Table 1
Resources for childhood cancer survivors, their parent and caregivers

Service and disability organizations	Service provided
National Childhood Cancer Foundation 440 E. Huntington Dr., Arcadia, CA 91066-6012, (800) 458-6223. http://www.curesearch.org	Provides information and resources for pediatric cancer survivors.
American Cancer Society 1599 Clifton Rd NE, Atlanta, GA 30329-4215, (800) ACS-2345. http://www.cancer.org	Programs include equipment and supplies, support groups, educational literature, and summer camps for childhood cancer survivors.
Canadian Cancer Society 565 W. 10th Ave., Vancouver, BC V5Z 4J4 Canada. http://www.bc.cancer.ca	Programs include those that the American Cancer Society provides.
Association of Cancer Online Resources http://www.acor.org	Online information and electronic support groups for pediatric cancer survivors and their caregivers.
Candlelighters Childhood Cancer Foundation 3910 Warner St., Kensington, MD 20895, (800) 366-CCCF. http://www.candlelighters.org	Provides resource guides, quarterly newsletters, referrals, information, and publishes books for pediatric cancer survivors, including *Educating the Child with Cancer*.
Candlelighters Childhood Cancer Foundation Canada 55 Eglington Ave. E., Suite 401, Toronto, Ontario M4P 1G8 Canada, (800) 363-1062. http://www.candlelighters.org.ca	Provides resource guides, newsletters, and information.
Childhood Cancer Ombudsman Program 27 Witch Duck Lane, Heathsville, VA 22473. gpmonaco@rivnet.net	Provides help for pediatric cancer survivors experiencing problems getting access to appropriate education, medical care, health care cost coverage, and employment.

Federation for Children with Special Needs
1135 Tremont St, Suite 420, Boston, MA 02120, (617) 236-7210.
http://www.fcsn.org

Lance Armstrong Foundation
P.O. Box 161150, Austin, TX 78716, (866) 235-7205. www.livestrong.org

National Center for Learning Disabilities
381 Park Ave. S., Suite 1401, New York, NY 10016, (888) 575-7373.
http://www.ncld.org

US Department of Justice
ADA Information Line, Civil Rights Division, PO Box 66738, Washington,
DC 20035, (800) 514-0301. http://www.usdoj.gov/crt/ada/adahom1.htm

Federally funded organization providing information on special education
rights and laws, conferences, referrals for services, parent training
workshops, publications, and advocacy information.

A nonprofit organization that offers extensive education, advocacy and
public health resources.

Offers extensive resources, referral services, and educational programs
related to learning disabilities.

Answers questions about the Americans with Disabilities Act, explains how
to file a complaint, and provides dispute resolution information.

Data from Nathan PC, Patel SK, Dilley K, et al. Guidelines for identification of, advocacy for, and intervention in neurocognitive problems in survivors of childhood cancer: a report from the Children's Oncology Group. Arch Pediatr Adolesc Med 2007;161(8):798–806.

In North America, the 240-institution Children's Oncology Group (COG) "Long-Term Follow-Up Guidelines for Survivors of Childhood, Adolescent, and Young Adult Cancers" (available at www.survivor shipguidelines.org) are widely used [55]. Recommendations for periodic evaluations are based upon different treatment exposures or therapeutic modalities and include modifying risk factors. For each late effect, a score of the quality of the evidence is provided, along with supporting references. In addition, over 40 different patient education handouts (Health Links) that discuss frequent problems or questions are accessible through the Web site. The guidelines are periodically reviewed by the COG Late Effects Committee and updated as new evidence becomes available.

In the Netherlands, 16 multidisciplinary teams summarized the evidence in existing guidelines, systematic reviews, books, and papers based on clinical questions regarding the magnitude of the risk of selected late effects, the efficacy of screening, and possible treatments. Ten nationwide meetings were held to define the final Dutch recommendations based on available evidence [134]. These recommendations led to standardization and improvement of patient care for survivors in the Netherlands [2].

Long-term follow up practices vary across the United States, Canada, and the Netherlands. In the United States, most COG institutions have a specialized long-term follow up (LTFU) program that delivers risk-based health care for survivors during their childhood years [135,136]. However, because of insurance limitations, travel distances, and other barriers, survivors are gradually lost to follow-up over time. Moreover, very few LTFU programs in the United States provide care for childhood cancer survivors who are in their adult years. In Canada, Ontario is the only province with a coordinated system of care for both pediatric and adult survivors of childhood cancer. The province funds a group of coordinated Aftercare Clinics, located in cancer centers in five major cities across the province (see http://www.pogo.ca/care/aftercareclinics/, accessed August 29, 2007). Although the majority of survivors receive their medical care in such a program during their childhood years, many adult survivors are not seen regularly in these Aftercare programs, despite such care being provided free of charge. The majority of adult survivors of childhood cancer in Canada report receiving care from a family physician [137]. In the Netherlands, all pediatric oncology centers have an LTFU program and most children are followed through these programs. As in the United States, financial support limits the care of adult survivors.

The majority of late effects become clinically apparent many years after the cancer therapy, generally when survivors are in their adult years [3]. This is the time period when most survivors in North America and Europe are no longer followed in a specialized LTFU program. Formal transition of survivors to their primary care physician, with proper communication, is rare. Instead, follow-up care tends to be haphazard for most survivors. If our common goal is to optimize the life-long health of survivors, it is imperative that LTFU programs implement strategies that efficiently allocate limited resources where they are most needed.

As illustrated in Fig. 1, one potential strategy is to integrate primary care physicians into a risk-stratified shared care model [11,138,139]. This strategy stratifies survivors into three groups based upon their risk of late effects (see Fig. 1 for potential groupings). Given their expertise in this area, the stratification would be determined by the LTFU staff. All survivors would continue to have their noncancer-related care delivered by the primary care physician. At the time of diagnosis, the primary oncologist would mail (or

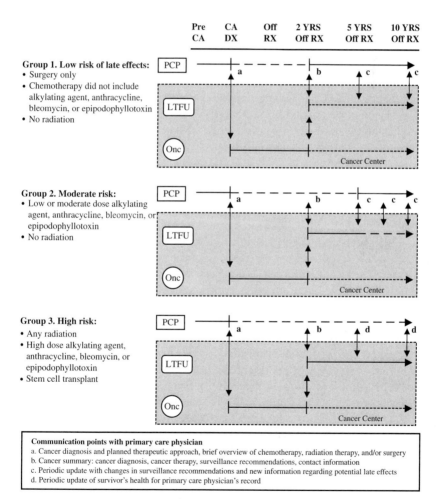

Fig. 1. Proposed risk-stratified shared care model for childhood cancer survivors. Solid line denotes primary responsibility for risk-based care; risk stratification based upon determination of the LTFU staff. CA, cancer; DX, diagnosis; Onc, Oncologist; PCP, primary care provider; RX, therapy. (*Adapted from* Oeffinger KC, McCabe MS. Models for delivering survivorship care. J Clin Oncol 2006;24(32):5119; with permission from the American Society of Clinical Oncology.)

fax) the primary care physician a summary of the cancer treatment plan. At 2 years following the completion of therapy, the survivor would be transitioned from the oncology team to the LTFU program for a single visit. At this visit, a cancer summary would be developed and include information about the cancer, cancer therapy, and recommended surveillance. A copy of the summary would be sent to the primary care physician, with a lay version provided to the survivor (and his or her family). After this single LTFU visit, the survivor at low risk would be transitioned to the primary care physician for periodic risk-based care. The LTFU staff would communicate with the primary care physician every 3 to 5 years and inquire about changes in the survivor's health and any new findings that might change surveillance recommendations. Survivors at moderate risk would be followed annually through the LTFU program for their risk-based care until 5 to 10 years after the completion of cancer therapy. During this time period, in addition to monitoring for late effects and surveillance for recurrence, age- and developmental stage-appropriate education and counseling highlighting the benefits of healthy lifestyles would be provided. At 5 to 10 years after cancer therapy, depending upon the program, the survivor would be transitioned to their primary care physician for the delivery of risk-based care. At the time of transition, the LTFU staff would provide the primary care physician with an updated treatment summary and surveillance plan, and then annually communicate with the primary care physician (and survivor if needed) to document any new late effects, changes in lifestyle behaviors and family history, and update the surveillance recommendations. The LTFU program would also serve in a consultative mode, as needed, for survivors at low or moderate risk who develop a late effect or need further evaluation. A survivor at high risk of developing late effects would continue to be monitored through the LTFU program, with continued communication with the primary care physician regarding any new health problems and planned surveillance (to avoid duplication of testing).

This strategy would allow LTFU programs to concentrate their resources on the survivors at highest risk and provide foundational education and counseling to those at moderate risk. Furthermore, the standardized and systematic communication between the LTFU staff and the primary care physician would serve to inform both groups of the evolving health and health care needs of the survivor. To implement this strategy, LTFU programs located at a children's hospital that restricts care of adult patients would need to develop an alternative strategy for the care of their high risk survivors.

Summary

Late effects of therapy for childhood cancer are frequent and serious. Fortunately, many late effects are also modifiable. Proactive and anticipatory risk-based care can reduce the frequency and severity of treatment-related morbidity. The primary care physician should be an integral component in risk-based care of survivors.

Acknowledgments

The authors would like to acknowledge Dr. Charles Sklar for his insightful comments with this review.

References

[1] Ries LAG, Melbert D, Krapcho M, et al. SEER cancer statistics review, 1975–2004. Bethesda (MD): National Cancer Institute; 2007. Available at: http://seer.cancer.gov/csr/1975_2004/. Based on November 2006 SEER data submission, posted to the SEER Web site. Accessed September 1, 2007.

[2] Geenen MM, Cardous-Ubbink MC, Kremer LC, et al. Medical assessment of adverse health outcomes in long-term survivors of childhood cancer. JAMA 2007;297(24):2705–15.

[3] Oeffinger KC, Mertens AC, Sklar CA, et al. Chronic health conditions in adult survivors of childhood cancer. N Engl J Med 2006;355(15):1572–82.

[4] Mertens AC, Yasui Y, Neglia JP, et al. Late mortality experience in five-year survivors of childhood and adolescent cancer: the Childhood Cancer Survivor Study. J Clin Oncol 2001; 19(13):3163–72.

[5] Moller TR, Garwicz S, Barlow L, et al. Decreasing late mortality among five-year survivors of cancer in childhood and adolescence: a population-based study in the Nordic countries. J Clin Oncol 2001;19(13):3173–81.

[6] Hudson MM, Mertens AC, Yasui Y, et al. Health status of adult long-term survivors of childhood cancer: a report from the Childhood Cancer Survivor Study. JAMA 2003; 290(12):1583–92.

[7] Ness KK, Mertens AC, Hudson MM, et al. Limitations on physical performance and daily activities among long-term survivors of childhood cancer. Ann Intern Med 2005;143(9): 639–47.

[8] Oeffinger KC. Longitudinal risk-based health care for adult survivors of childhood cancer. Curr Probl Cancer 2003;27(3):143–67.

[9] Hewitt M, Weiner SL, Simone JV, editors. Childhood cancer survivorship: improving care and quality of life. Washington, DC: National Academies Press; 2003.

[10] Oeffinger KC, Mertens AC, Hudson MM, et al. Health care of young adult survivors of childhood cancer: a report from the Childhood Cancer Survivor Study. Ann Fam Med 2004;2(1):61–70.

[11] Oeffinger KC, Wallace WH. Barriers to follow-up care of survivors in the United States and the United Kingdom. Pediatr Blood Cancer 2006;46(2):135–42.

[12] Kadan-Lottick NS, Robison LL, Gurney JG, et al. Childhood cancer survivors' knowledge about their past diagnosis and treatment: Childhood Cancer Survivor Study. JAMA 2002; 287(14):1832–9.

[13] Oeffinger KC, Hudson MM. Long-term complications following childhood and adolescent cancer: foundations for providing risk-based health care for survivors. CA Cancer J Clin 2004;54(4):208–36.

[14] Bhatia S, Landier W. Evaluating survivors of pediatric cancer. Cancer J 2005;11(4):340–54.

[15] Friedman DL, Meadows AT. Late effects of childhood cancer therapy. Pediatr Clin North Am 2002;49(5):1083–106.

[16] Wallace WH, Green DM, editors. Late effects of childhood cancer. London: Arnold Publishers; 2004.

[17] Schwartz CL, Hobbie WL, Constine LS, et al, editors. Survivors of childhood and adolescent cancer: a multidisciplinary approach. Berlin: Springer-Verlag; 2005.

[18] Nathan PC, Patel SK, Dilley K, et al. Guidelines for identification of, advocacy for, and intervention in neurocognitive problems in survivors of childhood cancer: a report from the Children's Oncology Group. Arch Pediatr Adolesc Med 2007;161(8):798–806.

[19] Kramer JH, Crittenden MR, DeSantes K, et al. Cognitive and adaptive behavior 1 and 3 years following bone marrow transplantation. Bone Marrow Transplant 1997;19(6): 607–13.

[20] Grill J, Renaux VK, Bulteau C, et al. Long-term intellectual outcome in children with posterior fossa tumors according to radiation doses and volumes. Int J Radiat Oncol Biol Phys 1999;45(1):137–45.

[21] Mulhern RK, Kepner JL, Thomas PR, et al. Neuropsychologic functioning of survivors of childhood medulloblastoma randomized to receive conventional or reduced-dose craniospinal irradiation: a Pediatric Oncology Group study. J Clin Oncol 1998;16(5): 1723–8.

[22] Ris MD, Packer R, Goldwein J, et al. Intellectual outcome after reduced-dose radiation therapy plus adjuvant chemotherapy for medulloblastoma: a Children's Cancer Group study. J Clin Oncol 2001;19(15):3470–6.

[23] Pui CH, Evans WE. Treatment of acute lymphoblastic leukemia. N Engl J Med 2006; 354(2):166–78.

[24] Moleski M. Neuropsychological, neuroanatomical, and neurophysiological consequences of CNS chemotherapy for acute lymphoblastic leukemia. Arch Clin Neuropsychol 2000; 15(7):603–30.

[25] Espy KA, Moore IM, Kaufmann PM, et al. Chemotherapeutic CNS prophylaxis and neuropsychologic change in children with acute lymphoblastic leukemia: a prospective study. J Pediatr Psychol 2001;26(1):1–9.

[26] Riva D, Giorgi C, Nichelli F, et al. Intrathecal methotrexate affects cognitive function in children with medulloblastoma. Neurology 2002;59(1):48–53.

[27] Brown RT, Madan-Swain A, Walco GA, et al. Cognitive and academic late effects among children previously treated for acute lymphocytic leukemia receiving chemotherapy as CNS prophylaxis. J Pediatr Psychol 1998;23(5):333–40.

[28] Waber DP, Carpentieri SC, Klar N, et al. Cognitive sequelae in children treated for acute lymphoblastic leukemia with dexamethasone or prednisone. J Pediatr Hematol Oncol 2000;22(3):206–13.

[29] Nand S, Messmore HL Jr, Patel R, et al. Neurotoxicity associated with systemic high-dose cytosine arabinoside. J Clin Oncol 1986;4(4):571–5.

[30] von der Weid N, Mosimann I, Hirt A, et al. Intellectual outcome in children and adolescents with acute lymphoblastic leukaemia treated with chemotherapy alone: age- and sex-related differences. Eur J Cancer 2003;39(3):359–65.

[31] Waber DP, Tarbell NJ, Kahn CM, et al. The relationship of sex and treatment modality to neuropsychologic outcome in childhood acute lymphoblastic leukemia. J Clin Oncol 1992;10(5):810–7.

[32] Christie D, Leiper AD, Chessells JM, et al. Intellectual performance after presymptomatic cranial radiotherapy for leukaemia: effects of age and sex. Arch Dis Child 1995;73(2): 136–40.

[33] Ronning C, Sundet K, Due-Tonnessen B, et al. Persistent cognitive dysfunction secondary to cerebellar injury in patients treated for posterior fossa tumors in childhood. Pediatr Neurosurg 2005;41(1):15–21.

[34] Palmer SL, Goloubeva O, Reddick WE, et al. Patterns of intellectual development among survivors of pediatric medulloblastoma: a longitudinal analysis. J Clin Oncol 2001;19(8): 2302–8.

[35] Copeland DR, deMoor C, Moore BD 3rd, et al. Neurocognitive development of children after a cerebellar tumor in infancy: a longitudinal study. J Clin Oncol 1999;17(11):3476–86.

[36] Packer RJ, Sutton LN, Atkins TE, et al. A prospective study of cognitive function in children receiving whole-brain radiotherapy and chemotherapy: 2-year results. J Neurosurg 1989;70(5):707–13.

[37] Radcliffe J, Bunin GR, Sutton LN, et al. Cognitive deficits in long-term survivors of childhood medulloblastoma and other noncortical tumors: age-dependent effects of whole brain radiation. Int J Dev Neurosci 1994;12(4):327–34.

[38] Radcliffe J, Packer RJ, Atkins TE, et al. Three- and four-year cognitive outcome in children with noncortical brain tumors treated with whole-brain radiotherapy. Ann Neurol 1992; 32(4):551–4.

[39] Kaleita TA, Reaman GH, MacLean WE, et al. Neurodevelopmental outcome of infants with acute lymphoblastic leukemia: a Children's Cancer Group report. Cancer 1999;85(8): 1859–65.

[40] Mabbott DJ, Spiegler BJ, Greenberg ML, et al. Serial evaluation of academic and behavioral outcome after treatment with cranial radiation in childhood. J Clin Oncol 2005;23(10): 2256–63.

[41] Mulhern RK, Palmer SL. Neurocognitive late effects in pediatric cancer. Curr Probl Cancer 2003;27(4):177–97.

[42] Butler RW, Copeland DR. Attentional processes and their remediation in children treated for cancer: a literature review and the development of a therapeutic approach. J Int Neuropsychol Soc 2002;8(1):115–24.

[43] Said JA, Waters BG, Cousens P, et al. Neuropsychological sequelae of central nervous system prophylaxis in survivors of childhood acute lymphoblastic leukemia. J Consult Clin Psychol 1989;57(2):251–6.

[44] Armstrong FD, Briery BG. Childhood cancer and the school. In: Brown RT, editor. Handbook of pediatric psychology in school settings. Mahwah (NJ): Lawrence Erlbaum Associates, Inc.; 2004. p. 263–81.

[45] Kingma A, van Dommelen RI, Mooyaart EL, et al. Slight cognitive impairment and magnetic resonance imaging abnormalities but normal school levels in children treated for acute lymphoblastic leukemia with chemotherapy only. J Pediatr 2001;139(3):413–20.

[46] Butler RW, Mulhern RK. Neurocognitive interventions for children and adolescents surviving cancer. J Pediatr Psychol 2005;30(1):65–78.

[47] Mulhern RK, Khan RB, Kaplan S, et al. Short-term efficacy of methylphenidate: a randomized, double-blind, placebo-controlled trial among survivors of childhood cancer. J Clin Oncol 2004;22(23):4743–51.

[48] Lipshultz SE, Lipsitz SR, Sallan SE, et al. Chronic progressive cardiac dysfunction years after doxorubicin therapy for childhood acute lymphoblastic leukemia. J Clin Oncol 2005;23(12):2629–36.

[49] Kremer LC, van Dalen EC, Offringa M, et al. Frequency and risk factors of anthracycline-induced clinical heart failure in children: a systematic review. Ann Oncol 2002;13(4): 503–12.

[50] Kremer LC, van der Pal HJ, Offringa M, et al. Frequency and risk factors of subclinical cardiotoxicity after anthracycline therapy in children: a systematic review. Ann Oncol 2002; 13(6):819–29.

[51] Lipshultz SE, Colan SD, Gelber RD, et al. Late cardiac effects of doxorubicin therapy for acute lymphoblastic leukemia in childhood. N Engl J Med 1991;324(12):808–15.

[52] Rammeloo LA, Postma A, Sobotka-Plojhar MA, et al. Low-dose daunorubicin in induction treatment of childhood acute lymphoblastic leukemia: no long-term cardiac damage in a randomized study of the Dutch Childhood Leukemia Study Group. Med Pediatr Oncol 2000;35(1):13–9.

[53] Hudson MM, Rai SN, Nunez C, et al. Noninvasive evaluation of late anthracycline cardiac toxicity in childhood cancer survivors. J Clin Oncol 2007;25(24):3635–43.

[54] van Dalen EC, van der Pal HJ, Kok WE, et al. Clinical heart failure in a cohort of children treated with anthracyclines: a long-term follow-up study. Eur J Cancer 2006; 42(18):3191–8.

[55] Landier W, Bhatia S, Eshelman DA, et al. Development of risk-based guidelines for pediatric cancer survivors: the Children's Oncology Group long-term follow-up guidelines from the Children's Oncology Group Late Effects Committee and nursing discipline. J Clin Oncol 2004;22(24):4979–90.

[56] Scottish Intercollegiate Guidelines Network (SIGN). Long term follow up of survivors of childhood cancer. Guideline no. 76. Available at: www.sign.ac.uk/pdf/sign76.pdf. Accessed September 1, 2007.

[57] van Dalen EC, Caron HN, Kremer LC. Prevention of anthracycline-induced cardiotoxicity in children: the evidence. Eur J Cancer 2007;43(7):1134–40.

[58] Silber JH, Cnaan A, Clark BJ, et al. Enalapril to prevent cardiac function decline in long-term survivors of pediatric cancer exposed to anthracyclines. J Clin Oncol 2004;22(5):820–8.

[59] Lipshultz SE, Lipsitz SR, Sallan SE, et al. Long-term enalapril therapy for left ventricular dysfunction in doxorubicin-treated survivors of childhood cancer. J Clin Oncol 2002; 20(23):4517–22.

[60] van Dalen EC, van der Pal HJ, Reitsma JB, et al. Management of asymptomatic anthracycline-induced cardiac damage after treatment for childhood cancer: a postal survey among Dutch adult and pediatric cardiologists. J Pediatr Hematol Oncol 2005;27(6):319–22.

[61] Wouters KA, Kremer LC, Miller TL, et al. Protecting against anthracycline-induced myocardial damage: a review of the most promising strategies. Br J Haematol 2005;131(5): 561–78.

[62] Swerdlow AJ, Higgins CD, Smith P, et al. Myocardial infarction mortality risk after treatment for Hodgkin disease: a collaborative British cohort study. J Natl Cancer Inst 2007; 99(3):206–14.

[63] Aleman BM, van den Belt-Dusebout AW, De Bruin ML, et al. Late cardiotoxicity after treatment for Hodgkin lymphoma. Blood 2007;109(5):1878–86.

[64] Reinders JG, Heijmen BJ, Olofsen-van Acht MJ, et al. Ischemic heart disease after mantlefield irradiation for Hodgkin's disease in long-term follow-up. Radiother Oncol 1999;51(1):35–42.

[65] Boivin JF, Hutchison GB, Lubin JH, et al. Coronary artery disease mortality in patients treated for Hodgkin's disease. Cancer 1992;69(5):1241–7.

[66] Constine LS, Schwartz RG, Savage DE, et al. Cardiac function, perfusion, and morbidity in irradiated long-term survivors of Hodgkin's disease. Int J Radiat Oncol Biol Phys 1997; 39(4):897–906.

[67] Hancock SL, Tucker MA, Hoppe RT. Factors affecting late mortality from heart disease after treatment of Hodgkin's disease. JAMA 1993;270(16):1949–55.

[68] Heidenreich PA, Schnittger I, Strauss HW, et al. Screening for coronary artery disease after mediastinal irradiation for Hodgkin's disease. J Clin Oncol 2007;25(1):43–9.

[69] Hull MC, Morris CG, Pepine CJ, et al. Valvular dysfunction and carotid, subclavian, and coronary artery disease in survivors of Hodgkin lymphoma treated with radiation therapy. JAMA 2003;290(21):2831–7.

[70] King V, Constine LS, Clark D, et al. Symptomatic coronary artery disease after mantle irradiation for Hodgkin's disease. Int J Radiat Oncol Biol Phys 1996;36(4):881–9.

[71] Bowers DC, McNeil DE, Liu Y, et al. Stroke as a late treatment effect of Hodgkin's disease: a report from the Childhood Cancer Survivor Study. J Clin Oncol 2005;23(27): 6508–15.

[72] Meeske KA, Nelson MD, Lavey RS, et al. Premature carotid artery disease in long-term survivors of childhood cancer treated with neck irradiation: a series of 5 cases. J Pediatr Hematol Oncol 2007;29(7):480–4.

[73] Florin TA, Fryer GE, Miyoshi T, et al. Physical inactivity in adult survivors of childhood acute lymphoblastic leukemia: a report from the Childhood Cancer Survivor Study. Cancer Epidemiol Biomarkers Prev 2007;16(7):1356–63.

[74] Reilly JJ, Ventham JC, Ralston JM, et al. Reduced energy expenditure in preobese children treated for acute lymphoblastic leukemia. Pediatr Res 1998;44(4):557–62.

[75] Jarfelt M, Lannering D, Bosaeus I, et al. Body composition in young adult survivors of childhood acute lymphoblastic leukaemia. Eur J Endocrinol 2005;153(1);81–9.

[76] Oeffinger KC, Mertens AC, Sklar CA, et al. Obesity in adult survivors of childhood acute lymphoblastic leukemia: a report from the Childhood Cancer Survivor Study. J Clin Oncol 2003;21(7):1359–65.

[77] Janiszewski PM, Oeffinger KC, Church TS, et al. Abdominal obesity, liver fat and muscle composition in survivors of childhood acute lymphoblastic leukemia. J Clin Endocrinol Metab 2007;92:3816–21.

[78] Gurney JG, Ness KK, Sibley SD, et al. Metabolic syndrome and growth hormone deficiency in adult survivors of childhood acute lymphoblastic leukemia. Cancer 2006; 107(6):1303–12.

[79] Trimis G, Moschovi M, Papassotiriou I, et al. Early indicators of dysmetabolic syndrome in young survivors of acute lymphoblastic leukemia in childhood as a target for preventing disease. J Pediatr Hematol Oncol 2007;29(5):309–14.

[80] Moschovi M, Trimis G, Apostolakou F, et al. Serum lipid alterations in acute lymphoblastic leukemia of childhood. J Pediatr Hematol Oncol 2004;26(5):289–93.

[81] van Brussel M, Takken T, Lucia A, et al. Is physical fitness decreased in survivors of childhood leukemia? A systematic review. Leukemia 2005;19(1):13–7.

[82] Heikens J, Ubbink MC, van der Pal HP, et al. Long term survivors of childhood brain cancer have an increased risk for cardiovascular disease. Cancer 2000;88(9):2116–21.

[83] Baker KS, Ness KK, Steinberger J, et al. Diabetes, hypertension, and cardiovascular events in survivors of hematopoietic cell transplantation: a report from the Bone Marrow Transplantation Survivor Study. Blood 2007;109(4):1765–72.

[84] Neville KA, Cohn RJ, Steinbeck KS, et al. Hyperinsulinemia, impaired glucose tolerance, and diabetes mellitus in survivors of childhood cancer: prevalence and risk factors. J Clin Endocrinol Metab 2006;91(11):4401–7.

[85] Lee SJ, Schover LR, Partridge AH, et al. American Society of Clinical Oncology recommendations on fertility preservation in cancer patients. J Clin Oncol 2006;24(18):2917–31.

[86] Schover LR. Sexuality and fertility after cancer. Hematology Am Soc Hematol Educ Program 2005;1:523–7.

[87] Critchley H, Thomson AB, Wallace WH. Ovarian and uterine function and reproductive potential. In: Wallace WH, Green DM, editors. Late effects of childhood cancer. London: Arnold Publishers; 2004. p. 225–38.

[88] Thomson AB, Wallace WH, Sklar CA. Testicular function. In: Wallace WH Green DM, editors. Late effects of childhood cancer. London: Arnold Publishers; 2004. p. 239–53.

[89] Chemaitilly W, Mertens AC, Mitby P, et al. Acute ovarian failure in the Childhood Cancer Survivor Study. J Clin Endocrinol Metab 2006;91(5):1723–8.

[90] Sklar C. Maintenance of ovarian function and risk of premature menopause related to cancer treatment. J Natl Cancer Inst Monogr 2005;34:25–7.

[91] Sklar C. Growth and endocrine disturbances after bone marrow transplantation in childhood. Acta Paediatr Suppl 1995;411:57–61 [discussion: 62].

[92] Michel G, Socie G, Gebhard F, et al. Late effects of allogeneic bone marrow transplantation for children with acute myeloblastic leukemia in first complete remission: the impact of conditioning regimen without total-body irradiation—a report from the Societe Francaise de Greffe de Moelle. J Clin Oncol 1997;15(6):2238–46.

[93] Thibaud E, Rodriguez-Macias K, Trivin C, et al. Ovarian function after bone marrow transplantation during childhood. Bone Marrow Transplant 1998;21(3):287–90.

[94] Sklar CA, Mertens AC, Mitby P, et al. Premature menopause in survivors of childhood cancer: a report from the Childhood Cancer Survivor Study. J Natl Cancer Inst 2006; 98(13):890–6.

[95] Larsen EC, Muller J, Schmiegelow K, et al. Reduced ovarian function in long-term survivors of radiation- and chemotherapy-treated childhood cancer. J Clin Endocrinol Metab 2003;88(11):5307–14.

[96] Constine LS, Woolf PD, Cann D, et al. Hypothalamic-pituitary dysfunction after radiation for brain tumors. N Engl J Med 1993;328(2):87–94.

[97] Rappaport R, Brauner R, Czernichow P, et al. Effect of hypothalamic and pituitary irradiation on pubertal development in children with cranial tumors. J Clin Endocrinol Metab 1982;54(6):1164–8.

[98] Sklar CA, Constine LS. Chronic neuroendocrinological sequelae of radiation therapy. Int J Radiat Oncol Biol Phys 1995;31(5):1113–21.

[99] Bisharah M, Tulandi T. Laparoscopic preservation of ovarian function: an underused procedure. Am J Obstet Gynecol 2003;188(2):367–70.

[100] Williams RS, Littell RD, Mendenhall NP. Laparoscopic oophoropexy and ovarian function in the treatment of Hodgkin disease. Cancer 1999;86(10):2138–42.

[101] Blumenfeld Z, Dann E, Avivi I, et al. Fertility after treatment for Hodgkin's disease. Ann Oncol 2002;13(Suppl 1):138–47.

[102] Oktay K, Cil AP, Bang H. Efficiency of oocyte cryopreservation: a meta-analysis. Fertil Steril 2006;86(1):70–80.

[103] Green DM, Whitton JA, Stovall M, et al. Pregnancy outcome of female survivors of childhood cancer: a report from the Childhood Cancer Survivor Study. Am J Obstet Gynecol 2002;187(4):1070–80.

[104] Rovo A, Tichelli A, Passweg JR, et al. Spermatogenesis in long-term survivors after allogeneic hematopoietic stem cell transplantation is associated with age, time interval since transplantation, and apparently absence of chronic GvHD. Blood 2006;108(3):1100–5.

[105] Howell SJ, Shalet SM. Spermatogenesis after cancer treatment: damage and recovery. J Natl Cancer Inst Monogr 2005;34:12–7.

[106] Sklar CA, Robison LL, Nesbit ME, et al. Effects of radiation on testicular function in long-term survivors of childhood acute lymphoblastic leukemia: a report from the Children Cancer Study Group. J Clin Oncol 1990;8(12):1981–7.

[107] Mansky P, Arai A, Stratton P, et al. Treatment late effects in long-term survivors of pediatric sarcoma. Pediatr Blood Cancer 2007;48(2):192–9.

[108] Ginsberg JP, Ogle SK, Tuchman LK, et al. Sperm banking for adolescent and young adult cancer patients: sperm quality, patient, and parent perspectives. Pediatr Blood Cancer 2007, in press.

[109] Kenney LB, Laufer MR, Grant FD, et al. High risk of infertility and long term gonadal damage in males treated with high dose cyclophosphamide for sarcoma during childhood. Cancer 2001;91(3):613–21.

[110] Clarke SA, Eiser C. Health behaviours in childhood cancer survivors: a systematic review. Eur J Cancer 2007;43(9):1373–84.

[111] Larcombe I, Mott M, Hunt L. Lifestyle behaviours of young adult survivors of childhood cancer. Br J Cancer 2002;87(11):1204–9.

[112] Bauld C, Toumbourou JW, Anderson V, et al. Health-risk behaviours among adolescent survivors of childhood cancer. Pediatr Blood Cancer 2005;45(5):706–15.

[113] Rourke MT, Hobbie WL, Schwartz L, et al. Posttrauamatic stress disorder (PTSD) in young adult survivors of childhood cancer. Pediatr Blood Cancer 2007;49(2):177–82.

[114] Schwartz L, Drotar D. Posttraumatic stress and related impairment in survivors of childhood cancer in early adulthood compared to healthy peers. J Pediatr Psychol 2006;31(4): 356–66.

[115] Alderfer MA, Cnaan A, Annunziato RA, et al. Patterns of posttraumatic stress symptoms in parents of childhood cancer survivors. J Fam Psychol 2005;19(3):430–40.

[116] Kazak AE, Alderfer M, Rourke MT, et al. Posttraumatic stress disorder (PTSD) and posttraumatic stress symptoms (PTSS) in families of adolescent childhood cancer survivors. J Pediatr Psychol 2004;29(3):211–9.

[117] Alderfer MA, Labay LE, Kazak AE. Brief report: does posttraumatic stress apply to siblings of childhood cancer survivors? J Pediatr Psychol 2003;28(4):281–6.

[118] Barakat LP, Alderfer MA, Kazak AE. Posttraumatic growth in adolescent survivors of cancer and their mothers and fathers. J Pediatr Psychol 2006;31(4):413–9.

[119] Parry C, Chesler MA. Thematic evidence of psychosocial thriving in childhood cancer survivors. Qual Health Res 2005;15(8):1055–73.

[120] Zebrack BJ, Chesler MA. Quality of life in childhood cancer survivors. Psychooncology 2002;11(2):132–41.

[121] Zebrack BJ, Zevon MA, Turk N, et al. Psychological distress in long-term survivors of solid tumors diagnosed in childhood: a report from the Childhood Cancer Survivor Study. Pediatr Blood Cancer 2007;49(1):47–51.

[122] Zebrack BJ, Gurney JG, Oeffinger K, et al. Psychological outcomes in long-term survivors of childhood brain cancer: a report from the Childhood Cancer Survivor Study. J Clin Oncol 2004;22(6):999–1006.

[123] Langeveld NE, Stam H, Grootenhuis MA, et al. Quality of life in young adult survivors of childhood cancer. Support Care Cancer 2002;10(8):579–600.

[124] Langeveld NE, Grootenhuis MA, Voute PA, et al. Quality of life, self-esteem and worries in young adult survivors of childhood cancer. Psychooncology 2004;13(12):867–81.

[125] Rauck AM, Green DM, Yasui Y, et al. Marriage in the survivors of childhood cancer: a preliminary description from the Childhood Cancer Survivor Study. Med Pediatr Oncol 1999; 33(1):60–3.

[126] Langeveld NE, Ubbink MC, Last BF, et al. Educational achievement, employment and living situation in long-term young adult survivors of childhood cancer in the Netherlands. Psychooncology 2003;12(3):213–25.

[127] Frobisher C, Lancashire ER, Winter DL, et al. Long-term population-based marriage rates among adult survivors of childhood cancer in Britain. Int J Cancer 2007;121(4):846–55.

[128] Koch SV, Kejs AM, Engholm G, et al. Leaving home after cancer in childhood: a measure of social independence in early adulthood. Pediatr Blood Cancer 2006;47(1):61–70.

[129] Ross L, Johansen C, Dalton SO, et al. Psychiatric hospitalizations among survivors of cancer in childhood or adolescence. N Engl J Med 2003;349(7):650–7.

[130] Lim JW, Zebrack B. Social networks and quality of life for long-term survivors of leukemia and lymphoma. Support Care Cancer 2006;14(2):185–92.

[131] Keene N, Hobbie W, Ruccione K. Childhood cancer survivors: a practical guide to your future. Sebastopol (CA): O'Reilly & Associates; 2007.

[132] Keene N. Educating the child with cancer: a guide for parents and teachers. Bethesda (MD): Candlelighters Childhood Cancer Foundation; 2003.

[133] Skinner R, Wallace WHB, Levitt GA, editors. Therapy based long term follow up. 2nd edition. Leicester (UK): United Kingdom Children's Cancer Study Group: Late effects group; 2005.

[134] Kremer LCM, Jaspers MWM, van Leeuwen FE, et al. [Landelijke richtlijnen voor follow-up van overlevenden van kinderkanker]. Tijdschrift voor Kindergeneeskunde 2006;74: 214–8 [in Dutch].

[135] Aziz NM, Oeffinger KC, Brooks S, et al. Comprehensive long-term follow-up programs for pediatric cancer survivors. Cancer 2006;107(4):841–8.

[136] Friedman DL, Freyer DR, Levitt GA. Models of care for survivors of childhood cancer. Pediatr Blood Cancer 2006;46(2):159–68.

[137] Shaw AK, Pogany L, Speechley KN, et al. Use of health care services by survivors of childhood and adolescent cancer in Canada. Cancer 2006;106(8):1829–37.

[138] Oeffinger KC, McCabe MS. Models for delivering survivorship care. J Clin Oncol 2006; 24(32):5117–24.

[139] Skinner R, Wallace WH, Levitt GA. Long-term follow-up of people who have survived cancer during childhood. Lancet Oncol 2006;7(6):489–98.

Index

Note: Page numbers of article titles are in **boldface** type.

0031-3955/08/$ - see front matter © 2008 Elsevier Inc. All rights reserved.
doi:10.1016/S0031-3955(08)00010-2   *pediatric.theclinics.com*

HOX11L2 gene mutations, acute
lymphoblastic leukemia in, 5

Human leukocyte antigens
in cancer immune response, 153
matching of, for stem cell
transplantation, 85–87

Hutchinson syndrome, in neuroblastoma,
104

Hyperdiploidy, in acute lymphoblastic
leukemia, 4

I

Idarubicin, for acute myeloid leukemia,
25, 28

Idarubicinol, for acute myeloid leukemia, 25

Imatinib, for acute lymphoblastic leukemia,
12–13

Immune escape, in cancer immunotherapy,
153

Immunization. *See* Vaccines.

Immunotherapy, for cancer, **147–167**
clinical experience with, 157–162
B-cell therapy, 161–162
natural killer cell therapy,
160–161
T-cell therapy, 157–160
history of, 147
principles of, 148–157
B cells, 149–150
immune escape, 153
immune suppression, 155–156
lymphocyte migration, 156–157
natural killer cells, 150–153
T cells, 149–150
tumor recognition, 153–155
tumor susceptibility, 155

Individualized care planning and
coordination model, for palliative care,
224–226, 228–229

Induction therapy, for acute lymphoblastic
leukemia, 6–8

Infections, in chemotherapy, 38–39

Infertility, in long-term survivors, 257–260

Influenza vaccination, for
immunocompromised cancer patients,
172, 176, 179

Informed consent
for clinical trials, 192–193
versus assent, 213

Institutional review board, 191–193, 195,
197

Interleukin-2, for neuroblastoma, 114

International Berlin-Frankfurt-Münster
trial, of acute lymphoblastic leukemia
treatment, 73, 76

*International Classification of Disease, Ninth
Revision, Clinical Modification* codes,
241, 244–245

International Conference on
Harmonization, 188, 192–193

International Neuroblastoma Staging
System, 103–107

Intrathecal therapy
for acute lymphoblastic leukemia, 6, 8
for acute myeloid leukemia, 28–29

Investigational New Drug application,
189–191, 204–205

Investigational products, in clinical trials,
195–196

Investigator, in clinical trials, 191–192

Isotretinoin, for neuroblastoma, 114

J

Janus kinases, defects of, myeloid leukemia
of Down syndrome in, 65

Juvenile myelomonocytic leukemia, stem
cell transplantation for, 82

Juvenile pilocytic astrocytomas, 133

K

Kefauver-Harris Amendment of 1962, 205

Kerner-Morrison syndrome, in
neuroblastoma, 104

Killer immunoglobulin-like receptors,
151–153

kit gene mutations
acute myeloid leukemia in, 34–35
myeloid leukemia of Down syndrome
in, 65

L

Learning disabilities, in long-term survivors,
252–254

Leukemias
acute lymphoblastic. *See* Acute
lymphoblastic leukemia.
acute myeloid. *See* Acute myeloid
leukemia.
acute promyelocytic, 31